DEVICE THERAPY IN HEART FAILURE

CONTEMPORARY CARDIOLOGY

CHRISTOPHER P. CANNON, MD
SERIES EDITOR
ANNEMARIE M. ARMANI, MD
EXECUTIVE EDITOR

DEVICE THERAPY
IN HEART FAILURE

Edited by

WILLIAM H. MAISEL, MD, MPH

Beth Israel Deaconess Medical Center,
Boston, MA, USA

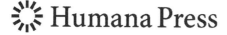 Humana Press

Editor
William H. Maisel
Harvard Medical School
Beth Israel Deaconess Medical Center
Cardiovascular Division
185 Pilgrim Road
Boston MA 02215
Baker 4
USA
wmaisel@bidmc.harvard.edu

ISBN 978-1-58829-994-9   e-ISBN 978-1-59745-424-7
DOI 10.1007/978-1-59745-424-7

Library of Congress Control Number: 2009934685

Printed on acid-free paper

springer.com

Preface

Heart failure affects close to five million patients in the United States and causes substantial morbidity and mortality. It is often a chronic and debilitating disease that results in mortality rates after initial diagnosis that approach or exceed mortality rates of many common malignancies. While a number of pharmacologic therapies have demonstrated efficacy, many recent advances in the treatment of heart failure patients have focused on device-based therapies. This book is designed to provide a comprehensive overview of current and developing technologies used to treat heart failure patients.

Contents

Contributors

AMI BHATT, MD • *Cardiovascular Division, Brigham and Women's Hospital, Boston, MA*

ARIE BLITZ, MD • *Department of Surgery, Case Western Reserve University School of Medicine, Cleveland, OH*

JOSEPH P. CARROZZA JR., MD • *Chief, Cardiology Division, St. Elizabeth Medical Center, Brighton, MA*

ERIC A. CHEN, MSE • *US Food and Drug Administration, Rockville, MD*

JOSHUA M. COOPER, MD • *Division of Cardiovascular Medicine, University of Pennsylvania Health System, Philadelphia, PA*

AKSHAY DESAI, MD • *Heart Failure Service, Cardiovascular Division, Brigham and Women's Hospital, Boston, MA*

JAMES C. FANG, MD • *Heart and Vascular Institute, University Hospitals/Case Medical Center, Case Western Reserve University School of Medicine, Cleveland, OH*

OWEN P. FARIS, PHD • *US Food and Drug Administration, Rockville, MD*

DANIEL FRISCH, MD • *Division of Cardiology, Jefferson Medical College, Thomas Jefferson University, Philadelphia, PA*

LAWRENCE A. GARCIA, MD • *Director, Cardiac Catheterization Laboratory, St. Elizabeth Medical Center, Boston, MA*

ZACHARY GOLDBERGER, MD • *Division of Cardiology, University of Washington School of Medicine, Seattle, WA*

MATTHEW G. HILLEBRENNER, MSE • *Division of Cardiovascular Devices, Center for Devices and Radiological Health, US Food and Drug Administration, Rockville, MD*

MARK E. JOSEPHSON, MD • *Chief, Division of Cardiology, Beth Israel Deaconess Medical Center, Boston, MA*

DANIEL B. KRAMER, MD • *Associate Editor, Division of Cardiology, Beth Israel Deaconess Medical Center, Boston, MA*

ROGER J. LAHAM, MD • *Interventional Cardiology Section, Division of Cardiology, Beth Israel Deaconess Medical Center/Harvard Medical School, Boston, MA*

NEAL K. LAKDAWALA, MD • *Heart Failure Service, Cardiovascular Division, Brigham and Women's Hospital, Boston, MA*

RACHEL LAMPERT, MD • *Section of Cardiology, Yale University School of Medicine, New Haven, CT*

WARREN K. LASKEY, MD • *Robert S. Flinn Professor of Medicine, Division of Cardiology, Department of Internal Medicine, University of New Mexico School of Medicine, Albuquerque, NM*

RENEE MANRING-DAY, RN, MSN, ACNP • *University of New Mexico School of Medicine, Albuquerque, NM*

ANJU NOHRIA, MD • *Heart Failure Service, Cardiovascular Division, Brigham and Women's Hospital, Boston, MA*

KATHRYN M. O'CALLAGHAN • *US Food and Drug Administration, Rockville, MD*

MOBEEN A. SHEIKH, MD • *Department of Cardiology, Beth Israel Deaconess Medical Center, Boston, MA*

NANCY K. SWEITZER, MD, PHD • *Division of Cardiovascular Medicine, University of Wisconsin School of Medicine and Public Health, Madison, WI*

MAURICIO VELEZ, MD • *Department of Medicine, University of Wisconsin School of Medicine and Public Health, Madison, WI*

JOANNA J. WYKRZYKOWSKA, MD • *Department of Cardiology, Beth Israel Deaconess Medical Center, Boston, MA*

JOHN V. WYLIE, MD • *Director, Clinical Cardiac Electrophysiology, St. Elizabeth's Medical Center, Brighton, MA*

CLYDE W. YANCY, MD • *Division of Cardiothoracic Transplantation, Baylor Heart and Vascular Institute, Baylor University Medical Center, Dallas TX*

PETER J. ZIMETBAUM, MD • *Director, Clinical Cardiology Cardiovascular Institute, Beth Israel Deaconess Medical Center, Boston, MA*

1

Pathophysiology of Heart Failure

Mauricio Velez, MD and Nancy K. Sweitzer, MD, PhD

CONTENTS

Abstract

Heart failure (HF) is a clinical syndrome resulting from structural or functional disorders that impair the heart's ability to fill with or eject blood. The pathophysiologic mechanisms leading to HF are complex and encompass hemodynamic alterations and neurohormonal changes that contribute to the chronic, progressive nature of the disease. This chapter reviews the pathophysiologic mechanisms that underlie the clinical manifestations of the HF syndrome, primarily focusing on HF due to left ventricular systolic dysfunction. Cardiac compensatory mechanisms, hemodynamic adjustments, neurohormonal activation, ventricular remodeling, and arrhythmogenesis will be reviewed.

Key Words: Pathophysiology; Heart failure; Systolic dysfunction; Mechanisms; Hemodynamics; Neurohormones; Remodeling.

Heart failure (HF) is a clinical syndrome resulting from any structural or functional cardiac disorder that impairs the ability of the ventricle to fill with or eject blood *(1)*. In its best understood form, systolic dysfunction HF can result from virtually any cardiac disease and typically progresses from being a compensated, asymptomatic condition to a decompensated, symptomatic

From: *Contemporary Cardiology: Device Therapy in Heart Failure*
Edited by: W.H. Maisel, DOI 10.1007/978-1-59745-424-7_1
© Humana Press, a part of Springer Science+Business Media, LLC 2010

state characterized by fatigue and dyspnea. The underlying pathophysiologic mechanisms leading to HF are complex. The pathophysiology encompasses symptom-causing hemodynamic alterations resulting from decreased cardiac output or increased filling pressures as well as numerous neurohormonal changes that contribute to the chronic, progressive nature of the disease. It is now clear that most compensatory mechanisms triggered by an initial insult to the heart, if unchecked, lead to chronic myocardial remodeling and dysfunction *(2)*. Ultimately, the majority of patients with HF die a cardiac death, with deaths being evenly split between progressive pump failure and sudden arrhythmic death. Patients with milder HF symptoms (NYHA Class I/II) are more likely to die of sudden cardiac death (SCD), while those with more advanced symptomatic heart failure (NYHA Class III/IV) die more often of pump failure *(3)*.

In this chapter, we discuss the pathophysiologic mechanisms that underlie the clinical manifestations of the HF syndrome, focusing on systolic dysfunction HF. Because of their contribution to the pathophysiology of systolic dysfunction HF, attention will be focused on cardiac compensatory mechanisms, from early hemodynamic adjustments to neurohormonal activation and ventricular remodeling. The pathophysiology of arrhythmogenesis in HF will also be reviewed.

1. THE PATHOPHYSIOLOGY OF COMPENSATORY SYSTEMS IN HEART FAILURE

1.1. Normal Cardiac Function

In order to understand compensatory mechanisms fully, basic concepts need to be reviewed. Cardiac output (CO) represents the amount of blood ejected per unit time (L/min) and is the product of heart rate (HR) and stroke volume (SV):

$$CO = HR \times SV$$

Mean arterial pressure (MAP) is the product of CO and systemic vascular resistance (SVR):

$$MAP = CO \times SVR$$

While heart rate is controlled by the autonomic nervous system, stroke volume is dependent on variations in preload, afterload, and contractility. By the Frank–Starling mechanism, increases in myocardial contractile force result from increases in preload. As myocardial fibers stretch, the number of effective cross-bridges between thick and thin filaments increases, augmenting contractile force. In normal hearts, small increases in left ventricular end-diastolic pressure (LVEDP) cause large increases in cardiac output.

In clinical settings, both LVEDP and its surrogate, the pulmonary capillary wedge pressure (PCWP), allow dynamic assessment of preload.

Afterload is a more complex concept best appreciated as a sum of all the forces that impede ejection of blood from the ventricle. SVR is a major determinant of afterload. In patients with LV systolic dysfunction, there is an inverse relationship between afterload (SVR) and stroke volume such that increases in SVR cause decreases in SV and, therefore, CO (Fig. 1) (4, 5).

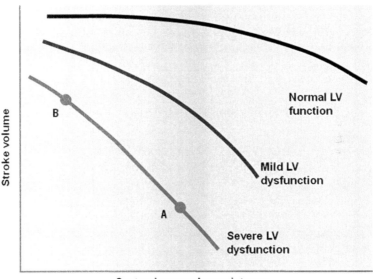

Fig. 1. Relationship between stroke volume and systemic vascular resistance. In an individual with normal left ventricular (LV) function, increasing systemic vascular resistance has little effect on stroke volume. As the extent of LV dysfunction increases, the effect of increases in systemic vascular resistance to decrease stroke volume becomes significant (B to A). [Adapted from Johnson et al. (4), with permission.]

1.2. The Frank–Starling Mechanism in HF

Following ventricular injury, preload increases due to decreased contractility and resultant increases in end-systolic volume and pressure. This decreases cardiac output and renal blood flow, activating juxtaglomerular cells in the afferent arterioles of nephrons. The resulting renal production of angiotensin II and aldosterone promotes sodium and fluid reabsorption in the renal tubules to increase intravascular volume, further increasing cardiac filling pressures. In addition, decreased renal blood flow leads to sympathetic nervous system (SNS) activation, initiating a cascade of events including venoconstriction to increase preload, arteriolar vasoconstriction to help maintain blood pressure and to shift blood flow away from non-vital organs, and an intrinsic increase in cardiac contractility to maintain stroke volume. The neurohormonally-mediated increase in preload should increase contractility by the Frank–Starling mechanism.

However, failing hearts have a right-shifted and flattened Starling curve at rest. In this clinical situation, a rise in left ventricular volume leads instead to increased ventricular wall tension, higher filling pressures, and HF symptoms, without a significant rise in cardiac output (Fig. 2). These events contribute to ventricular dilation and development of mitral regurgitation (6). Because of the profound effect of afterload on the failing left ventricle, increased preload has minimal effects on cardiac output. This leads to increased filling pressure and decreased cardiac output, the quintessential HF phenotype (4, 7).

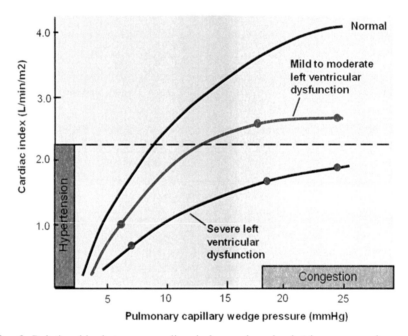

Fig. 2. Relationship between cardiac index and preload (shown as pulmonary capillary wedge pressure). In left ventricular dysfunction, there is a blunted Frank–Starling relationship, with smaller increases in stroke volume for a given rise in preload. Congestion can result in the patient with severe left ventricular dysfunction, despite adequate cardiac output. [Adapted from Johnson et al. (4), with permission.]

1.3. Chronic Ventricular Remodeling

The term ventricular remodeling describes a series of genetic, molecular, cellular, and interstitial cardiac changes resulting in global alterations in the shape, size, and function of the heart after injury (8). Ventricular remodeling can be triggered by any combination of pressure or volume overload, or by myocyte injury and necrosis as seen in myocardial infarction or myocarditis *(9)*. Although remodeling may be compensatory in some situations such as chronic valvular disease, remodeling associated with symptomatic heart failure is associated with a uniformly adverse prognosis and carries an increased risk of both pump failure and sudden cardiac death *(10)*. This is true of both ischemic and non-ischemic remodeling.

1.3.1. MYOCARDIAL HYPERTROPHY AND REMODELING

Hypertrophy is a response to pressure- or volume-induced stress, mutations of sarcomeric (or other) proteins, or loss of contractile mass from injury or infarction. In animal models, hypertrophy precedes ventricular dilation and failure, and is accompanied by shifts in myocardial gene expression. This shift results in a decrease in α-myosin heavy chain, increases in α-skeletal actin and β-tropomyosin, and the expression of other genes typical of fetal cardiac development *(11)*. In concert with the switch in gene expression, increases in expression of atrial natriuretic peptide (ANP) are also seen *(12)*. Important signaling pathways in myocardial hypertrophy include H-Ras, MAP kinase, and Akt pathways *(13–18)*.

Three primary patterns of hypertrophy, occurring in response to specific types of overload or injury, have been described: hypertrophy due to pressure overload, volume overload, or post-infarction remodeling (Fig. 3). Most HF patients exhibit a mixture of these pure types. In concentric hypertrophy due to pressure overload, new sarcomeres are added in parallel to existing ones, increasing myocyte width and ventricular wall thickness. In contrast, chronic volume overload leads to myocyte lengthening due to the addition of new sarcomeres in series and predominant ventricular dilation with normal wall thickness, labeled eccentric hypertrophy. If these adaptive mechanisms are appropriate, cardiac performance may remain in a compensated state. Post-infarction remodeling incorporates elements of both pressure overload hypertrophy and volume overload hypertrophy *(9)*.

Pressure overload-induced concentric hypertrophy is seen in its most pure form in aortic stenosis or hypertension. This type of remodeling is thought to be partially compensatory, diminishing myocardial wall stress and oxygen consumption *(11, 19)*. However, myocardial pressure overload leads to the release of neurohormonal mediators that may promote apoptosis, fibrosis, and ventricular dilation in addition to myocyte hypertrophy and survival. In the presence of chronic pressure overload, angiotensin-converting enzyme (ACE) is upregulated in myocardial tissue, resulting in local production of angiotensin II (A-II) *(20)*. A-II increases aldosterone levels and promotes the transcription of transforming growth factor-β (TGF-β), a well-characterized profibrotic cytokine. Both contribute to myocardial interstitial fibrosis *(21)*. Matrix metalloproteinases (MMPs) and tissue inhibitors of metalloproteinases (TIMPs) are also upregulated in response to A-II

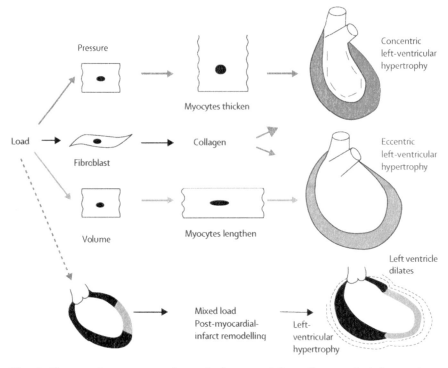

Fig. 3. Three major patterns of ventricular remodeling. Concentric left ventricular hypertrophy occurs when a pressure load leads to growth in cardiomyocyte thickness (*dotted lines* represent left ventricle growing inward); eccentric hypertrophy develops when a volume load produces myocyte lengthening; and post-infarct remodeling occurs when the stretched and dilated infarcted tissue increases the left ventricular volume with a combined volume and pressure load on the non-infarcted zones (*dotted lines* represent combined effects of concentric and eccentric hypertrophy). Fibrosis contributes to all three patterns. [From Opie et al. *(9)*, with permission.]

and promote increased collagen turnover. In patients with chronic pressure overload, these structural changes correlate directly with macroscopic morphologic changes in the size of the left ventricle, as well as with deterioration of its contractile performance *(22)*. Fibrosis contributes to diastolic dysfunction, decreased systolic performance, and arrhythmogenesis. Persistence of pressure overload conditions results ultimately in derangement of the extracellular matrix (ECM) via the above processes, altering myocardial architecture and promoting ventricular dilation (Fig. 4) *(23, 24)*.

Volume overload-induced eccentric hypertrophy is seen in its most pure form in mitral regurgitation. This type of remodeling is also compensatory, as a dilated ventricle has increased stroke volume for any given level of contractility. Eccentric hypertrophy occurs as myocyte stretch stimulates the addition of new sarcomeres in series, resulting in ventricular dilation

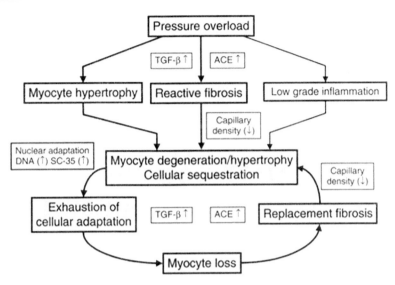

Fig. 4. Schematic illustration of continuous remodeling in pressure overload hypertrophy. [From Hen et al. *(128)*, with permission.]

with normal wall thickness *(25, 26)*. Although myocardial contractile protein levels increase in response to a pure volume load, the increase is slower and of lower magnitude than that seen in pressure overload, leading to a smaller increase in myocardial mass for a given increase in stroke work *(27, 28)*. This suggests that wall stress is the primary stimulus for increased protein synthesis. Passive myocyte stretch is associated with increased expression of TNF-α in animal models and in individuals with mitral regurgitation. Initially, TNF-α contributes to increased protein synthesis. Prolonged elevation in TNF-α may lead to degeneration of the extracellular matrix due to overexpression of matrix metalloproteinases with denaturation of collagen and myocyte apoptosis *(9, 29)*, promoting decompensation of the dilated ventricle.

In humans, remodeling secondary to myocardial damage is most commonly secondary to myocardial infarction (MI). The remodeling process in this setting is complex and results from combined pressure- and volume-induced hypertrophic stimuli, in addition to the neurohormonal and cytokine responses initiated by the abnormal hemodynamic state, as well as the injury. In post-MI remodeling, the infarcted area becomes akinetic and increased local wall stresses lead to local enlargement and extension of the infarct. Volume overload results in an associated pressure overload component. Compensatory physiologic responses aimed at reducing wall stress are generally ineffective. When unchecked, these damaging compensatory processes contribute to a larger akinetic area and increased wall stress, creating a vicious cycle. As scar forms, further ventricular dilation occurs due to

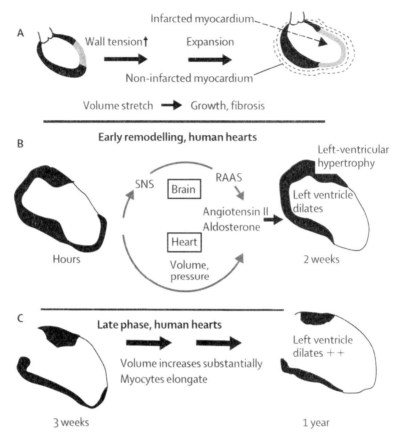

Fig. 5. Post-infarct left ventricular remodeling patterns. (**A**) Simplified overall pattern based on animal models. There is potential for substantial remodeling of the infarct zone and increased volume of the non-infarcted zone. Endocardial wall motion of two different infarcted human hearts in (**B**) early post-infarct phase and (**C**) late post-infarct phase, derived from contrast ventriculography. *Black* = extent of preserved movement of endocardial surface in non-infarcted zone. Note substantial remodeling in accordance with the animal models, with emphasis on progressively increased volume of left ventricle. RAAS = renin–angiotensin–aldosterone system. SNS = sympathetic nervous system. [From Opie et al. *(9)*, with permission.]

lengthening of the remaining myocytes as they try to compensate for chronic volume overload (Fig. 5) *(9, 30)*.

1.4. Neurohormones in Heart Failure

Following cardiac injury, neurohormonal systems are activated in an attempt to restore normal circulatory function. Sustained activation of these mechanisms, however, leads to a paradoxical worsening of cardiac function. These substances modulate vascular tone, sodium and fluid retention, and cardiac contractility. The sympathetic nervous system (SNS) and the renin–angiotensin–aldosterone system (RAAS) constitute the principal neurohormonal systems involved in this process and are primary targets of therapy. Other signaling systems have been implicated in chronic myocardial injury and progression to heart failure including arginine vasopressin, natriuretic peptides, endothelin-1, the nitric oxide system, and proinflammatory cytokines, although their specific roles are not fully understood and intervening in these pathways currently has a minimal role in routine therapy of HF *(31, 32)*. Neurohormonal activation occurs at early stages of the disease. Even in the absence of HF symptoms, continued activation promotes progressive adverse remodeling and ultimately clinical worsening (Fig. 6).

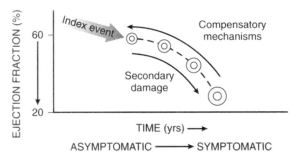

Fig. 6. Pathogenesis of heart failure. Heart failure begins after an index event produces an initial decline in pumping capacity of the heart. Following this initial decline in pumping capacity of the heart, a variety of compensatory mechanisms are activated, including the adrenergic nervous system, the renin–angiotensin system, and the cytokine system. In the short term, these systems are able to restore cardiovascular function to a normal homeostatic range with the result that the patient remains asymptomatic. However, with time, the sustained activation of these systems can lead to secondary damage within the ventricle, with worsening LV remodeling and subsequent cardiac decompensation. As a result of worsening LV remodeling and cardiac decompensation, patients undergo the transition from asymptomatic to symptomatic heart failure. [From Colucci and Braunwald *(26)*, with permission.]

1.4.1. THE SYMPATHETIC NERVOUS SYSTEM

The earliest neurohormonal change detectable following cardiac injury is sympathetic nervous system (SNS) activation. The mechanisms that trigger acute sympathetic activation of the normal heart are not fully understood. While desensitization of baroreceptors may lead to lack of tonic inhibition of the SNS in chronic heart failure, recent experimental data show that elevated pulmonary artery and wedge pressures induce high levels of circulating catecholamines, suggesting a direct relationship between cardiopulmonary baroreflex stimulation and efferent SNS activity *(33)*. In addition, increased input from peripheral chemoreceptors and cardiac receptors that traverse sympathetic pathways may lead to persistent excitation of the SNS, although human evidence for these mechanisms is inconclusive *(34)*. SNS activation increases heart rate and myocardial contractility. However, failing myocardium, with its diminished contractile reserve, has a limited response to sympathetic activation.

SNS activation leads to release of norepinephrine from synapses in the myocardium. Norepinephrine binds to β_1-adrenergic receptors, stimulating adenylate cyclase via a G-protein-dependent mechanism, which converts ATP into cAMP. Protein kinase A, activated by cAMP, phosphorylates multiple intracellular proteins, including Ca^{2+} regulatory proteins. This results in increased Ca^{2+} influx into the cell, accumulation of Ca^{2+} in the sarcoplasmic reticulum, an increased cross-bridge cycling rate, and an increased magnitude of the systolic Ca^{2+} transient with decreased duration. The net effect is an increase in the rate and magnitude of force generation and faster relaxation (35).

While SNS activation may effectively improve contractility in early systolic dysfunction, chronic adrenergic stimulation of the myocytes has been shown to have toxic effects on cultured myocytes and may be responsible for direct cell damage via cAMP-mediated Ca^{2+} overload (36), increased energy consumption, hypertrophy, and induction of apoptosis (37). The sustained sympathetic response seen in chronic LV systolic dysfunction causes significant changes in β-adrenergic receptor signaling, including downregulation of β_1-adrenergic receptors and desensitization of β_1 and β_2-receptors by uncoupling them from downstream regulatory proteins. Although these changes protect the myocardium by preventing sustained β-adrenergic stimulation and its consequences, they also blunt adrenergic responsiveness and result in an inability of the heart to react to increased workload demands (35, 38).

The prognosis of patients with HF is directly related to the degree of SNS activation; patients with the highest plasma levels of norepinephrine have increased mortality (39). Randomized controlled trials of β-blocker therapy in HF patients have demonstrated significant reductions not only in SCD but also in pump failure death (40–46), primarily through reverse remodeling and improved contractility (47–49). Elevated heart rate itself may be a poor prognostic factor in chronic heart failure, particularly in those with ischemic cardiomyopathy (50).

1.4.2. THE RENIN–ANGIOTENSIN–ALDOSTERONE SYSTEM

Renin release from the juxtaglomerular cells is triggered by multiple stimuli found in HF including decreased renal perfusion, increased SNS activity, chronic diuretic use, and dietary sodium restriction. Renin converts angiotensinogen to angiotensin I, which interacts with angiotensin-converting enzyme (ACE) to produce angiotensin II (A-II), a potent vasoconstrictor (51). Systemically, A-II activity results in vasoconstriction, glomerular hypertension, and thirst (26, 52). Persistent RAAS and SNS activation are associated with progressive LV remodeling, may facilitate the evolution from hypertrophy to failure, and have been associated with increased mortality (53, 54). AT_1 receptor activation by A-II results in the proliferation of non-myocyte cell types in the heart, increasing collagen synthesis and fibrosis. Although A-II promotes cell growth in neonatal cardiac myocytes, this effect is not seen in adult myocytes, suggesting that myocardial fibrosis is the main mechanism of A-II-induced remodeling *(55)*.

A-II is a potent stimulator of other neurohormonal pathways, including the SNS, aldosterone, and mediators of oxidative stress and inflammation. Use of ACE inhibitors in HF results in decreased systemic vascular resistance, afterload reduction, and augmentation of cardiac output, reducing morbidity and mortality *(56–58)*. Interestingly, there is only a small effect of ACE inhibitor therapy to reduce sudden cardiac death; most of the benefits of these agents appear to be due to effects on progressive pump failure *(57, 59)*. Although some effects of ACE inhibition are due to decreased levels of circulating A-II, many of the beneficial effects of these drugs may be due to other effects, such as decreased SNS activation and increased levels of bradykinin, explaining the differential effects of ACE inhibitors and AT1 blocking drugs in HF *(60, 61)*. Levels of A-II rise slowly in some HF patients despite ACE inhibitor therapy, suggesting synthesis through non-ACE pathways, such as tissue chymase *(62, 63)*.

Aldosterone is also implicated in HF progression. Aldosterone actions are mediated through nuclear mineralocorticoid receptors (MR) and gene activation, leading to cellular hypertrophy, fibrosis, impaired metabolism, and altered sodium balance, both in the myocardium and the vasculature *(64)*. Aldosterone production in HF is mediated by A-II, corticotrophin, elevations in serum potassium, and alterations in renal water and sodium handling. High A-II levels in HF patients promote sodium reabsorption in the proximal renal tubules, while aldosterone leads to sodium reabsorption in the distal tubule. Thus the combination of A-II plus aldosterone leads to avid renal sodium reabsorption in HF. In addition to mineralocorticoid properties that may cause hypokalemia and hypomagnesemia, aldosterone also induces endothelial dysfunction *(65)*. In the myocardium, aldosterone causes increased fibrillar collagen deposition and fibrosis *(66, 67)*.

Aldosterone blockade improves morbidity and mortality in both symptomatic heart failure patients being treated with ACE inhibitors *(68)* and post-MI patients with left ventricular dysfunction *(69)*. There is evidence that much of the benefits of aldosterone antagonism are due to antifibrotic effects. In a substudy of the RALES trial, a group of patients had serial measurements of the N-terminal propeptide of type III pro-collagen, a marker of collagen synthesis that correlates with myocardial fibrosis in humans. Treatment with spironolactone was associated with decreased levels of this pro-collagen precursor and was correlated with decreased mortality compared with those treated with placebo *(66, 68, 70)*. The addition of spironolactone to therapy with angiotensin II receptor blockade in patients with chronic systolic heart failure produced LV reverse remodeling by measurements of LV mass, LV ejection fraction, and tissue Doppler parameters *(71)*. In addition to an overall mortality benefit, aldosterone antagonist therapy has been shown to significantly reduce the risk of sudden cardiac death *(68, 69)*.

1.4.3. ARGININE VASOPRESSIN

Arginine vasopressin (AVP) is synthesized in the hypothalamus and secreted by the posterior pituitary. By binding to its V_{1a} and V_2 receptors, AVP increases body fluid volume, increases vascular tone, and decreases cardiac contractility. AVP release follows osmoreceptor activation in response to changes in plasma osmolality. Vascular baroreceptors also trigger AVP release when they sense low intravascular pressure. Even slight decreases in pressure result in elevation of SVR via V_{1a} receptor activation. In HF patients, AVP is persistently elevated due to carotid baroreceptor activation in the setting of low cardiac output and low blood pressure (72). This mechanism overrides the hypothalamic osmoreceptors. Inappropriate elevation of AVP leads to overexpression of aquaporin water channels in the renal collecting duct, excessive water reabsorption, and hyponatremia, even in the presence of hypoosmolality (73).

AVP can increase SVR without elevating blood pressure due to simultaneous V_2 receptor-induced bradycardia and decreased cardiac output. Elevations in blood pressure are evident only with supraphysiologic levels of AVP, which cause hyperactivation of V_{1a} receptors that overwhelms V_2 receptor effects. The reduced myocyte contractility seen with AVP is believed to result from impaired coronary flow due to V_{1a}-mediated vasoconstriction (74). In the kidneys, V_2 receptor activation increases cAMP in renal tubular cells, increasing expression of aquaporin channels and reabsorption of water in the collecting duct (73). There are no specific data linking AVP levels and cardiac arrhythmia. Ongoing clinical trials are exploring selective inhibition of AVP receptors as a therapeutic target in heart failure (75–77).

1.4.4. ENDOTHELIN

Endothelin-1 (ET-1) is a vasoconstrictor peptide synthesized by vascular endothelial cells. Although additional endothelins have been described, ET-1 is the major cardiovascular isoform. ET-1 is synthesized by a neutral endopeptidase, and stimuli for its release include shear stress, pulsatile stretch, epinephrine, A-II, thrombin, several inflammatory cytokines, and hypoxia. ET-1 effects occur via two G-protein-coupled receptor types, ET_A and ET_B, found on vascular smooth muscle cells, endothelial cells, and cardiac myocytes (78). ET-1 regulates basal vascular tone and myocardial contractility, as well as renal sodium excretion. ET_A receptor stimulation leads to vasoconstriction, while ET_B receptors cause vasodilation via nitric oxide and prostacyclin release. ET_B receptors are also responsible for the plasma clearance of ET-1 in the pulmonary and renal circulation (78, 79).

Plasma and myocardial tissue ET-1 levels are elevated in HF patients. ET-1 contributes to the vasoconstriction seen in HF, particularly pulmonary vasoconstriction. ET_A receptors are upregulated in failing ventricular muscle, and antagonism of these receptors results in improvement of LV dysfunction *(80)*. However, selective antagonism of ET_B increases pulmonary and diastolic pressures and decreases cardiac output *(81)*. Thus, it is believed that local production and local concentrations are important in mediating effects of ET-1 in HF. Circulating levels of ET-1 increase late in the course of heart failure, and there is evidence that most of this increase is due to biologically less-active big endothelin-1 *(82)*. ET-1 production by elevated filling pressures in HF contributes to excessive pulmonary hypertension in some patients. Therapy with β-blockers and ACE inhibitors has been shown to decrease ET-1 levels in plasma *(79)*. Blockade of the ET-1 system with endothelin antagonists has not been shown to be an effective treatment for HF *(83–85)*.

1.4.5. NITRIC OXIDE

Nitric oxide (NO) is a messenger molecule with wide-ranging physiologic effects. Both protective and deleterious cardiovascular effects of NO have been described *(84, 86)*. The physiologic effects of NO vary depending on the intracellular compartment where it is synthesized (Fig. 7). According to this paradigm, NOS isoforms demonstrate regional localization such that endothelial NOS (eNOS, NOS3) is found in sarcolemmal caveolae and neuronal NOS (nNOS, NOS1) is segregated to the SR and mitochondria. NO interacts with local effectors with responses based on the site of action. NOS1 and NOS3 appear to be cardioprotective, while inducible NOS (iNOS, NOS2) can cause myocardial toxicity *(87)*.

NOS1 mediates calcium release from the SR via the RyR, contributing to increased inotropy by β-adrenergic stimulation. Conversely, NOS3, found on the membrane of cardiac myocytes in close proximity to $β_3$-adrenergic receptors, causes blunting of β-adrenergic-induced increases in contractility by inactivation of L-type calcium channels (LTCC), resulting in decreased intracellular calcium levels *(87, 88)*.

Decreased NOS1 and NOS3 function leads to production of reactive oxygen species (ROS) and an altered NO/ROS ratio (nitroso-redox imbalance). ROS alone have been implicated in cardiac hypertrophy and myocyte apoptosis, suppressed LTCC currents, decreased SERCA2a activity, MMP activation, decreased myofilament calcium sensitivity, activation of inflammatory cytokines, and impaired cardiac energetics. It has been suggested that these abnormalities may result from nitroso-redox imbalance, rather than just oxidative stress *(87, 88)*. Modulation of nitroso-redox balance may have clinical benefits, as seen with the combination of isosorbide dinitrate (ISDN) and hydralazine to treat African-Americans with HF *(90)*. ISDN has NO-donor properties, and hydralazine acts as a ROS and peroxynitrite scavenger. This combination can restore nitroso-redox balance toward normal in failing ventricular muscle *(87, 89)*. No direct evidence ties the NO system or the nitroso-redox balance to risk for sudden cardiac death.

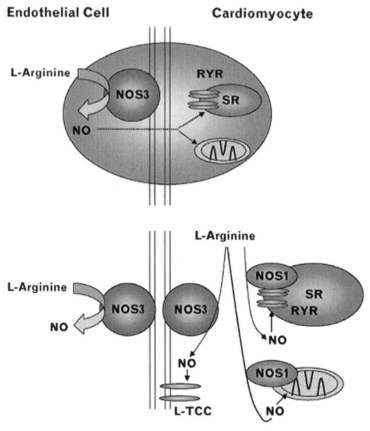

Fig. 7. The *upper panel* shows the classic paradigm that nitric oxide (NO) derived from endothelial NO synthase (NOS3) localized within endothelial cells diffuses to underlying myocardial cells. The *lower panel* depicts an alternative view that NOS isoforms are expressed in both endothelial cells and cardiomyocytes. Moreover, NOS isoforms are expressed in specific organelles in proximity to mediators of effector signaling pathways. NOS3 localizes to the sarcolemma, where it is involved in *S*-nitrosylation of the L-type calcium channel (LTCC), and neuronal NOS (NOS1) localizes to the sarcoplasmic reticulum (SR) and participates in regulating the ryanodine receptor (RYR) calcium channel and to mitochondria, where it contributes to the regulation of oxygen consumption. [From Saraiva and Hare *(87)*, with permission.]

1.4.6. NATRIURETIC PEPTIDES

The natriuretic peptide system is a counterregulatory system to the many upregulated vasoconstrictor neurohormonal systems in HF. The two major natriuretic peptides are atrial natriuretic peptide (ANP) and B-type natriuretic peptide (BNP). ANP and BNP decrease RAAS activation, promote natriuresis, are vasodilatory, and inhibit hypertrophy and fibrosis *(91)*. They exert their effects by binding the natriuretic peptide receptor-A (NPR-A), which uses cyclic GMP (cGMP) as its intracellular messenger *(92)*. BNP is synthesized primarily in the LV in response to increased wall stress. Its precursor protein proBNP is cleaved to form BNP and the metabolically active peptide N-terminal proBNP (NT-proBNP) *(93)*. BNP is cleared from the circulation by C-type receptors in the renal tubules, but is also partly degraded by neutral endopeptidases (NEP) *(92)*. Serum levels of ANP and BNP generally increase as ventricular dysfunction progresses, and increased levels are highly correlated with risk of sudden cardiac death *(94–96)*. Despite this correlation, it is not thought that BNP plays a role in exacerbating cardiac arrhythmia, but rather that it is a marker for HF disease severity.

1.4.7. INFLAMMATORY CYTOKINES

Proinflammatory cytokines are not constitutively expressed in the heart; however, they are found at significant concentrations in patients with chronic HF *(97)*. Rather than being related to specific insults, these molecules are expressed in all forms of cardiac injury, suggesting that they are part of an intrinsic response of the heart to damage. While expression of proinflammatory cytokines in the short term may be beneficial, sustained production or dysregulated expression can contribute to cardiac decompensation *(29)*.

Tumor necrosis factor-α (TNF-α) and interleukin-1 (IL-1) play important roles in protecting the myocardium against acute oxidative damage, especially during ischemia and reperfusion injury *(29)*. The deleterious effects of TNF-α and IL-1 on the myocardium were first described in neonatal cardiac myocytes, where continuous exposure for 72 hours resulted in blunting of the inotropic response of these cells to isoproterenol. TNF-α, IL-1, interleukin-6 (IL-6), and interleukin 2 (IL-2) decrease contractility and heart rate. The underlying mechanism may be related to impaired calcium cycling, as TNF-α affects calcium handling by the sarcoplasmic reticulum *(29)*. In addition to rapidly changing cardiac contractility, proinflammatory cytokines contribute to both hypertrophy and apoptosis. In particular, TNF-α alters the balance in activity of MMPs and TIMPs, leading to fibrosis and adverse remodeling *(29, 98)*.

The presence of elevated levels of TNF-α in HF and these suggested pathophysiologic mechanisms led to HF trials of the TNF-α inhibitors etanercept and infliximab for HF therapy. These studies found no clinical benefit of these agents in HF, but rather trends toward increased mortality and HF-related hospitalizations in the treatment groups when compared to placebo *(99–101)*.

2. MOLECULAR MECHANISMS AFFECTING CARDIAC ARRHYTHMOGENESIS

Sudden cardiac death (SCD) is a major cause of mortality in HF and is responsible for up to 50% of deaths in heart failure patients *(102, 103)*. Both ventricular tachyarrhythmias [pulseless ventricular tachycardia and ventricular fibrillation (VT/VF)] and bradyarrhythmias/pulseless electrical activity may occur, and the incidence of SCD increases as HF becomes more severe *(102)*. Although an unstable electrical substrate in the diseased myocardium is the direct cause, the situation is complex, as illustrated by the fact that drugs that alter the neurohormonal and hemodynamic state of failing myocardium without direct electrophysiologic actions have been shown to be effective in preventing SCD, including β-blockers, ACE inhibitors, ARBs, statins, spironolactone, thrombolytics, and antithrombotic agents. The direct triggers of arrhythmogenesis in HF are still unknown, but it is believed that a series of structural and functional changes in the heart, including impaired Ca^{2+} cycling, neurohormonal activation, and genetic factors, lead to increased risk of SCD *(104, 105)*.

Ventricular tachyarrhythmias are the result of one of three basic mechanisms: abnormal automaticity, triggered activity, or reentry. Normal ventricular myocytes maintain a steady negative transmembrane resting potential and depolarize only when stimulated by activation of neighboring cells. In HF, the presence of ischemia may lead to abnormal automaticity of ventricular cells, particularly Purkinje cells. Triggered arrhythmias are the result of premature activation of ventricular cells either during (early afterdepolarization, EAD) or just after (delayed afterdepolarization, DAD) the repolarization phase of the ventricular action potential. EADs are bradycardia dependent, occurring in the setting of a prolonged QT interval, and typically lead to polymorphic VT. DADs result from abnormal oscillation and accumulation of calcium in the diseased myocardium. Re-entrant arrhythmias occur around lines of electrical block, typically in HF due to scar or fibrosis.

2.1. Calcium Cycling in Normal and Failing Cardiac Myocytes

Contraction in cardiac muscle is the result of increased intracellular calcium during systole in cardiac myocytes. The magnitude of Ca^{2+} release is normally controlled to maintain a constant cardiac output and can increase to augment contractility, but is decreased in HF. Small amounts of calcium enter the cytoplasm through L-type Ca^{2+} channels (LTCC), increasing the local concentration of Ca^{2+} between the cell membrane and the SR (Fig. 8). This leads to RyR opening and Ca^{2+} efflux from the SR into the cytoplasm. Calcium then binds to the contractile proteins and permits interaction of myosin with actin to generate force. For effective diastolic relaxation to occur, Ca^{2+} must be removed from the cytosol by the SR Ca^{2+}-ATPase (SERCA) or the Na^+–Ca^{2+} exchanger (NCX) *(106)*.

The magnitude of the Ca^{2+} transient increases with faster heart rates. This force–frequency response is deranged in HF, resulting in unchanged or even decreased contractility with rising heart rates *(35)*. Failing hearts demonstrate abnormal intracellular calcium handling as heart rate increases *(107)*, although the exact molecular mechanisms of this failed response are unknown *(35)*.

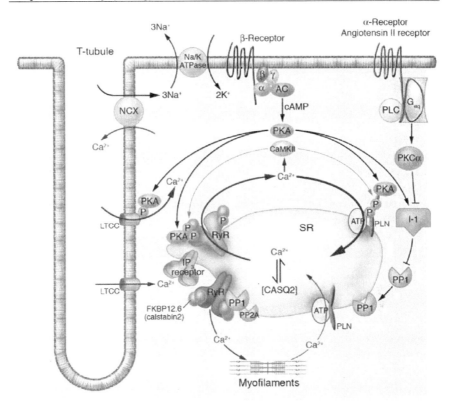

Fig. 8. Schematic illustration of intracellular Ca^{2+} cycling and associated second messenger pathways in cardiomyocytes. AC, adenylyl cyclase; α, G-protein subunit α; α-receptor, α-adrenergic receptor; β, G-protein subunit β; β-receptor, β-adrenergic receptor; γ, G-protein subunit γ; LTCC, L-type Ca^{2+} channel; CAMKII, Ca^{2+}-calmodulin kinase II; I-1, inhibitor 1; NCX, Na^+/Ca^{2+} exchanger; P, phosphate group; PLC, phospholipase C; PLN, phospholamban; PP1, protein phosphatase 1; PP2A, protein phosphatase 2A; SERCA2a, SR Ca^{2+}-ATPase isoform 2a; T-tubule, transverse tubule. [From Rubart and Zipes (*104*), with permission.]

During diastole, SERCA2a is responsible for Ca^{2+} reaccumulation in the SR. Decreases in the expression or the function of SERCA2a have been implicated in HF (*108, 109*). However, failing myocardium can manifest impaired calcium handling even in the presence of normal SERCA2a activity (*110, 111*), which suggests that other mechanisms are important. Normal SERCA2a function is dependent on cytosolic and SR Ca^{2+} concentrations and is regulated by phospholamban (PBL). Abnormalities in PBL function may result in abnormal SERCA2a activity, even when the latter is abundant and properly functional (*112*). Elevated NCX activity may decrease cytoplasmic Ca^{2+} levels and indirectly reduce SR Ca^{2+} content, even in the presence of normal SERCA2a activity.

The RyR may also play a role in the dysregulation of calcium handling in HF. The RyR functions as a Ca^{2+}-release channel from the SR in its phosphorylated state. Animal studies suggest that a "hyperphosphorylated" RyR is present in heart failure, increasing the probability of an open RyR and leading to persistent leaking of Ca^{2+} from the SR (113). This phenomenon has been demonstrated in humans, where a hyperphosphorylated RyR is associated with RyR uncoupling, which in fact induces SR Ca^{2+} leak and decreases the amount of calcium available for release after LTCC-induced RyR channel activation. Increased SR calcium leak may also lead to increased diastolic stiffness (112). In addition, Ca^{2+} leak can induce DADs, directly triggering ventricular arrhythmias (104, 113). Lastly, the persistent calcium leak may lead to increases in ATP consumption by SERCA2a to maintain SR Ca^{2+} content, contributing to systolic dysfunction.

Catecholamines are arrhythmogenic, and β-blocker therapy clearly reduces SCD risk in HF patients. Persistent SNS activation in HF stimulates SERCA2a to replete SR calcium and may actually lead to relative SR calcium overload, with increases in RyR calcium permeability and local Ca^{2+} release, producing Ca^{2+} sparks. Ca^{2+} sparks may cause delayed afterdepolarizations, which then trigger reentrant arrhythmias. Constant stimulation of calcium cycling pathways by high norepinephrine levels may serve as a mechanism for the high frequency of arrhythmia in HF.

2.2. Prolongation of the Cardiac Action Potential

Failing myocytes have prolonged action potentials (AP), regardless of the etiology of HF. AP prolongation is heterogeneous in the myocardium, varying across the thickness of the myocardial wall and in different regions of the heart. This exaggerated dispersion and heterogeneity of the AP in failing myocardium provide the substrate for reentrant ventricular arrhythmias (103).

Electrical remodeling describes changes that occur in ion channel biology in the failing myocardium, including downregulation of transient outward potassium (K) current (I_{to}) and inward rectifier K current (I_{K1}), decreased responsiveness to β-adrenergic stimulation, and alterations of intracellular Ca^{2+} handling (114), resulting in prolongation of AP duration (Fig. 9). Potassium currents are involved in every phase of the cardiac action potential, and downregulation of K currents is consistently observed in hypertrophied and failing ventricles (115, 116). The inward rectifier K current (I_{K1}) maintains resting membrane potential and contributes to the terminal phase of repolarization. The delayed rectifier K current (I_K) is important in phase 3 repolarization and is composed of distinct rapid (I_{Kr}) and slow (I_{Ks}) components. The calcium-independent transient outward current (I_{to}) is crucial in early phase depolarization, and its downregulation is the predominant ionic current change isolated from myocardium in animal models of cardiac hypertrophy and terminal HF (105). While I_{to} is a transient current and its

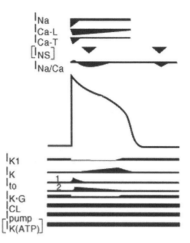

Fig. 9. Currents and channels involved in generating resting and action potentials. The time course of a stylized action potential of atrial and ventricular cells is shown. Above and below are the various channels and pumps that contribute the currents underlying the electrical events. Where possible, the approximate time courses of the currents associated with the channels or pumps are shown symbolically, without trying to represent their magnitudes relative to each other. I_K incorporates at least two currents I_{K-R} and I_{K-S}. The channels identified by brackets (I_{NS} and $I_{K(ATP)}$) are active only under pathological conditions. I_{NS} may represent a swelling-activated cation current. [Adapted from Rubart and Zipes *(117)*, with permission.]

downregulation does not affect AP duration directly, its role in early phase depolarization affects other ionic currents that become active later in the AP. I_{to} density varies significantly in different regions of the myocardium in HF, and this phenomenon is thought to be due to differential K channel gene expression regionally within failing myocardium *(103)*. Changes in other currents have been described, although not with the same frequency as I_{to}.

Purkinje fibers are specialized myocardial cells that connect with the ends of the bundle branches to form interweaving networks on the endocardial surface of both ventricles. They transmit the cardiac impulse almost simultaneously to the entire right and left ventricular endocardium *(118)*. Purkinje fibers are thought to be a potential source of automaticity in diseased hearts. These cells have been shown to undergo significant remodeling of potassium and calcium currents, with prolongation of the action potential, labile repolarization, and functional reentry *(105, 118)*.

2.3. Abnormalities in Conduction

Abnormalities in conduction and ventricular activation result in disorganized repolarization in failing myocardium, facilitating reentrant excitation and ventricular tachyarrhythmias *(105)*. The principal determinants of conduction in ventricular myocardium are availability of Na current, the size and shape of ventricular myocytes, the quantity and distribution of fibrous tissue, and cellular coupling by gap junction channels. The contribution of alterations in the Na currents is controversial, as abnormalities in Na current kinetics are not a consistent feature of dilated cardiomyopathy. Fibrosis can alter a number of conduction features through the myocardium, leading to conduction block and reentry *(119)*. Fibrosis impacts profoundly on cardiac electrophysiology and the risk of sudden death *(105)*. Differences in the distribution of gap junctions are also important in the development of ventricular arrhythmias. Connexin 43 (Cx43), an important component of gap junctions, is downregulated in hypertrophic myocardium. These changes contribute to slowed conduction and increase the likelihood of reentrant VT *(120)*.

Prolonged QRS duration (>120 ms) occurs in approximately 30% of HF patients, with left bundle branch block (LBBB) being the predominant variant. QRS duration lengthens as LV systolic function decreases and is associated with worse mortality and increased risk of SCD *(121)*.

3. ATRIAL FIBRILLATION IN HF

HF results in atrial stretch, fibrosis and hypertrophy, sympathetic activation, and abnormal ion currents, all of which promote the occurrence of atrial tachyarrhythmias *(122)*. Atrial fibrillation (AF) is the most common sustained cardiac arrhythmia, and HF is associated with an 18-fold increased risk of AF in men and 6-fold in women *(123)*. Many of the cellular mechanisms underlying atrial fibrillation are similar to those involved in ventricular arrhythmias. AF is the result of multiple reentrant wavelets propagating in abnormal atrial tissue. Abnormalities in potassium and calcium currents seen in HF patients result in shorter action potential duration, while atrial stretch leads to lengthened atrial refractoriness and increased dispersion of refractoriness *(124)*. AF decreases cardiac output due to a loss of atrial–ventricular synchrony, an irregularity of ventricular rhythm, and occasionally through tachycardia-mediated cardiomyopathy *(122)*. While atrial fibrillation predicts a poor outcome in patients with systolic heart failure *(125)*, strategies directed at restoring sinus rhythm through pharmacologic means have not proved beneficial *(126)*. Whether interventional approaches to restore sinus rhythm will yield improved long-term results remains to be determined *(127)*.

4. CONCLUSIONS

Hemodynamic alterations resulting from decreased cardiac output and/or increased filling pressures underscore the pathophysiologic changes of HF, classically characterized by complex neurohormonal changes that contribute to the chronic, progressive nature of the disease. An increased understanding of this pathophysiology has led to the development of pharmacologic interventions that have improved quality of life, reduced symptoms and heart failure hospitalizations, and improved mortality. Similarly, devices designed to improve outcomes in heart failure patients typically do so by having a beneficial effect on the underlying HF pathophysiology. Additional insight into the pathophysiology of HF will undoubtedly lead to novel therapeutic interventions.

REFERENCES

1. Hunt SA, Abraham WT, Chin MA, et al. ACC/AHA 2005 Guideline update for the diagnosis and management of chronic heart failure in the adult – Summary article. Journal of the American College of Cardiology 2005;46:1114–1142.
2. Jessup M, Brozena S. Heart Failure. New England Journal of Medicine 2003;348: 2007–2018.
3. Sweeney MO, Ellison KE, Stevenson WG. Implantable cardioverter defibrillators in heart failure. Cardiology Clinics 2001;19(4):653–667.
4. Johnson JA, Parker RB, Patterson JH. Heart failure. In: DiPiro JT, Talbert RL, Yee GC, Matzke GR, Wells BG, Posey LM, eds. Pharmacotherapy: A Pathophysiologic Approach. 5th ed. New York: McGraw-Hill; 2002:185–218.
5. Opie LH. Mechanisms of cardiac contraction and relaxation. In: Zipes DP, Libby P, Bonow RO, Braunwald E, eds. Braunwald's Heart Disease: A Textbook of Cardiovascular Medicine. Philadelphia: Elsevier Saunders; 2005:457–489.
6. Stevenson LW, Bellil D, Grover-McKay M, et al. Effects of afterload reduction (diuretics and vasodilators) on left ventricular volume and mitral regurgitation in severe congestive heart failure secondary to ischemic or idiopathic dilated cardiomyopathy. American Journal of Cardiology 1987;60:654–658.
7. Banasik JL, Copstead LC. Heart failure and dysrhythmias: Common sequelae of cardiac diseases. In: Copstead LC, Banasik JL, eds. Pathophysiology. 3rd ed. St. Louis: Elsevier Saunders; 2005:499–526.
8. Cohn JN, Ferrari R, Sharpe N. Cardiac remodeling - concepts and clinical implications: A consensus paper from an international forum on cardiac remodeling. Journal of the American College of Cardiology 2000;35:569–582.
9. Opie LH, Commerford PJ, Gersh BJ, Pfeffer MA. Controversies in ventricular remodelling. Lancet 2006;367:356–367.
10. Udelson JE, Konstam MA. Relation between left ventricular remodeling and clinical outcomes in heart failure patients with left ventricular systolic dysfunction. Journal of Cardiac Failure 2002;8(6 Suppl):S465–471.
11. Yousef ZR, Redwood SR, Marber MS. Postinfarction left ventricular remodelling: where are the theories and trials leading us? Heart 2000;83:76–80.
12. Chien KR, Knowlton KU, Zhu H, Chien S. Regulation of cardiac gene expression during myocardial growth and hypertrophy: Molecular studies of an adaptive physiologic response. FASEB Journal 1991;5:3037–3046.
13. Aoki H, Richmond M, Izumo S, Sadoshima J. Specific role of the extracellular signal-regulated kinase pathway in angiotensin II-induced cardiac hypertrophy in vitro. The Biochemical Journal 2000;347:275–284.
14. Chien KR, Zhu H, Knowlton KU, et al. Transcriptional regulation during cardiac growth and development. Annual Review of Physiology 1993;55:77–95.
15. Ruwhof C, van der Laarse A. Mechanical stress-induced cardiac hypertrophy: mechanisms and signal transduction pathways. Cardiovascular Research 2000;47:23–37.
16. Sugden PH. Signaling pathways in cardiac myocyte hypertrophy. Annals of Medicine 2001;33:611–622.

17. Thorburn A, Thorburn J, Chen SY, et al. HRas-dependent pathways can activate morphological and genetic markers of cardiac muscle cell hypertrophy. Journal of Biological Chemistry 1993;268:2244–2249.
18. Shiojima I, Walsh K. Regulation of cardiac growth and coronary angiogenesis by the Akt/PKB signaling pathway. Genes & Development 2006;20(24):3347–3365.
19. Frey N, Katus HA, Olson EN, Hill JA. Hypertrophy of the heart: A new therapeutic target? Circulation 2004;109:1580–1589.
20. Serneri N, Modesti PA, Boddi M, et al. Cardiac growth factors in human hypertrophy: relations with myocardial contractility and wall stress. Circulation Research 1999;85:57–67.
21. Schultz JJ, Witt SA, Glascock BJ, et al. TGF-?1 mediates the hypertrophic cardiomyocyte growth induced by angiotensin II. Journal of Clinical Investigation 2002;109:787–796.
22. Hein S, Amon E, Kostin S, et al. Progression from compensated hypertrophy to failure in the pressure-overloaded human heart: Structural deterioration and compensatory mechanisms. Circulation 2003;107:984–991.
23. Iwanaga Y, Aoyama T, Kihara Y, Onozawa Y, Yoneda T, Sasayama S. Excessive activation of matrix metalloproteinases coincides with left ventricular remodeling during transition from hypertrophy to heart failure in hypertensive rats. Journal of the American College of Cardiology 2002;39:1384–1391.
24. Lopez B, Gonzalez A, Querejeta R, Larman M, Diez J. Alterations in the pattern of collagen deposition may contribute to the deterioration of systolic function in hypertensive patients with heart failure. Journal of the American College of Cardiology 2006;48: 89–96.
25. Carabello BA. Concentric versus eccentric remodeling. Journal of Cardiac Failure 2002;8(6 Suppl):S258–263.
26. Colucci WS, Braunwald E. Pathophysiology of heart failure. In: Zipes DP, Libby P, Bonow RO, Braunwald E, eds. Braunwald's Heart Disease: A Textbook of Cardiovascular Medicine. 7th ed. Philadelphia: Elsevier Saunders; 2005:509–538.
27. Imamura T, McDermott PJ, Kent RL, Nagatsu M, Cooper Gt, Carabello BA. Acute changes in myosin heavy chain synthesis rate in pressure versus volume overload. Circulation Research 1994;75(3):418–425.
28. Matsuo T, Carabello BA, Nagatomo Y, et al. Mechanisms of cardiac hypertrophy in canine volume overload. American Journal of Physiology 1998;275(1 Pt 2): H65–74.
29. Mann DL. Stress-activated cytokines and the heart: From adaptation to maladaptation. Annual Review of Physiology 2003;65:81–101.
30. Mitchell GF, Lamas GA, Vaughan DE, Pfeffer MA. Left ventricular remodeling in the year after first anterior myocardial infarction: A quantitative analysis of contractile segment length and ventricular shape. Journal of the American College of Cardiology 1992;19:1136–1144.
31. Baig MK, Mahon N, McKenna WJ, et al. The pathophysiology of advanced heart failure. American Heart Journal 1999;28(2):87–101.
32. Braunwald E. Biomarkers in heart failure. New England Journal of Medicine 2008;358(20):2148–2159.
33. Esler M, Kaye D, Lambert G, Esler D, Jennings G. Adrenergic nervous system in heart failure. American Journal of Cardiology 1997;80:7L–14L.
34. Zucker I. Novel mechanisms of sympathetic regulation in chronic heart failure. Hypertension 2006;48:1005–1011.
35. Houser SR, Margulies KB. Is depressed myocyte contractility centrally involved in heart failure? Circulation Research 2003;92:350–358.
36. Mann DL, Kent RL, Parsons B, Cooper G. Adrenergic effects on the biology of the adult mammalian cardiocyte. Circulation 1992;85:790–804.

37. Singh K, Xiao L, Remondino A, Sawyer DB, Colucci WS. Adrenergic regulation of cardiac myocyte apoptosis. Journal of Cellular Physiology 2001;189(3):257–265.

38. Lohse MJ, Engelhardt S, Eschenhagen T. What is the role of adrenergic signaling in heart failure? Circulation Research 2003;93:896–906.

39. Cohn JN, Levine TB, Olivari MT, et al. Plasma norepinephrine as a guide to prognosis in patients with chronic congestive heart failure. New England Journal of Medicine 1984;311:819–823.

40. The Cardiac Insufficiency Bisoprolol Study (CIBIS). A randomized trial of beta-blockade in heart failure. CIBIS Investigators and Committees. Circulation 1994;90(4):1765–1773.

41. CIBIS-II. The Cardiac Insufficiency Bisoprolol Study II (CIBIS-II): a randomised trial. Lancet 1999;353(9146):9–13.

42. MERIT-HF. Effect of metoprolol CR/XL in chronic heart failure: Metoprolol CR/XL Randomised Intervention Trial in Congestive Heart Failure (MERIT-HF). Lancet 1999;353(9169):2001–2007.

43. Dargie HJ. Effect of carvedilol on outcome after myocardial infarction in patients with left-ventricular dysfunction: the CAPRICORN randomised trial. Lancet 2001;357(9266):1385–1390.

44. Packer M, Bristow MR, Cohn JN, et al. The effect of carvedilol on morbidity and mortality in patients with chronic heart failure. U.S. Carvedilol Heart Failure Study Group. New England Journal of Medicine 1996;334(21):1349–1355.

45. Packer M, Coats AJ, Fowler MB, et al. Effect of carvedilol on survival in severe chronic heart failure. New England Journal of Medicine 2001;344(22):1651–1658.

46. Poole-Wilson PA, Swedberg K, Cleland JG, et al. Comparison of carvedilol and metoprolol on clinical outcomes in patients with chronic heart failure in the Carvedilol Or Metoprolol European Trial (COMET): randomised controlled trial. Lancet 2003;362(9377):7–13.

47. Dubach P, Myers J, Bonetti P, et al. Effects of bisoprolol fumarate on left ventricular size, function, and exercise capacity in patients with heart failure: Analysis with magnetic resonance myocardial tagging. American Heart Journal 2002;143(4):676–683.

48. Lowes BD, Gill EA, Abraham WT, et al. Effects of carvedilol on left ventricular mass, chamber geometry, and mitral regurgitation in chronic heart failure. American Journal of Cardiology 1999;83(8):1201–1205.

49. Waagstein F, Strömblad O, Andersson B, et al. Increased exercise ejection fraction and reversed remodeling after long-term treatment with metoprolol in congestive heart failure: a randomized, stratified, double-blind, placebo-controlled trial in mild to moderate heart failure due to ischemic or idiopathic dilated cardiomyopathy. Eur J Heart Fail 2003;5(5):679–691.

50. Fox K, Ford I, Steg PG, Tendera M, Robertson M, Ferrari R; BEAUTIFUL investigators. Lancet 2008;372(9641):817–821.

51. Kim S, Ohta K, Hamaguchi A, Yukimura T, Miura K, Iwao H. Angiotensin II induces cardiac phenotypic modulation and remodeling in vivo in rats. Hypertension 1995;25:1252–1259.

52. Kim S, Iwao H. Molecular and cellular mechanisms of angiotensin II-mediated cardiovascular and renal disease. Pharmacological Reviews 2000;52:11–34.

53. Latini R, Masson S, Anand I, et al. The comparative prognostic value of plasma neurohormones at baseline in patients with heart failure enrolled in Val-HeFT. European Heart Journal 2004;25:292–299.

54. Swedberg K, Eneroth P, Kjekshus J, Wilhelmsen L. Hormones regulating cardiovascular function in patients with severe congestive heart failure and their relation to mortality. CONSENSUS Trial Study Group. Circulation 1990;82(5):1730–1736.

55. Rosenkranz S. TGF-beta1 and angiotensin networking in cardiac remodeling. Cardiovascular Research 2004;63(3):423–432.

56. CONSENSUS. Effects of enalapril on mortality in severe congestive heart failure. Results of the Cooperative North Scandinavian Enalapril Survival Study (CONSENSUS). The CONSENSUS Trial Study Group. New England Journal of Medicine 1987;316(23):1429–1435.

57. Cohn JN, Johnson G, Ziesche S, et al. A comparison of enalapril with hydralazine–isosorbide dinitrate in the treatment of chronic congestive heart failure. New England Journal of Medicine 1991;325(5):303–310.

58. Pfeffer MA, Braunwald E, Moye LA, et al. Effect of captopril on mortality and morbidity in patients with left ventricular dysfunction after myocardial infarction. Results of the survival and ventricular enlargement trial. The SAVE Investigators. New England Journal of Medicine 1992;327(10):669–677.

59. The SOLVD Investigators. Effect of enalapril on survival in patients with reduced left ventricular ejection fractions and congestive heart failure. New England Journal of Medicine 1991;325(5):293–302.

60. Pitt B, Poole-Wilson PA, Segal R, et al. Effect of losartan compared with captopril on mortality in patients with symptomatic heart failure: randomised trial–the Losartan Heart Failure Survival Study ELITE II. Lancet 2000;355(9215):1582–1587.

61. Spinale FG, de Gasparo M, Whitebread S, et al. Modulation of the renin–angiotensin pathway through enzyme inhibition and specific receptor blockade in pacing-induced heart failure: I. Effects on left ventricular performance and neurohormonal systems. Circulation 1997;96(7):2385–2396.

62. Miyazaki M, Takai S. Tissue angiotensin II generating system by angiotensin-converting enzyme and chymase. Journal of Pharmacology Science 2006;100(5): 391–397.

63. Re RN. Mechanisms of disease: local renin–angiotensin–aldosterone systems and the pathogenesis and treatment of cardiovascular disease. Nature Clinical Practice. Cardiovascular Medicine 2004;1(1):42–47.

64. Rajagopalan S, Pitt B. Aldosterone as a target in congestive heart failure. Medical Clinics of North America 2003;87(2):441–457.

65. Farquharson C, Struthers AD. Spironolactone increases nitric oxide bioactivity, improves endothelial vasodilator dysfunction, and suppresses vascular angiotensin I/angiotensin II conversion in patients with chronic heart failure. Circulation 2000;101:594–597.

66. Weber KT. Aldosterone in congestive heart failure. New England Journal of Medicine 2001;345:1689–1697.

67. Zannad F, Radauceanu A. Effect of MR blockade on collagen formation and cardiovascular disease with a specific emphasis on heart failure. Heart Failure Reviews 2005;10(1):71–78.

68. Pitt B, Zannad F, Remme WJ, et al. The effect of spironolactone on morbidity and mortality in patients with severe heart failure. New England Journal of Medicine 1999;341:709–717.

69. Pitt B, Remme W, Zannad F, et al. Eplerenone, a selective aldosterone blocker, in patients with left ventricular dysfunction after myocardial infarction. New England Journal of Medicine 2003;348(14):1309–1321.

70. Zannad F, Alla F, Dousset B, Perez A, Pitt B. Limitation of excessive extracellular matrix turnover may contribute to survival benefit of spironolactone therapy in patients with congestive heart failure. Circulation 2000;102:2700–2706.

71. Chan AK, Sanderson JE, Wang T, Lam W, Yip G, Wang M, Lam YY, Zhang Y, Yeung L, Wu EB, Chan WW, Wong JT, So N, Yu CM. Aldosterone receptor antagonism induces reverse remodeling when added to angiotensin receptor blockade in chronic heart failure. Journal of the American College of Cardiology 2007;50(7):597–599.

72. Schrier RW, Abraham WT. Hormones and hemodynamics in heart failure. New England Journal of Medicine 1999;341(8):577–585.

73. Lee CR, Watkins ML, Patterson H, et al. Vasopressin: A new target for the treatment of heart failure. American Heart Journal 2003;146:9–18.

74. Chatterjee K. Neurohormonal activation in congestive heart failure and the role of vaso-pressin. American Journal of Cardiology 2005;95(9A):8B–13B.

75. Sanghi P, Uretsky BF, Schwarz ER. Vasopressin antagonism: a future treatment option in heart failure. European Heart Journal 2005;26(6):538–543.

76. Konstam MA, Gheorghiade M, Burnett JC Jr, Grinfeld L, Maggioni AP, Swedberg K, Udelson JE, Zannad F, Cook T, Ouyang J, Zimmer C, Orlandi C. Effects of oral tolvaptan in patients hospitalized for worsening heart failure: the EVEREST Outcome Trial. JAMA 2007;297(12):1319–1331.

77. Gheorghiade M, Konstam MA, Burnett JC Jr, Grinfeld L, Maggioni AP, Swedberg K, Udelson JE, Zannad F, Cook T, Ouyang J, Zimmer C, Orlandi C. Effects of oral tolvaptan in patients hospitalized for worsening heart failure: the EVEREST Clinical Status Trials. JAMA 2007;297(12):1332–1343.

78. Attina T, Camidge R, Newby DE, Webb DJ. Endothelin antagonism in pul-monary hypertension, heart failure, and beyond. Heart (British Cardiac Society) 2005;91(6):825–831.

79. Spieker LE, Luscher TF. Will endothelin receptor antagonists have a role in heart fail-ure? Medical Clinics of North America 2003;87:459–474.

80. Cowburn PJ, Cleland JG. Endothelin antagonists for chronic heart failure: do they have a role? European Heart Journal 2001;22(19):1772–1784.

81. Wada A, Tsutamoto T, Fukai D, et al. Comparison of the effects of selective endothelin ETA and ETB receptor antagonists in congestive heart failure. Journal of the American College of Cardiology 1997;30(5):1385–1392.

82. Wei CM, Lerman A, Rodeheffer RJ, et al. Endothelin in human congestive heart failure. Circulation 1994;89(4):1580–1586.

83. Kelland NF, Webb DJ. Clinical trials of endothelin antagonists in heart failure: a ques-tion of dose? Experimental Biology & Medicine 2006;231(6):696–699.

84. Malinski T. Understanding nitric oxide physiology in the heart: a nanomedical approach. American Journal of Cardiology 2005;96(7B):13i–24i.

85. Anand I, McMurray J, Cohn JN, Konstam MA, Notter T, Quitzau K, Ruschitzka F, Luscher TF. Long-term effects of darusentan on left-ventricular remodeling and clinical outcomes in the EndothelinA Receptor Antagonist Trial in Heart Failure (EARTH): randomized, double-blind, placebo-controlled trial. Lancet 2004;364(9421):347–54.

86. Wollert KC, Drexler H. Regulation of cardiac remodeling by nitric oxide: focus on cardiac myocyte hypertrophy and apoptosis. Heart Failure Reviews 2002;7(4): 317–325.

87. Saraiva RM, Hare JM. Nitric oxide signaling in the cardiovascular system: Implications for heart failure. Current Opinion in Cardiology 2006;21:221–228.

88. Khan SA, Skaf MW, Harrison RW, et al. Nitric oxide regulation of myocardial contrac-tility and calcium cycling: independent impact of neuronal and endothelial nitric oxide synthases. Circulation Research 2003;92(12):1322–1329.

89. Hare JM. Nitroso-redox balance in the cardiovascular system. New England Journal of Medicine 2004;351(20):2112–2114.

90. Taylor AL, Ziesche S, Yancy C, et al. Combination of isosorbide dinitrate and hydralazine in blacks with heart failure. New England Journal of Medicine 2004;351 (20):2049–2057.

91. Cataliotti A, Burnett JC, Jr. Natriuretic peptides: novel therapeutic targets in heart fail-ure. Journal of Investigative Medicine 2005;53(7):378–384.

92. Nishikimi T, Maeda N, Matsuoka H. The role of natriuretic peptides in cardioprotec-tion. Cardiovascular Research 2006;69(2):318–328.

93. McKie PM, Burnett JC, Jr. B-type natriuretic peptide as a biomarker beyond heart fail-ure: speculations and opportunities. Mayo Clinic Proceedings 2005;80(8):1029–1036.

94. Berger R, Huelsman M, Strecker K, et al. B-type natriuretic peptide predicts sudden death in patients with chronic heart failure. Circulation 2002;105(20):2392–2397.

95. Latini R, Masson S, Wong M, et al. Incremental prognostic value of changes in B-type natriuretic peptide in heart failure. American Journal of Medicine 2006;119(1):70.e23–70.e30.

96. Logeart D, Thabut G, Jourdain P, et al. Predischarge B-type natriuretic peptide assay for identifying patients at high risk of re-admission after decompensated heart failure. Journal of the American College of Cardiology 2004;43(4):635–641.

97. Torre-Amione G. Immune activation in chronic heart failure. American Journal of Cardiology 2005;95(11A):3C–8C.

98. Bradham WS, Bozkurt B, Gunasinghe H, Mann D, Spinale FG. Tumor necrosis factor-alpha and myocardial remodeling in progression of heart failure: a current perspective. Cardiovascular Research 2002;53(4):822–830.

99. Chung ES, Packer M, Lo KH, Fasanmade AA, Willerson JT, Anti TNFTACHFI. Randomized, double-blind, placebo-controlled, pilot trial of infliximab, a chimeric monoclonal antibody to tumor necrosis factor-alpha, in patients with moderate-to-severe heart failure: results of the anti-TNF Therapy Against Congestive Heart Failure (ATTACH) trial. Circulation 2003;107(25):3133–3140.

100. Khanna D, McMahon M, Furst DE. Anti-tumor necrosis factor alpha therapy and heart failure: what have we learned and where do we go from here? Arthritis & Rheumatism 2004;50(4):1040–1050.

101. Mann DL, McMurray JJ, Packer M, et al. Targeted anticytokine therapy in patients with chronic heart failure: results of the Randomized Etanercept Worldwide Evaluation (RENEWAL). Circulation 2004;109(13):1594–1602.

102. Stevenson WG, Ellison KE, Sweeney MO, Epstein LM, Maisel WH. Management of arrhythmias in heart failure. Cardiology in Review 2002;10(1):8–14.

103. Tomaselli GF, Marban E. Electrophysiological remodeling in hypertrophy and heart failure. Cardiovascular Research 1999;42:270–283.

104. Rubart M, Zipes DP. Mechanisms of sudden cardiac death. Journal of Clinical Investigation 2005;115:2305–2315.

105. Tomaselli GF, Zipes DP. What causes sudden death in heart failure? Circulation Research 2004;95:754–763.

106. Eisner DA, Choi HS, Diaz ME, O'Neill SC, Trafford AW. Integrative analysis of calcium cycling in cardiac muscle. Circulation Research 2000;87(12):1087–1094.

107. Pieske B, Kretschmann B, Meyer M, et al. Alterations in intracellular calcium handling associated with the inverse force–frequency relation in human dilated cardiomyopathy. Circulation 1995;92(5):1169–1178.

108. del Monte F, Harding SE, Schmidt U, et al. Restoration of contractile function in isolated cardiomyocytes from failing human hearts by gene transfer of SERCA 2a. Circulation 1999;100(23):2308–2311.

109. Schmidt U, Hajjar RJ, Kim CS, Lebeche D, Doye AA, Gwathmey JK. Human heart failure: cAMP stimulation of SR Ca(2+)-ATPase activity and phosphorylation level of phospholamban. American Journal of Physiology 1999;277(2 Pt 2): H474–480.

110. Boluyt MO, O'Neill L, Meredith AL, et al. Alterations in cardiac gene expression during the transition from stable hypertrophy to heart failure. Marked upregulation of genes encoding extracellular matrix components. Circulation Research 1994;75(1): 23–32.

111. Williams RE, Kass DA, Kawagoe Y, et al. Endomyocardial gene expression during development of pacing tachycardia-induced heart failure in the dog. Circulation Research 1994;75(4):615–623.

112. Hasenfuss G, Burkert P. Calcium cycling in congestive heart failure. Journal of Molecular & Cellular Cardiology 2002;34(8):951–969.

113. Marks AR, Reiken S, Marx SO. Progression to heart failure: Is protein kinase a hyperphosphorylation of the ryanodine receptor a contributing factor? Circulation 2002;105:272–275.
114. Bodi I, Muth JN, Hahn HS, et al. Electrical remodeling in hearts from a calcium-dependent mouse model of hypertrophy and failure: complex nature of K+ current changes and action potential duration. Journal of the American College of Cardiology 2003;41(9):1611–1622.
115. Kaab S, Dixon J, Duc J, et al. Molecular basis of transient outward potassium current downregulation in human heart failure: a decrease in Kv4.3 mRNA correlates with a reduction in current density. Circulation 1998;98(14):1383–1393.
116. Tomita F, Bassett AL, Myerburg RJ, Kimura S. Diminished transient outward currents in rat hypertrophied ventricular myocytes. Circulation Research 1994;75(2):296–303.
117. Rubart M, Zipes DP. Genesis of cardiac arrhythmias: Electrophysiological considerations. In: Zipes DP, Libby P, Bonow RO, Braunwald E, eds. Braunwald's Heart Disease: A Textbook of Cardiovascular Medicine. 7th ed. Philadelphia: Elsevier Saunders; 2005:653–687.
118. Weiss JN, Chen PS, Qu Z, Karagueuzian HS, Garfinkel A. Ventricular fibrillation: how do we stop the waves from breaking? Circulation Research 2000;87(12):1103–1107.
119. Kawara T, Derksen R, de Groot JR, et al. Activation delay after premature stimulation in chronically diseased human myocardium relates to the architecture of interstitial fibrosis. Circulation 2001;104(25):3069–3075.
120. Spach MS, Heidlage JF, Dolber PC, Barr RC. Electrophysiological effects of remodeling cardiac gap junctions and cell size: experimental and model studies of normal cardiac growth. Circulation Research 2000;86(3):302–311.
121. Kashani A, Barold SS. Significance of QRS complex duration in patients with heart failure. Journal of the American College of Cardiology 2005;46(12):2183–2192.
122. Knight BP. Atrial fibrillation in patients with congestive heart failure. Pacing & Clinical Electrophysiology 2003;26(7 Pt 2):1620–1623.
123. Kannel WB, Abbott RD, Savage DD, McNamara PM. Epidemiologic features of chronic atrial fibrillation: the Framingham study. New England Journal of Medicine 1982;306(17):1018–1022.
124. Markides V, Peters NS. Mechanisms underlying the development of atrial arrhythmias in heart failure. Heart Failure Reviews 2002;7:243–253.
125. Dries DL, Exner DV, Gersh BJ, Domanski MJ, Waclawiw MA, Stevenson LW. Atrial fibrillation is associated with an increased risk for mortality and heart failure progression in patients with asymptomatic and symptomatic left ventricular systolic dysfunction: a retrospective analysis of the SOLVD trials: Studies of Left Ventricular Dysfunction. J Am Coll Cardiol 1998:32:695–703.
126. Roy D, Talajic M, Nattel S, Wyse DG, Dorian P, Lee KL, Bourassa MG, Arnold JM, Buston AE, Camm AJ, Connolly SJ, Dubuc M, Ducharme A, Guerra PG, Hohnloser SH, Lambert J, Le Heuzey JY, O'Hara G, Pedersen OD, Rouleau JL, Singh BN, Stevenson LW, Stevenson WG, Thibault B, Waldo AL. Atrial Fibrillation and Congestive Heart Failure investigators. Rhythm control versus rate control for atrial fibrillation and heart failure. New England Journal of Medicine 2008;358(25)2667–2677.
127. Khan MN, Jais P, Cummings J, Di Biase L, Sanders P, Martin DO, Kautzner J, Hao S, Themistoclakis S, Fanelli R, Potenza D, Massaro R, Wazni P, Schweikert R, Saliba W, Wang P, Al-Ahmad A, Behiery S, Santarelli P, Starlin RC, Dello Russo A, Pelargonio G, Brachmann J, Schibgilla V, Bonso A, Casella M, Raveile A, Haissaguerre M, Natala A, PABA-CHF investigators. Pulmonary-vein isolation for atrial fibrillation in patients with heart failure. New England Journal of Medicine 2008;359(17):1778–1785.
128. Hen S, Amon E, Kostin S, et al. Progression from compensated hypertrophy to failure in the pressure-overloaded human heart: Structural deterioration and compensatory mechanisms. Circulation 2003;107:984–991.

2

Medical Therapy for Heart Failure

Neal K. Lakdawala, MD
and Akshay Desai, MD

CONTENTS

Abstract

Heart failure due to a decline in cardiac performance initiates compensatory neurohormonal mechanisms in an effort to maintain systemic perfusion. Ongoing neurohormonal activation may have deleterious consequences for cardiac performance, ventricular remodeling, myocardial function, and heart failure progression. The fundamental objective of modern medical therapy for heart failure is to relieve symptoms (largely through relief of volume overload) and to stall (or even reverse) disease progression through combined utilization of neurohormonal antagonists that help to restore normal hemodynamics, maintain normal plasma volume, and prevent ventricular enlargement. This chapter focuses on the key elements of medical therapy for heart failure.

Key Words: Heart failure; Medical therapy; Neurohormones; Renin–angiotensin system; Digitalis; Systolic dysfunction; Remodeling; Hemodynamics.

From: *Contemporary Cardiology: Device Therapy in Heart Failure*
Edited by: W.H. Maisel, DOI 10.1007/978-1-59745-424-7_2
© Humana Press, a part of Springer Science+Business Media, LLC 2010

1. INTRODUCTION

Heart failure begins from a primary myocardial injury (for example, myocardial infarction) that precipitates a decline in cardiac performance and initiates a variety of compensatory neurohormonal mechanisms in an effort to maintain systemic perfusion. Chief among these mechanisms is activation of the renin–angiotensin–aldosterone system (RAAS) and sympathetic nervous system (SNS) which promotes salt and water retention as well as peripheral vasoconstriction that helps to increase plasma volume, restore cardiac output, and preserve mean arterial pressure. While beneficial in the short term, ongoing neurohormonal activation generates sustained increases in ventricular preload and afterload that may have deleterious consequences for cardiac performance, fueling a vicious cycle of ventricular remodeling, further decline in myocardial function, additional neurohormonal activation, and heart failure progression. The fundamental objective of modern medical therapy for heart failure is to relieve heart failure symptoms (largely through relief of volume overload) and to stall (or even reverse) this cycle of myocardial remodeling and heart failure progression through combined utilization of neurohormonal antagonists that help to restore normal hemodynamics, maintain normal plasma volume, and prevent ventricular enlargement. Our focus in this chapter will be on the key pharmacologic elements of this approach, highlighting the evidence supporting the utilization of digitalis glycosides, diuretics, RAAS antagonists, other vasodilators, and beta-blockers in the management of patients with chronic heart failure. It should be noted that medical therapy for heart failure described in this chapter applies to patients with heart failure with decreased (<40%) systolic ejection fraction (EF), including patients with ischemic heart disease and idiopathic dilated cardiomyopathy. Currently, there are few large-scale trials that inform the management of the syndrome of heart failure with preserved systolic function (i.e., diastolic heart failure); thus, we limit the scope of this chapter to only those patients with demonstrated systolic dysfunction.

2. DIGITALIS GLYCOSIDES

Digitalis and its derivatives have been used in the therapy of heart failure dating to William Withering's description of the use of foxglove in 1785 *(1)*. Digoxin is the prototypical drug in this class, and the only one currently in widespread use. By reversibly inhibiting Na^+/K^+ ATPase pump in the cell membrane of the cardiac myocyte, digoxin increases intracellular Na^+ and potentiates calcium influx via the membrane-associated Na^+/Ca^+ exchanger. Enhanced cytosolic calcium in turn enhances calcium loading of the sarcoplasmic reticulum, increasing calcium release during systole and enhancing the force of myocyte contraction. As well, digoxin has important effects on the autonomic nervous system, including a vagotonic property that accounts for its slowing of heart rate and slowing of conduction velocity through the atrioventricular node, and a sympatholytic effect resulting from diminished sensitivity of carotid baroreceptors. As it is a relatively weak inotropic agent in the doses utilized in clinical practice, the primary mechanism of digoxin benefit in heart failure patients is thought to be related to its ability to modulate the activity of the autonomic nervous system and to limit downstream activation of the renin–angiotensin–aldosterone system *(2, 3)*.

Extensive evidence from randomized clinical trials exists to support the use of digoxin for relief of symptoms in patients with chronic heart failure, though there is no evidence of an impact on cardiovascular mortality. The Randomized Assessment of Digoxin on Inhibitors of the Angiotensin-Converting Enzyme Study (RADIANCE) randomly assigned 178 patients to continued digoxin therapy or digoxin withdrawal. The study population was made up of patients with NYHA class II–III heart failure and sinus rhythm, who were clinically stable on a regimen of digoxin, diuretics, and an ACE inhibitor. The result was a sixfold (RR 5.9, 95% CI 2.1–17.2) excess in worsening heart failure symptoms when digoxin was withdrawn from these otherwise stable patients *(4)*. These results were extended by the Digitalis Investigators Group (DIG) trial, which prospectively randomized 6800 patients with mild–moderate heart failure (54% class II and 31% class III) to standard medical therapy with or without digoxin. In this trial, patients randomized to digoxin experienced a 28% reduction in the risk of hospitalization for heart failure and an 8% relative risk reduction in all-cause hospitalization, but no difference in mortality relative to those assigned to placebo (Fig. 1). Although there was a trend toward fewer deaths from progressive pump failure in the digoxin group, this benefit was offset by deaths related to arrhythmia and coronary disease. Subgroup analysis suggested that patients

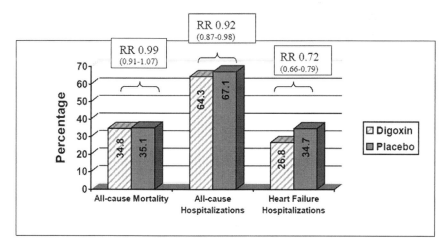

Fig. 1. Major outcomes in the Digitalis Investigators Group (DIG) Trial. Patients randomized to digoxin in the DIG trial experienced reductions in the risk of heart failure and all-cause hospitalizations but not mortality when compared to patients assigned to placebo.

with more advanced heart failure (class III, very low EF) derived a larger benefit from digoxin *(5)*.

The primary limitation to utilization of digoxin in heart failure patients is its narrow therapeutic index and its interaction with many other drugs that are commonly utilized in this population (Table 1). Digoxin toxicity is a potentially lethal complication characterized by atrial and ventricular arrhythmias, vomiting, visual disturbances, confusion, and potassium abnormalities that may be challenging to manage despite the availability of an antidote. The toxic effects of digoxin are more common in the setting of active ischemia, electrolyte disturbance, or hypothyroidism and may not be accurately predicted by the measured serum digoxin concentration. However, post hoc analyses of the DIG trial have suggested an increase in mortality in patients with plasma digoxin levels greater than 0.8 ng/mL *(6)*. Another post hoc analysis of the DIG trial suggested excess mortality in women in the digoxin-treated group (HR 1.23, $p = 0.014$) but was not adjusted for plasma digoxin level *(7)*; subsequent analysis that accounted for digoxin level failed to find this association *(8)*. Since the salutary effect of digoxin on ventricular function and neuroendocrine activation is evident

Table 1
Potential drug interactions with digoxin

Drug	Mechanism of digoxin interaction	Result
Non-potassium-sparing diuretics	Hypokalemia and/or hypomagnesemia	Increased risk of arrhythmias
Intravenous calcium	Increased myocyte calcium	Increased risk of arrhythmias
Quinidine, verapamil, amiodarone, propafenone, spironolactone	Reduced digoxin clearance	Increased serum digoxin concentration
Macrolides, tetracycline	Decreased intestinal digoxin metabolism and resultant increase in digoxin absorption	Increased serum digoxin concentration
Antacids, bran, cholestyramine, metoclopramide, neomycin	Decreased digoxin absorption	Decreased serum digoxin concentration
Thyroid medications	Increased metabolic state	Decreased serum digoxin concentration
Beta-blockers, non-dihydropyridine calcium channel blockers, flecainide	Decreased sinoatrial or atrioventricular node conduction	Increased risk of bradyarrhythmias and heart block

even at lower serum concentrations (0.5–1.0 ng/mL) *(9)*, efforts should be made to maintain serum digoxin concentrations <1.0 ng/mL and to avoid up-titration of digoxin dose for heart rate control, even in patients with atrial fibrillation.

Practically speaking, the use of digoxin is no longer mandated in heart failure and this was reflected in the guidelines which downgraded digoxin from a class I to a class IIa recommendation. In the language of the ACC/AHA guidelines, digoxin *may be considered* for persistent heart failure symptoms in patients already receiving therapy with diuretics, ACEi, and beta-blockers. In light of the results of RADIANCE and other digoxin withdrawal studies *(10)*, it is not recommended that digoxin be withdrawn from patients unless they are taking an ACEi and a beta-blocker *(11)*.

3. DIURETIC THERAPY FOR HEART FAILURE

Diuretics play an essential role in the medical management of heart failure patients. By interfering with the kidney's ability to reabsorb sodium, diuretics reduce extracellular fluid volume and rapidly relieve symptoms of congestion. There is universal acknowledgement of their utility in improving symptoms and functional capacity; however, increasing evidence suggests that diuretics may have detrimental vascular, hemodynamic, and neurohormonal effects. The net impact of diuretics on mortality in heart failure patients remains unknown, largely due to the ethical and practical considerations precluding conduct of a randomized, controlled clinical trial.

Diuretics are commonly classified by their site of action within the nephron, which is the primary determinant of their effect on the filtered sodium load *(12)* (Fig. 2). Agents active in the proximal tubule, such as carbonic anhydrase inhibitors (e.g., acetazolamide), are relatively ineffective natriuretic agents, since most of the sodium that escapes the proximal tubule is reabsorbed downstream in the loop of Henle. As well, these agents tend to enhance urinary bicarbonate loss, generating a metabolic acidosis that lessens their efficacy. As a consequence, carbonic anhydrase inhibitors are used infrequently in the management of heart failure patients. By contrast, loop-type diuretics, of which furosemide is a prototypical agent, are the cornerstone of heart failure therapy. These agents inhibit the $Na^+2Cl^-K^+$ co-transporter at the thick ascending limb of the loop of Henle and are extremely effective natriuretic agents, capable of increasing the fractional excretion of sodium (FENA) to 25% of the filtered sodium load. Thiazide-type diuretics (e.g., hydrochlorothiazide, metolazone) inhibit the Na^+Cl^- co-transporter in the distal convoluted tubule, and when used alone, they are associated with only a modest natriuretic effect (5–8% of filtered sodium load, 1/5–1/3 potency compared to loop diuretics). However, when used in combination with loop diuretics, they are a potent tool for enhancing natriuresis and diuresis, a property which is frequently exploited for the management of patients with refractory volume overload. Potassium-sparing

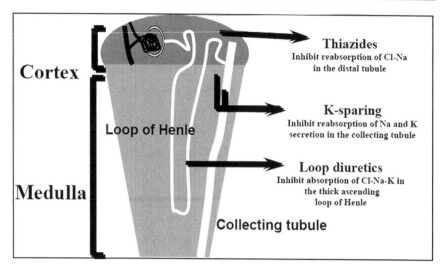

Fig. 2. Diuretics typically used in the treatment of heart failure: mechanism of action.

diuretics (e.g., spironolactone, triamterene, amiloride) inhibit sodium reabsorption either by inhibiting synthesis or by directly blocking the epithelial sodium channel in the principal cells of the collecting duct. These agents are weak natriuretic and diuretic agents, but may be useful as adjunctive agents to stem urinary potassium losses and prevent hypokalemia in patients receiving loop diuretics. The mineralocorticoid receptor antagonist spironolactone is a special case, as it is the only diuretic agent demonstrated to improve mortality in patients with advanced heart failure (see separate discussion below).

To be effective, diuretics must be delivered to their active sites in the renal tubule at the threshold concentration necessary to elicit a natriuretic response *(13)*. Loop diuretics exhibit a characteristic sigmoidal dose–response curve; this implies that for any given patient, the diuretic dose must be titrated to a therapeutic concentration before any significant diuretic effect can be achieved, and that beyond a certain "ceiling" dose, no further natriuresis will occur. In patients with congestive heart failure, the normal dose–response to loop diuretics is disturbed, and the maximal achievable sodium excretion is limited. This may be due in part to diminished renal blood flow (as a consequence of decreased cardiac output), which reduces the filtered sodium load, and as well to enhanced proximal tubule reabsorption of sodium in the face of sustained SNS and RAAS activation. Further, in the face of prolonged exposure to loop diuretics, there is hypertrophy of the distal tubule with resultant increase in sodium reabsorption (diuretic "resistance"). This can lead to a decrease in loop diuretic responsiveness and is occasionally remediable with the addition of a diuretic active in the distal tubule (e.g., thiazide). Intrinsic renal disease and progressive renal failure often further complicate the management of heart failure patients since even with optimal dosing and combination diuretic therapy, the maximal sodium excretion in response to full-dose diuretic may be limited to as little as 25 mmol of sodium excretion (300–400 cc of urine).

The effects of diuretics are not limited to an increase in sodium excretion. Relief of heart failure symptoms in patients receiving furosemide occurs prior to the onset of diuresis, perhaps due to acute preload reduction related to venodilation (14). Despite clear symptomatic benefits, several studies have shown that RAAS activation is markedly enhanced following loop diuretic administration with an associated increase in systemic vascular resistance and decrease in cardiac output. Long-term RAAS activation may have deleterious effects due to increased systemic vasoconstriction, enhanced sodium and water retention, and aldosterone-mediated myocardial fibrosis. These impacts on neurohormonal activation may account for the relationship between loop diuretic dose and mortality seen in both hospitalized heart failure patients (15) and those with chronic heart failure in the outpatient setting (16) though these studies are heavily confounded by the tight association between loop diuretic requirement and heart failure severity. Due to the potential adverse effects, however, maintenance diuretic therapy should be reserved for patients with symptomatic heart failure and clinical evidence of volume overload.

Choice of a diuretic, dose, and frequency of administration requires knowledge of the pharmacokinetics of the individual diuretic drugs, including the duration of effect and the bioavailability of the individual agents (Table 2). As it is familiar and inexpensive, furosemide is the most widely utilized loop diuretic agent, but it is considerably less potent and less bioavailable orally than bumetanide and torsemide. No large, randomized, blinded studies comparing different loop diuretics have been conducted to help inform the choice of one agent over another, although there are some discernible differences in effects on potassium excretion and neurohormonal activation that may impact on patient outcomes (17).

For patients who fail to respond to maximal doses of loop diuretics, combination diuretic therapy, particularly with addition of a thiazide diuretic, can enhance effective natriuresis due to "sequential blockade" of sodium reabsorption within the nephron. As well, for hospitalized patients, continuous intravenous infusions of loop diuretics may enhance urine output and sodium excretion, perhaps due to more constant maintenance of adequate serum levels. For patients refractory to conventional measures, mechanical fluid removal with ultrafiltration or hemodialysis may be necessary. A number of additional therapies have been investigated for the diuretic refractory patient including early ultrafiltration (18), natriuretic peptides (e.g., nesiritide) (19), vasopressin receptor antagonists (20), and adenosine receptor antagonists (21); these therapies are the subject of active, ongoing

Table 2
Diuretics typically used in the treatment of heart failure

Class	Daily oral dose (mg) Initial dose (mg)	Maximum dose[a] (mg/day)	Duration of action (hours)	Effect on FENA	Effect on serum sodium concentration	Oral bio-availability (%)
Loop diuretics						
Furosemide	20–40	600	6–8	↑20–	Increase	10–100[b]
Bumetanide	0.5–1.0	10	4–6	25%		80–100
Torsemide	10–20	200	12–16			80–100
Thiazide diuretics						
Chlorthalidone	12.5–25	100	6–12	↑5–10%	Decrease	65–75
HCTZ	25–50	200	6–12			ND
Metolazone	2.5–5	20	12–24			ND

FENA – Fractional excretion of filtered sodium; ND – No reliable data.

[a]The average starting dose is an increment of one- to twofold of the minimum effective dose, rarely the maximum dose will be indicated

[b]The average bioavailability is ∼50% but varies widely.

investigation and have not yet become part of the standard heart failure armamentarium. For all patients with refractory heart failure, dietary sodium restriction and limitation of agents which further diminish glomerular filtration (such as non-steroidal anti-inflammatory drugs, NSAIDs) must be emphasized.

The primary risks associated with diuretics are electrolyte disturbances (and associated arrhythmias) and hypovolemia, which can be prevented with careful monitoring. Hypokalemia is the most frequent complication and may enhance the risk of ventricular arrhythmias and sudden cardiac death. In fact, in retrospective analyses of large clinical trials (SOLVD), patients taking non-potassium-sparing diuretics appear to experience a higher risk of arrhythmic death than those taking potassium-sparing diuretics (22). However, widespread use of potassium-sparing diuretics such as spirono-lactone carries its own risk of life-threatening hyperkalemia (23). Careful monitoring of serum potassium during diuretic therapy is therefore critically important to maintain normal balance. Hyponatremia is another potential complication, more commonly observed with thiazide diuretics which enhance sodium excretion and impair maximal urinary dilution. However, because diuresis is usually iso-osmotic, true diuretic-induced hyponatremia is uncommon; most heart failure patients with hyponatremia have free water excess rather than salt depletion and actually improve with administration of additional loop diuretics and restriction of free water intake. Though hypo-magnesemia is also seen commonly in patients receiving chronic loop diuretics, the clinical significance of this is unclear, especially as serum magnesium levels do not reliably assess intracellular magnesium stores. Among patients with gout, both loop and thiazide-type diuretics appear to increase the risk of precipitating a flare by two- to threefold *(24, 25)*.

4. VASODILATOR THERAPY

4.1. Angiotensin-Converting Enzyme (ACE) Inhibitors

ACE inhibitors (ACEi) were established as the cornerstone of heart failure therapy after their efficacy was validated in several large clinical trials in the 1980s and 1990s. The primary action of ACE inhibitors is to block the conversion of angiotensin I to angiotensin II, attenuating myriad downstream consequences of RAAS activation (Fig. 3). Through signaling at the angiotensin type 1 receptor, angiotensin II promotes myocyte hypertrophy and apoptosis, enhances arteriolar tone, stimulates fibroblast and smooth muscle cell proliferation, and increases circulating levels of norepinephrine and aldosterone. Enhanced activation of the SNS further potentiates systemic vasoconstriction and increases the load on the failing heart. As has been well described in the post-infarction setting, persistent neurohormonal activation leads to maladaptive ventricular enlargement and remodeling, which in turn reduce myocardial reserve and enhance vulnerability to heart failure development. Within the kidney, activation of angiotensin II and aldosterone stimulates tubular reabsorption of salt and water, enhancing circulating plasma volume, and ultimately precipitating heart failure symp-

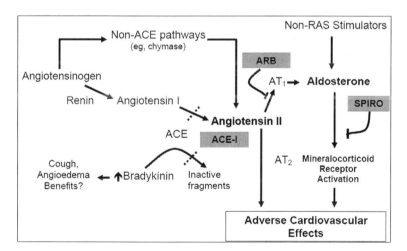

Fig. 3. The renin–angiotensin–aldosterone system (RAAS) and its inhibitors: angiotensin-converting enzyme inhibitors (ACEi), angiotensin receptor blockers (ARBs), and aldosterone antagonists. ACEi are active by blocking the conversion of angiotensin I to angiotensin II as well as by blocking the degradation of bradykinin. The pathologic effects of angiotensin II can be directly antagonized through the mechanism of selective AT1 blockers (ARBs).

toms including dyspnea and peripheral edema. Interruption of angiotensin II generation therefore retards myocardial hypertrophy and fibrosis, while simultaneously providing hemodynamic benefits to the failing heart by reducing ventricular preload and afterload *(26)*. ACEi also prevent the breakdown of bradykinin, with additional vasodilatory benefits.

A wealth of clinical trial evidence now supports the benefits of ACE inhibitors across the spectrum of patients with chronic heart failure, ranging from patients with asymptomatic left ventricular dysfunction to those with disabling class IV symptoms (Table 3). The Studies of Left Ventricular Dysfunction (SOLVD) enrolled a broad population of patients (NYHA I–III) with symptomatic heart failure and LVEF <35% and randomized them to treatment with enalapril or placebo *(27)*. Over 41 months, enalapril therapy was associated with a 16% relative risk reduction in all-cause mortality (HR 0.84, $p = 0.0036$). Patients with asymptomatic LV dysfunction were enrolled in an ancillary study (SOLVD-Prevention) and derived similar benefits from enalapril therapy (HR for death or HF with enalapril 0.80, $p < 0.001$ relative to placebo). The Cooperative North Scandinavian Enalapril Survival Study (CONSENSUS) extended the benefits of ACE inhibition to the population of patients with advanced heart failure, demonstrating potential for mortality benefit with enalapril among those with class III–IV heart failure despite a mortality rate of 52% at 1 year in the placebo arm *(28)*. In that study, overall mortality was reduced by 31% in the group treated with enalapril (HR 0.69, 95% CI, $p = 0.001$) largely due to a marked decrement in the incidence of progressive pump failure.

In addition to chronic heart failure, long-term studies of patients following myocardial infarction (Survival and Ventricular Enlargement: SAVE *(29)*, Acute Infarction Ramipril Study: AIRE *(30)*, and Trandolapril Cardiac Evaluation: TRACE *(31)*) have demonstrated the benefit of ACE inhibitors in heart failure prevention and mortality reduction. SAVE studied patients with little or no clinical heart failure, who were enrolled on the basis of a reduced LVEF ($\leq 40\%$). Among the post-MI ACEi trials, this was a less sick group, with an estimated 1-year mortality rate of 11% in the placebo group. In this study, initiation of captopril 3–16 days after myocardial infarction was associated with a 19% reduction in all-cause mortality, at a median of 42 months post-infarction. The AIRE trial studied a highly selected group (52,019 screened and 1986 enrolled) of patients with symptomatic heart failure, but without evidence of reduced perfusion, early (2–6 days) after an MI. In this population (slightly sicker than SAVE, with estimated 1-year mortality in the placebo arm of 20%), there was a 27% reduction in all-cause mortality in the ramipril group that became evident after several weeks. The TRACE study was an important contribution to the growing field of post-MI ACEi studies in that it had loosely defined inclusion criteria that more closely approximated "real-life" practice and enrolled 1749 patients of the 6676 screened (the majority excluded on the basis of EF>35%). There was a 22% reduction in mortality with trandolapril compared to placebo; and mor-

Table 3
Major angiotensin-converting enzyme inhibitor (ACEi) trials in heart failure

Trial name, date, and number of participants (N)	Drug (and control group in the case of active comparator)	NYHA or Killip classification	Effect on all-cause mortality HR[d]	Affect on hospitalizations	1-year mortality in the control group	Caveats
Chronic heart failure trials						
CONSENSUS 1987 N = 253	Enalapril Goal 10 mg BID[a] Achieved: 9.2 mg BID	IV 100%	0.69 (p = 0.002)[a]	Not reported	52%	
V-HeFT II 1991 N = 804	Hydralazine/isordil Goal 300 mg/160 mg Achieved: 270 mg/136 mg Vs Enalapril Goal 20 mg daily Achieved: 18.6 mg	I 6% II 51% III 43% IV <1%	0.72 (p = 0.016)[b]	None	No placebo group	
SOLVD 1991 N = 2569	Enalapril Goal 20 mg daily Achieved: NA		ARR 4.5%, RRR 16% (at 41 months)		16% est.	
Post-myocardial infarction trials						
SAVE 1992 N = 2231	Captopril Goal: 50 mg TID (reached by 79% of patients still taking captopril)	I 60%[c] II III IV	0.81 (0.68–0.97)	All-cause hospitalization not reported, 22% RRR in HF hospitalizations	11% est.	The mortality curves began to separate after 1 year.

(Continued)

Table 3
(Continued)

Trial name, date, and number of participants (N)	Drug (and control group in the case of active comparator)	NYHA or Killip classification	Effect on all-cause mortality HR[d]	Affect on hospitalizations	1-year mortality in the control group	Caveats
AIRE 1993 N = 1986	Ramipril Goal 5 mg BID Achieved: 4.1 mg BID	Not published	0.73 (0.60–0.89)		20% est.	Mortality curves separated almost immediately Broad inclusion criteria
TRACE 1995 N = 1749	Trandolapril Goal 4 mg daily		5.6% ARR 22% RRR NNT~18 (at 12 months)		26% est.	
Asymptomatic left ventricular dysfunction						
SOLVD-Prevention 1992 N = 4228	Enalapril Goal: 10 mg BID Achieved: 6.35 mg BID	I 67% II 33%	0.92 (0.79–1.08)	No difference in all-cause hospitalization, 36% RRR in HF hospitalization	5% est.	Enalapril was associated with a significant reduction in the development of HF: HR 0.71 (0.64–0.79)

[a]95% confidence interval not published.

[b]hazard ratio after 2 years of follow-up, 95% CI not published.

[c]baseline Killip class beyond class 1 was not published.

[d]HR – Hazard ratio provided except as noted in table.

NYHA – New York Heart Association., NA = not available

ARR – Absolute Risk Reduction; RRR – Relative Risk Reduction; NNT – Number Needed to Treat tality curves began to diverge within weeks. Taken together, the ACEi trials in diverse HF populations have found that beyond reducing all-cause mortality (26% risk reduction), ACEi have also decreased hospitalizations for heart failure (27% risk reduction), reduced re-infarction (20% risk reduction), and improved quality of life (32, 33). Moreover, ACEi have been shown to attenuate progressive LV remodeling in patients with heart failure, consistently improving LVEF and reducing left ventricular volumes (34).

Given demonstrated benefits of a range of different ACE inhibitors across the spectrum of heart failure patients, there is ample evidence supporting a class effect, rather than benefit particular to any given agent. The optimal dose of ACE inhibitor remains a subject of some controversy, even though several clinical trials have been designed to address this question (35–37). Since benefit is proven only at the doses achieved in clinical trials, the consensus recommendations support the use of any of the agents listed in Table 4, with titration targeted to the recommended dose (11). The consensus ACC/AHA guidelines give a strong recommendation (class I) for the use of ACEi across the spectrum of left ventricular dysfunction, in patients both with and without symptoms of heart failure (11).

Table 4
Angiotensin-converting enzyme inhibitor (ACEi) doses
recommended in the treatment of heart failure

Drug	Initial dose (mg)	Target dose (mg)
Captopril	3.125–6.25 TID	50 TID
Enalapril	2.5 BID	10–20 BID
Fosinopril	5–10 QD	40 QD
Lisinopril	2.5–5 QD	20–40 QD
Perindopril	2 QD	8–16 QD
Quinapril	5 BID	20 BID
Ramipril	1.25–2.5 QD	10 QD
Trandolapril	1 QD	4 QD

BID (twice daily), QD (once daily), TID (three times daily).

In general, ACEi are well tolerated. Hypotension and dizziness, cough, azotemia, and angioedema are more commonly reported with ACEi; and in trials, the incidence of each side effect tended to be twofold higher than that with placebo (38). In general, the risk of symptomatic hypotension is low but can be predicted by baseline hyponatremia, renal insufficiency, or a high requirement for potassium replacement; all surrogate measures of RAAS activation (39). In patients with these features, a brief period observation after administration of the first dose of ACEi should be considered. Practically speaking, most of these patients will receive their first dose of medicine in the hospital and can expect a 8–10 mmHg drop in mean blood pressure after the first dose of ACEi (40). The CONSENSUS II study demonstrated that when given immediately post-infarct, an intravenously administered ACEi may actually worsen the clinical course if it causes hypotension, highlighting the importance of proper patient selection before administration of ACEi *(41)*. Cough and angioedema in ACE-inhibitor-treated patients are thought to be related to inhibition of bradykinin breakdown and may in many circumstances be avoided by substitution of an angiotensin receptor blocking drug (see below) with comparable long-term benefits for the patient. Angioedema is rare, occurring in less than 1% of patients.

4.2. Angiotensin Receptor Blockers (ARBs)

Roughly 9% of patients of European ancestry are ACE-inhibitor intolerant due to development of cough or angioedema, and the intolerance related to cough may be threefold higher in patients of Asian ancestry *(42, 43)*. These side effects are thought to be related to simultaneous inhibition of bradykinin breakdown and may be circumvented through blockade of angiotensin II activity downstream at the receptor level using angiotensin receptor blocking drugs (Fig. 3). As well, it has been demonstrated that levels of circulating angiotensin II return to pre-ACE inhibitor treatment values in patients receiving chronic ACE inhibitor therapy. This increase in angiotensin II levels, or "ACE escape," is incompletely understood but thought to be associated with alternate synthesis pathways for angiotensin II. Enzymes such as cathepsin G and elastase are thought to directly convert angiotensinogen to angiotensin II, while chymases and cathepsin G are thought to provide an alternate pathway for conversion of angiotensin I to angiotensin II. This observation supports a rationale for more complete blockade of the RAAS through combined utilization of ACEi/ARB.

Several large-scale clinical trials of ARBs have now been conducted to assess whether or not these theoretical benefits are borne out in clinical practice. Broadly speaking, the trials can be divided into those that tested ARBs as an alternative to ACEi and those that added ARBs to patients already taking ACEi. Each strategy has been explored in both chronic heart failure patients and those with post-MI left ventricular dysfunction (Table 5).

The clearest indication for ARBs is in the patients who are ACE intolerant, a hypothesis examined in the Candesartan Assessment of Reduction in Mortality and Morbidity-Alternative study (CHARM-Alternative) *(44)*. CHARM-Alternative randomized 2028 patients with mild–moderate heart failure, who were previously unable to tolerate an ACEi (primarily because of cough) to treatment with the ARB candesartan or placebo. After a median of 33.7 months of follow-up, there was a significant 23% reduction in the primary outcome of cardiovascular death or heart failure hospitalization (HR 0.77; 95% CI 0.67–0.89, $p < 0.0001$) as well as a statistically significant 17% reduction in the covariate-adjusted rate of all-cause mortality (HR 0.83; 95% CI 0.70–0.99, $p = 0.033$) in patients randomized to ARB.

Taken as a whole, randomized trials of ARB vs ACEi as monotherapy in patients with chronic heart failure suggest no difference in major cardiovas-

Table 5
Major angiotensin receptor blocker (ARB) trials in heart failure

Trial name and publication date	Drug and control group	NYHA or Killip classification of participants	Effect on all-cause mortality HR and 95% CI	Affect on hospitalizations	1-year mortality in the control group	Caveats
Chronic heart failure trials – ARB compared to ACEi or placebo without ACEi						
ELITE II 2000 N = 3152	Losartan Goal: 50 mg QD Achieved: NA Captopril Goal: 50 mg TID Achieved: NA	NYHA II 52% III 43% IV 5%	None HR: 1.13 (0.95–1.35)	None HR 1.04 (0.94–1.16)	10.4%	Older population, mean age 71.5 years
CHARM-Alternative 2003 N = 2028	Candesartan Goal: 32 mg Achieved: 23 mg (59% at goal)	NYHA II 48% III 48% IV 4%	17% reduction HR: 0.83 (0.70–0.99)*	NS difference	ND	Associated with a 23% reduction in the primary outcome of CV death or hospital admission for HF
Chronic heart failure trials – ARB added to ACEi						
Val-HeFT 2001 N = 5010	Valsartan Goal: 160 mg BID Achieved: 127 mg BID (84% achieved goal)	NYHA II 62% III 36% IV 2%	One HR 1.02 (0.88–1.18)	NS difference	9% (est.)	

* = 0.003

(Continued)

Table 5
(Continued)

Trial name and publication date	Drug and control group	NYHA or Killip classification of participants	Effect on all-cause mortality HR and 95% CI	Affect on hospitalizations	1-year mortality in the control group	Caveats
CHARM-Added 2003 $N = 2548$	Candesartan Goal: 32 mg daily Achieved: 27 mg (73% achieved goal)	NYHA II 24% III 73% IV 3%	None HR 0.89 (0.77–1.02)	No difference in patients hospitalized, but 12% reduction in total admissions ($p = 0.023$)		Increased hyperkalemia, hypotension, and azotemia in the combination group 15% reduction in the 1° outcome of CV death or admission for HF
Post-myocardial infarction trials – ARB compared to ACE						
OPTIMAAL 2002 $N = 5477$	Losartan Goal: 50 mg daily Achieved: NA Captopril Goal: 50 mg TID Achieved: NA	Killip I 32% II 57% III 10% IV 1.6%	None HR 1.13 (0.99–1.28)		9% (est.)	Non-inferiority criteria were **not** met.
Post-myocardial infarction trials – ARB added to ACEi						
VALIANT	Captopril 25 mg TID (control)	Killip I 28% II 48% III 17% IV 6%	No difference compared to control. HR 1.00 (0.90–1.11)	62.8%	13.3%	Non-inferiority criteria **were** met.
	Valsartan 80 mg BID			62.5% NS difference		
	Valsartan 40 mg BID and Captopril TID		HR 0.98 (0.89–1.09)	61.3% NS difference		

cular outcomes. Death, cardiovascular death, and hospitalizations for heart failure are no different between patients treated with an ACEi or ARB alone. The largest of these, the Evaluation of Losartan In The Elderly Study (ELITE II) trial, compared an ARB with an ACE inhibitor in patients at least 60 years of age with NYHA class II–IV heart failure, who had not been previously treated with either an ACE inhibitor or an ARB *(45)*. After a mean follow-up of 1.5 years, there were no significant differences in all-cause mortality (11.7% vs 10.4% average annual mortality rate) or in sudden death or resuscitated arrest (9.0% vs 7.3%) between the two treatment groups. Although ARB treatment was not clinically superior to ACE-inhibitor therapy, it was significantly better tolerated, with a withdrawal rate of 9.4%, as compared with 14.5% for ACE-inhibitor therapy ($p < 0.001$). Losartan was also tested in the post-infarction population in the Optimal Trial in Myocardial Infarction with the Angiotensin II Antagonist losartan (OPTIMAAL) *(46)*. Here 5477 patients not already taking an ACEi were randomized to either losartan or captopril 3 days after a myocardial infarction with associated heart failure or left ventricular dysfunction. There was a non-significant trend toward *increased* all-cause mortality in the losartan group (HR 1.13, 95% CI 0.99–1.28, $p = 0.07$), and for this primary outcome, losartan did not satisfy criteria for non-inferiority to captopril. Similar to the results of ELITE II, losartan was better tolerated, with significantly fewer discontinuations for cough, dysgeusia, and angioedema.

In the post-MI population, the Valsartan in Acute Myocardial Infarction (VALIANT) trial compared three different regimens, captopril, valsartan, or both, in 14,703 patients who had post-infarction heart failure and/or left ventricular dysfunction *(47)*. There was no significant difference in primary or secondary outcomes between any of the treatment groups. After a median follow-up of little over 2 years, the mortality rate was not statistically different between the groups: 19.5% in the captopril group, 19.9% in the valsartan group, and 19.3% in the valsartan and captopril groups (compared to captopril, HR 1.00; CI 0.90–1.11 and HR 0.98; CI 0.89–1.09). The study authors concluded that valsartan was noninferior to captopril in the post-myocardial infarction setting, and that the combination of ACE/ARB offered no significant mortality advantage over monotherapy in this population. Subgroup analysis found no variation in the effect of these three regimens in any subgroup, including those receiving background beta-blocker therapy.

Building on the notion that more effective ARBs might potentiate ACEi-induced blockage of angiotensin II, several trials have been conducted to examine the benefits of ARB and ACEi in combination in patients with chronic heart failure. The earliest of these, the Valsartan Heart Failure Trial (Val-HeFT), randomized 5010 patients with NYHA class II–IV heart failure to valsartan or placebo, in addition to the existing heart failure regimen (93% were already receiving an ACEi). After a mean follow-up of 23 months, no difference was observed in all-cause mortality. However, patients treated with valsartan showed a significant 13.2% reduction in the combined mortality and morbidity endpoint. This was primarily due to a significant ($p<0.001$) 24% reduction in hospitalizations for worsening heart failure. A subgroup analysis of Val-HeFT showed that among the 35% of trial participants that were taking an ACEi and a beta-blocker, there was statistically significant excess mortality in the valsartan group ($p = 0.009$), raising concern that excessive neurohormonal inhibition with ACEi/ARB/beta-blocker might be harmful in patients with heart failure; however, this finding was not borne out in subsequent studies. CHARM-Added randomized 2548 patients already taking an ACEi (~100%) to placebo or candesartan *(48)*. The treatment group received a 15% reduction in the primary outcome of death or heart failure hospitalization. Compared to Val-HeFT, a higher percentage (55%) of this population was also taking a beta-blocker and these patients received the same benefit from candesartan administration as did patients not previously taking beta-blockers ($p = 0.14$ for treatment interaction), highlighting the safety of adding an ARB to optimal medical therapy with ACEi/beta-blocker.

A meta-analysis of 17 trials comparing ARB with either placebo or an ACE inhibitor in patients with heart failure found that although ARBs were not superior to ACE inhibitors in reducing mortality or hospitalizations for heart failure, the combination of an ARB and an ACE inhibitor was superior to ACE-inhibitor monotherapy in reducing hospitalizations for heart failure but not mortality *(49)*. In addition, in patients not receiving an ACE inhibitor (but receiving other heart failure drugs), there was a nonsignificant trend favoring ARBs over placebo for both reductions in all-cause mortality (OR 0.68, 95% CI 0.38–1.22) and hospitalizations for heart failure (OR 0.67, 95% CI 0.29–1.51). In this context, the ACC/AHA heart failure guidelines state that while ACEi remain first-line therapy for patients with heart failure (both chronic and post-MI), ARBs are a suitable substitute in ACE-intolerant patients, and may be considered as add-on therapy in patients who are already optimally treated with an ACEi and a beta-blocker. However, the guidelines state that an ARB should not be used in patients receiving ACEi and aldosterone antagonist because of a perceived high risk of hyperkalemia and a lack of clinical trial data to support this strategy *(11)*.

With regard to side effects, one benefit of ARBs that has been consistently demonstrated in ACEi/ARB comparison studies has been the lower rate of drug discontinuation in the ARB group related to less cough, dysgeusia, and angioedema. Although the reported incidence and severity of angioedema are much lower with ARBs, these medicines should be used with great caution in patients with a history of life-threatening ACEi-induced angioedema. The composite of these studies that added an ARB to patients taking an ACEi showed that azotemia, hyperkalemia, and hypotension were significantly and substantially more common in patients randomized to dual ACEi and ARB therapy. Common ARBs and their suggested doses are displayed in Table 6.

Table 6
Angiotensin receptor blocker (ARB) doses recommended in
the treatment of heart failure

Drug	Initial dose (mg)	Target dose (mg)
Candesartan	4–8 QD	32 mg QD
Losartan	25–50 QD	50–100 QD
Valsartan	20–40 BID	160 BID

BID (twice daily), QD (once daily).

4.3. Other Vasodilators

Other than ACE inhibitors and ARBs, the only additional "vasodilator" regimen shown to be effective in chronic heart failure is the combination of hydralazine and isosorbide dinitrate (Hyd-Iso). Though other vasodilators have been tested, most (e.g., felodipine *(50)*, amlodipine *(51)*, and prazosin *(52)*) have been ineffective in improving cardiovascular outcomes, despite doses causing measurable reductions in blood pressure consistent with systemic hemodynamic effects. This raises the possibility that there are unique properties to Hyd-Iso that are beneficial and independent of the physiologic vasodilator properties of these medications. It is hypothesized that this combination works by reducing oxidant stress (hydralazine) and improving nitric oxide availability (isosorbide dinitrate); changes in both are felt to be part of the pathophysiology of heart failure *(53, 54)*.

In 1986, the seminal Vasodilator therapy in Heart Failure study (V-HeFT I) showed that when compared with placebo (or prazosin) the combination of hydralazine and isosorbide dinitrate caused a reduction in all-cause mortality in patients with advanced heart failure *(52)*. After 2 years of follow-up, there was a 34% reduction in mortality in the Hyd-Iso group (HR 0.66, 95% CI 0.46–0.96, $p < 0.028$) but over the entire period of follow-up, the survival difference was of marginal statistical significance. This was the first large trial to show that any particular pharmacotherapy could reduce mortality in chronic heart failure, but the role of Hyd-Iso was quickly supplanted by ACE inhibitors following the publication of V-HeFT II. This second V-HeFT study directly compared enalapril to Hyd-Iso (without a placebo group) and had identical enrollment criteria as V-HeFT I. It found that enalapril was associated with a significant 33.6% reduction in mortality by 1 year ($P = 0.016$), but this difference waned with time and by the end of the trial the mortality reduction was no longer statistically significant ($p = 0.08$). The improved survival with enalapril was driven by a significant reduction in sudden cardiac death that was not seen with Hyd-Iso. Subgroup analysis showed that the 179 patients with advanced heart failure (NYHA III and IV) fared no better on enalapril than on Hyd-Iso (RR 0.99, 0.72–1.35). Between the treatment arms there was no significant difference in hospitalizations and somewhat paradoxically, Hyd-Iso was associated with a larger improvement in ejection fraction and exercise capacity *(55)*. Based on ease of administration, less side effects, and improved efficacy, ACEi became the preferred agent for management of heart failure patients, with the combination of isordil/hydralazine being reserved for patients who were intolerant of ACE inhibitors and ARBs *(56)*.

A provocative post hoc analysis of pooled data from V-HeFT I and II suggested that the benefits of Hyd-Iso varied by patient race. In this analysis, nearly all of the benefit seen in the overall trial was attributable to a reduction in mortality seen in patients who self-identified themselves as black *(57)*. The observation that race may have influenced the efficacy of the Hyd-Iso combination fueled the design of the African-American Heart Failure Trial *(54)* (A-HeFT). This trial randomized 1050 black patients with symptomatic HF (NYHA class II–III) who were already receiving established therapies for heart failure (86% with ACEi or ARB, 74% βB, 39% spironolactone) to additional therapy with Hyd-Iso (goal dose: hydralazine 225 mg/isosorbide dinitrate 120 mg divided three times daily). They found that the fixed-dose combination of Hyd-Iso was associated with a 43% improvement in survival at an average follow-up of 10 months (HR 0.57, $p = 0.01$) as well as significant improvements in quality of life and need for heart failure associated hospitalization (Fig. 4). As a result of A-HeFT, the FDA approved the fixed-dose combination of Hyd-Iso for the therapy of advanced heart failure in self-identified black patients, though this decision has met with some controversy *(58 – 60)*.

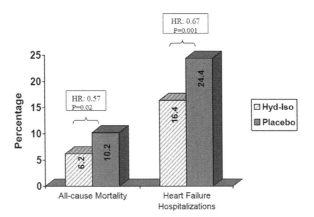

Fig. 4. Major outcomes in the A-HeFT trial. The combination of hydralazine and isosorbide dinitrate (Hyd-Iso) was associated with a significant reduction in mortality, improvement in QOL, and reduction in heart failure hospitalizations compared to placebo in the A-HeFT trial. Heart failure hospitalizations were defined as the rate of first hospitalization for heart failure.

Therapy with the combination of hydralazine and isosorbide dinitrate is associated with two principal side effects: headache and dizziness. These symptoms were extremely common in clinical trials of Hyd-Iso but rarely caused study medication withdrawal. Hyd-Iso caused a small but significant decrease in blood pressure in clinical trials, but the survival benefit was present regardless of blood pressure and thus it is recommended that asymptomatic low blood pressure should not contraindicate the use of Hyd-Iso *(61)*.

The consensus of the heart failure guideline writing committee is that Hyd-Iso is an option for patients who do not tolerate ACEi therapy but should not be given in the place of an ACEi in patients who would otherwise be expected to tolerate ACEi *(11)*. Hyd-Iso can also be considered in patients who remain symptomatic in spite of maximal therapy with beta-blockers and ACEi (class IIa recommendation). The guidelines do not identify race as a factor in selecting Hyd-Iso as a therapy but do acknowledge the results of the A-HeFT trial.

More recently, strategies targeting secondary pulmonary hypertension in heart failure with phosphodiesterase inhibitors such as sildenafil have received increasing attention. Secondary pulmonary hypertension is common in chronic severe left ventricular dysfunction, and may offer an important therapeutic target in this patient population facing high morbidity and mortality. In small trials, PDE-5 inhibition improved exercise capacity, 6-minute walk tests, and quality of life measurements *(62 – 64)*. Larger studies are needed to better define the long-term safety of effectiveness of this approach.

5. ALDOSTERONE RECEPTOR ANTAGONISTS

The importance of aldosterone in the pathogenesis of the volume retention of various disease states has been recognized for decades (Fig. 3). Since its isolation in the urine of heart failure patients, aldosterone has been recognized to contribute to the pathogenesis of heart failure. It either directly or indirectly contributes to heart failure progression (or ventricular arrhythmias) via volume retention, hypertension, hypokalemia, hypomagnesemia, secondary hyperparathyroidism, and myocardial fibrosis *(65, 66)*. ACEi and ARBs can cause upstream inhibition of aldosterone secretion but this inhibition is not complete ("aldosterone escape"), and, moreover, increased aldosterone levels are maintained due to decreased hepatic aldosterone clearance in the setting of heart failure *(67)*. Sustained aldosterone receptor activation in heart failure patients treated with optimal medical therapy provided the rationale for direct aldosterone inhibition as an additional therapeutic target in heart failure. On the basis of two well-designed trials published within the past decade (Fig. 5), aldosterone antagonists now have an established role in the treatment of certain patients with heart failure.

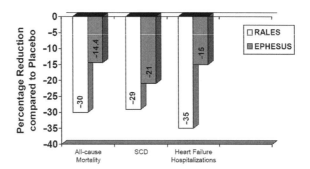

Fig. 5. Relative risk reduction in key outcomes in the major trials of aldosterone antagonism. Compared to placebo, both spironolactone (in RALES) and eplerenone (in EPHESUS) were associated with reductions in major cardiovascular outcomes. All results met statistical significance. SCD: sudden cardiac death.

The Randomized Aldactone Evaluation Study (RALES) randomized 1663 patients who had moderate to severe heart failure and a left ventricular ejection fraction not greater than 35% to either spironolactone (25 mg daily) or placebo against a background of ACEi and diuretics (few patients were taking beta-blockers) *(68)*. RALES was stopped early because of a strongly significant survival advantage in the spironolactone group. There was a striking 11% absolute risk reduction and a 31% relative risk reduction in all-cause mortality by 2 years (HR 0.70, 95% CI 0.60–0.82) that was attributable to both a reduction in sudden death (36% reduction) and progressive pump failure (29% reduction). There was also a 30% reduction in cardiac hospitalizations and a significant improvement in functional status *(68)*. The Eplerenone Post-Acute Myocardial Infarction Heart Failure Efficacy and Survival Study (EPHESUS) was a larger ($n = 6632$) one of patients immediately after a myocardial infarction who had reduced EF (average LVEF 33%) and signs of heart failure *(69)*. Here patients were randomized to the aldosterone antagonist eplerenone (25–50 mg daily) or placebo against a similar therapeutic background as RALES with the notable exception of much larger beta-blocker usage (75%). Eplerenone caused a 15% reduction in mortality at 1 year (HR 0.85, 95% CI 0.75–0.96) and there were similar reductions in sudden death and heart failure hospitalizations *(69)*.

In clinical trials the aldosterone antagonists were well tolerated, without significant hemodynamic effects; hyperkalemia and gynecomastia (10% with spironolactone and none with eplerenone) were the most frequent major adverse reactions. Although the entry criteria to both major aldosterone antagonist studies enrolled patients with a serum creatinine less than 2.5 mg/dL, there were few patients enrolled with a creatinine greater than 1.5 mg/dL *(11)*. This low prevalence of renal insufficiency, along with the careful monitoring and resources that the clinical trial was able to afford, could explain the wide discrepancy between the amount of symptomatic hyperkalemia seen in the trials and what has been observed in subsequent community-based studies. Serious hyperkalemia was seen in only 2% of spironolactone-treated subjects in RALES (compared to 1% of patients receiving placebo; *p* not significant for comparison), but in a population-based study of Canadian patients with heart failure there was a dramatic 4.6-fold increase in hospitalizations for hyperkalemia and 6.7-fold increase in hyperkalemic deaths after the publication of the RALES study *(70)*. As a consequence, the most recent heart failure guidelines highlight the imperative for careful patient selection and monitoring when using aldosterone antagonists, particularly in older patients who often have diminished baseline creatinine clearance, in other patients with baseline renal insufficiency, in those using other RAAS inhibitors, or in the presence of comorbidities which impair potassium excretion (e.g., diabetes).

Aldosterone antagonists should be considered for patients with NYHA class III and IV symptoms or post-MI LV dysfunction who do not have significant renal impairment (Cr < 2–2.5 and CrCl > 30–50) or a history of hyperkalemia. The serum potassium should be monitored frequently after starting aldosterone (after 3 days, after 1 week, then monthly for 3 months) and the starting dose should be low (12.5 mg–25 mg daily). This is reflected in the recent heart failure guidelines which gave a class I recommendation for the use of aldosterone antagonists; specifically they stated their use is "reasonable" provided that the risk of hyperkalemia is not high *(11)*. Based on a perceived high risk of hyperkalemia, it is advised that aldosterone inhibitors should not be given to patients already receiving an ACEi *and* an ARB.

6. BETA-ADRENERGIC RECEPTOR BLOCKERS

Beta-adrenergic receptor antagonists (beta-blockers, βB) inhibit the downstream consequences of sustained catecholamine activation in patients with heart failure. The degree of sympathetic nervous system activation has been shown to be an extremely powerful predictor of outcome in patients with heart failure, even better than other clinical (e.g., wedge pressure, pulse) and biochemical factors (e.g., serum sodium) *(71)*; beta-blockers, however, were initially considered to be contraindicated in patients with heart failure due to their negative inotropic activity. Nevertheless, a broad range of clinical studies beginning in the mid-1970s showed these agents to be useful in patients with dilated cardiomyopathy *(72, 73)* (Table 7). The exact mechanism of beta-blocker-induced benefit is not known, but putative effects include antagonism of cardiotoxic levels of circulating catecholamines *(74)* and improvement in systolic function associated with favorable patterns of contractile protein gene expression *(75)*.

Beta-blockers are capable of causing reverse remodeling, causing a *decrease* in left ventricular dimensions, *improvement* in systolic function (as measured by ejection fraction or fractional shortening), and a *return* to

Table 7
Major beta-blocker trials in heart failure[a]

Trial name and date	Drug and control group	NYHA or Killip classification of participants	Effect on all-cause mortality HR and 95% CI:	Change in all-cause hospitalizations	1-year mortality in the control group	Caveats
Chronic heart failure trials						
Carvedilol 1996 N = 1197	Carvedilol Goal: 25–50 mg BID Achieved: 23 mg BID (80% achieved goal)	II 53% III 44% IV 3%	HR: 0.35 (0.20–0.61)	All-cause hospitalization not published CV Hospitalization: HR: 0.73 (0.55–0.97)	11%[c]	no change in BP with carvedilol
MERIT-HF 1999 N = 3991	Metoprolol succinate Goal: 200 mg QD Achieved: 159 mg (64% reached goal)	II 41% III 55% IV 4%	HR: 0.66 (0.52–0.81)	HR: 0.88 P = 0.004[b]	11.0%	
CIBIS-II 1999 N = 2647	Bisoprolol Goal: 10 mg QD Achieved: 5.7 mg (43% reached goal)	III 83% IV 17%	HR: 0.66 (0.54–0.81)	HR: 0.80 (0.71–0.91)	13.2%	

Trial	Drug/Dose		Mortality		
Copernicus 2001 N = 2289	Carvedilol Goal: 25 mg BID Achieved: 18 mg BID (65% reached goal)	IV 100%	HR: 0.65 (0.52–0.81)	HR: 0.85 $P = 0.003$	19.7%	Carvedilol remained highly effective in the sickest subgroups
Post-myocardial infarction trial					
CAPRICORN 2001 N = 1959	Carvedilol 20 mg BID (74% reached target 25 mg BID)	Killip class I 66% II 31% III 3%	HR:0.77 (0.60–0.98)	NS 14% RRR in HF admissions	11%[c]

[a]The scope of the table is limited to large studies of beta-blockers *approved* for heart failure therapy and in all of these trials, ACEi was the required background therapy if tolerated.

[b]95% confidence interval not published.

[c]Mortality rates estimated from published Kaplan–Meier curves. RRR = Relative Risk Reduction

an elliptical shape *(76)*. Clinical trial results have shown that compared to placebo, beta-blockers may improve left ventricular ejection fraction by as much as 10% (e.g., EF 25–35%) *(77)*. These effects are seen at very low doses but incremental reverse remodeling is seen in a dose-dependent fashion *(78)*.

Though initially felt to be contraindicated in heart failure due to their negative inotropic effects, beta-blockers are now recognized as a critical component of standard heart failure therapy. In 1996 the US Carvedilol Heart Failure Study Group published the results of several prospective trials comparing carvedilol to placebo *(79)*. When the separate studies were combined, the patients randomized to carvedilol were 65% less likely to die than those randomized to placebo. Published 3 years later, the second Cardiac Insufficiency Bisoprolol Study (CIBIS II) randomized 2647 patients with class III–IV heart failure to placebo or bisoprolol *(86)*. Because of the emergence of a highly statistically significant decrease in mortality, this study was stopped early. After a mean of 1.3 years of follow-up, patients randomized to bisoprolol had a highly significant 34% reduction in all-cause mortality. Subgroup analysis showed a homogenous treatment effect and there was an associated 32% decrease in hospitalizations for worsening heart failure. Also published in 1999, but studying a slightly less sick group than CIBIS II, the Metoprolol CR/XL Randomized Intervention Trial in Congestive Heart Failure (MERIT-HF) randomized 3991 patients with primarily class II and III heart failure to either long-acting metoprolol or placebo *(80)*. MERIT-HF was also stopped early, after a mean follow-up time of 1 year, because of a highly significant 34% reduction in all-cause mortality in the metoprolol group.

Patients with severe heart failure were relatively underrepresented in the aforementioned trials and there remained a concern that patients with the advanced heart failure would not tolerate the addition of a beta-blocker to their regimen. To address the utility of beta-blockers in this population, the Carvedilol Prospective Randomized Cumulative Survival Study Group (COPERNICUS) randomized 2289 patients with NYHA class IV symptoms and left ventricular ejection fraction less than 25% to therapy with carvedilol or placebo *(81)*. The trial was terminated early after interim analyses found that patients randomized to carvedilol experienced a statistically significant 35% reduction in all-cause mortality. Moreover, in a prespecified subgroup analysis of the patients deemed to be at most risk (LVEF $\leq$ 15%, recurrent hospitalizations, any prior use of inotropic agents), there was a 39% reduction in all-cause mortality, indicating benefit to beta-blocker therapy even in the sickest heart failure patients. In aggregate, beta-blockers are associated with roughly a 30% relative risk reduction in 1-year mortality across the spectrum of patients with chronic heart failure due to LV dysfunction. Beta-blockers reduce cardiovascular hospitalizations, improve functional capacity *(82, 83)*, and reduce mortality by decreasing progressive pump failure and lowering the incidence of sudden death *(84–86)*. Since some beta-blockers have not been clearly associated with successful mortality reductions in heart failure patients *(87, 88)*, preference should be given to those agents with proven efficacy in prospective clinical trials (bisoprolol, carvedilol, and metoprolol succinate) *(89)*. Recommended dosing regimens for recommended beta-blockers for the treatment of heart failure are displayed in Table 8. The unique metabolic and vasodilatory effects of carvedilol (perhaps a consequence of its mixed alpha- and beta-adrenergic blocking properties) have fueled some enthusiasm about its potential advantages in heart failure patients. At least one trial (COMET) suggested clinical benefits to carvedilol exceeding those of metoprolol tartrate, but these results have been challenged due to concerns about the relative dosing of the two agents *(90)*. Since no head-to-head trials comparing carvedilol, metoprolol succinate, and bisoprolol have been conducted, there is at present little evidenced-based rationale for favoring one agent over another *(11)*.

Table 8
Beta-blocker doses recommended in the treatment of heart failure

Drug	Initial dose (mg)	Target dose (mg)
Bisoprolol	1.25 QD	10 QD
Carvedilol	3.125–6.25 BID	25[a] BID
Metoprolol succinate	12.5–25 QD	200 QD

BID (twice daily), QD (once daily).

[a]In patients weighing > 85 kg, the recommended target dose of carvedilol is 50 mg BID.

Since both ACE inhibitors and beta-blockers are associated with important clinical benefits in heart failure patients, and since most beta-blocker trials have demonstrated therapeutic efficacy on the background of ACE-inhibitor therapy, there has been some discussion of which agent should be initiated first. Recently, the CIBIS III investigators showed that beta-blocker initiation could precede ACEi initiation in patients with mild to moderate heart failure without evidence of hypervolemia. In that study of 1010 elderly patients who had previously not received a neuroendocrine antagonist, a "bisoprolol first" strategy was non-inferior to starting with enalapril *(91)*. Nevertheless, others have cautioned the more widespread application of these data, especially in more severely ill patients who would otherwise derive an immediate clinical benefit from vasodilators (e.g., ACEi) *(92)*.

Initiation of beta-blockade should occur in patients with no or minimal signs of volume overload, who demonstrate adequate tissue perfusion. In contrast to patients without heart failure who may have a different indication for beta-blockade (e.g., angina, hypertension), patients with heart failure require careful dose up-titration starting at low doses. In accordance with the experience in clinical trials, patients should be reassessed frequently and the dose is typically doubled every 2 weeks until the target dose is reached. If patients develop mild or moderate symptoms of congestion with beta-blockade, it is recommended that adjustments in other medications (diuretics, ACEi) precede a decrease or cessation of beta-blockers *(93)*. The most common adverse effect of beta-blockers has been symptomatic bradycardia, but this rarely results in need for hospitalization, and a meta-analysis from multiple trials has shown that if 153 patients were treated with beta-blockers for 1 year, only one patient would need to be withdrawn because of symptomatic bradycardia *(94)*. The effect on blood pressure has ranged from a modest decrease (−1.1/1.6 mmHg in COPERNICUS *(95)*) to no affect (in the U.S. Carvedilol study *(79)*) to a surprising *increase* in blood pressure relative to the placebo group in MERIT-HF and CIBIS-II *(85, 86)*. This is felt to reflect an improvement in stroke volume and is paralleled in the sustained and significant improvement in left ventricular ejection fraction. Even in patients with the most advanced disease (class IV, requiring recent hospitalization or treatment with intravenous inotropes or vasodilators), treatment with carvedilol was tolerated by most subjects and was associated with a significant mortality benefit that began after only 2–3 weeks of treatment. Although dose down-titration was more common with carvedilol (as opposed to placebo) in the most advanced disease subgroup, these patients were no more likely to require hospitalization and were less likely to be withdrawn from the study *(95)*. Target doses were often reached in clinical trials (65–80% of the time) but this has proven more difficult in practice outside of clinical trials, where patients tend to be older and have more comorbidities *(96)*. Although there are situations where the use of beta-blockers is either proscribed or potentially dangerous (e.g., high grade AV block, profound resting bradycardia), it may be needlessly withheld from patients with chronic obstructive pulmonary disease or stable mild asthma in spite of demonstrated safety in these populations *(97)*. Similarly, recent analysis from the OPTIMIZE-HF registry *(98)* suggests that beta-blocker therapy withdrawal in patients hospitalized with decompensated heart failure may actually be harmful, although this hypothesis has not yet been tested prospectively. Provided that there are not contraindications as described above, the consensus guidelines strongly support the use of beta-blockers across the spectrum of left ventricular dysfunction (class I recommendation) *(11)*.

7. ANTICOAGULATION

A multitude of patients have benefited from the reduced cardiovascular events associated with the appropriate use of anticoagulant and anti-platelet medications. Many patients with heart failure have pre-existing coronary artery disease, an indication for life-long aspirin therapy, or atrial fibrillation, which in most is an indication for anticoagulation with warfarin. Venous thromboembolism (VTE) is common in chronically ill patients, and heart failure is considered a risk factor for VTE *(99)*. Though the duration and intensity of anticoagulation for patients with a history of VTE continue to be modified, there remains no question that therapeutic anti-coagulation is a fundamental part of therapy for VTE. Nevertheless, in the large number of patients with heart failure and without another indication for anti-thrombotic medications, the role of anticoagulants and anti-platelet agents remains unsettled. Some reports have highlighted the increased relative risk of stroke in heart failure patients (particularly among those with severely reduced ejection fraction), but much of this risk may have been confounded by concomitant atrial fibrillation *(100)*. Data from prospective, randomized trials of prophylactic anticoagulation for prevention of thrombotic events in heart failure patients, however, are lacking. Three trials were designed to guide our strategies to prevent thromboembolism in heart failure patients: Warfarin and Antiplatelet Therapy in Chronic CHF (WATCH), Warfarin and Antiplatelet Therapy in Chronic CHF (WASH), and the ongoing Warfarin–Aspirin Reduced Cardiac Ejection Fraction (WARCEF). The WATCH study was stopped early due to poor recruitment *(101)* and the WASH study was a small pilot study intended to test the *feasibility* of anticoagulation *(102)*. The WARCEF trial is sponsored by the National Institute of Neurologic Disorders and Stroke (NINDS) and looks to enroll 2860 patients with LVEF $\leq$ 35%, on ACEi and without another accepted indication for anticoagulation (e.g., atrial fibrillation, mechanical heart valve). This trial began enrolling in 2002 and the primary outcome will be time to first ischemic stroke, intracerebral hemorrhage, or death from any cause *(103)*. Pending more definitive data, however, the recent AHA/ACC guidelines acknowledge the uncertainty regarding the necessity of prophylactic anticoagulation for prevention of embolic events in patients with heart failure and LV dysfunction, and advise initiation only when an accepted indication exists *(11)*.

8. STATINS

Inhibition of HMG coenzyme – a reductase with statins – has been shown to benefit patients across a wide spectrum of vascular diseases. The pleiotropic effects of these medications are frequently cited to explain apparent improvements in clinical outcomes independent of lipid-lowering effects. Data derived from post hoc analyses initially suggested a possible benefit of statins in patients with systolic heart failure *(104, 105)*. The largest prospective, randomized assessment of this hypothesis was the CORONA Trial *(106)*, which randomized 5011 patients with NYHA class II–IV heart failure to rosuvastatin 10 mg vs placebo. There were no significant differences in the primary composite outcome of cardiovascular death, nonfatal myocardial infarction, or nonfatal stroke at a median follow-up of 33 months. Thus, there is no clear evidence supporting the use of statins in patients with heart failure who are not considered to be candidates for this therapy based on established indications.

9. MEDICATIONS TO AVOID

The importance of a careful review of all medications cannot be overlooked. Ensuring that potentially harmful medicines have been avoided complements the prescription of medicines known to be efficacious in the treatment of heart failure (Table 9). The AHA/ACC heart failure guidelines specifically recommend the general avoidance of most antiarrhythmic medications, all non-dihydropyridine calcium channel blockers, and all nonsteroidal anti-inflammatory medications (NSAIDs) *(11)*. In addition, there are other classes of widely used medications that should also be avoided; among these are the thiazolidinediones *(107)* (e.g., pioglitazone) and the type 3 phosphodiesterase inhibitors (cilostazol) *(108)*. Class I antiarrhythmic medications have inherently negative inotropic effects that are more pronounced in the presence of left ventricular systolic dysfunction, and these agents have been shown to be proarrhythmic and associated with an increased risk of mortality in patients with structural heart disease. Two class III agents, amiodarone and dofetilide, have been demonstrated to be safe in this patient population, but other agents in this class, sotalol and ibutilide, have been shown to have high proarrhythmic effects in patients with left ventricular systolic dysfunction. A newer class III agent, dronedarone, was recently shown to increase mortality in patients with severe heart failure and left ventricular dysfunction *(109)*.

L-type calcium channel blockers (e.g., verapamil and diltiazem) exhibit a negative inotropic and chronotropic effect. The limited published experience with these drugs has shown them to be harmful to patients with symptomatic or asymptomatic LV dysfunction. A post hoc analysis of the Diltiazem Multicenter Postinfarction Study (MDPIT) showed that compared to placebo, diltiazem was associated with a highly significant 75% increase in symptomatic heart failure ($p = 0.0017$) when given to patients with an LVEF < 40% *(110)*. Due to a shared pharmacologic effect, and smaller studies suggesting harm, verapamil is also to be avoided in this patient population. Though nifedipine acts at a different calcium channel than diltiazem and verapamil, a small study of short-acting nifedipine showed that when added to stable patients treated with diuretics and digoxin, an ~25% absolute excess risk of decompensated heart failure was observed compared to patients receiving isosorbide dinitrate *(111)*. Two other dihydropyridine calcium channel blockers have been studied in heart failure in large, well-designed clinical trials. Both amlodipine *(51)* and felodipine *(112)* have been shown to be safe in this population but neither was associated with an improvement in mortality or other important endpoints. On this basis, these two agents can be considered for control of blood pressure in patients with heart failure who continue to be hypertensive.

The beneficial and harmful effects of NSAIDs are related to their inhibition of prostaglandin synthesis. The hemodynamic consequence of which is an increase in systemic vascular resistance and decrease in renal perfusion,

Table 9
Commonly used medicines that are potentially harmful to patients with heart failure

Drug	Example	Mechanism of harm	Caveats
Class I antiarrhythmics	Procainamide Flecainide Quinidine	Pro-arrhythmia Negative Inotropy	
Class III antiarrhythmics	Sotalol Ibutilide	Pro-arrhythmia Negative Inotropy (sotalol, amiodarone)	Amiodarone and dofetilide have an acceptable risk profile in patients with heart failure
Calcium channel blockers	Diltiazem Verapamil Nifedipine	Bradyarrhythmia Negative inotropy	Amlodipine and felodipine have an acceptable risk profile in patients with heart failure
NSAIDs[a]	Ibuprofen Diclofenac Celecoxib	Increased SVR Decreased renal perfusion Increased atherothrombotic events	
Thiazolidinediones	Rosiglitazone Pioglitazone	Fluid retention	Can be used cautiously in patients with NYHA class I and II heart failure and should be avoided in more advanced heart failure.
Cilostazol	Pletal	Increased heart rate and ventricular ectopy	

Antiarrhythmic classification based on the Vaughn–Williams schemata.
SVR – systemic vascular resistance.
[a]Does not include ASA, which is not proscribed in this population.

both of which have obvious negative implications for patients with heart failure. Moreover, NSAIDs increase the risk of atherothrombotic events *(113)*, which is a key risk factor for heart failure. One population-based study showed that NSAID use was associated with a twofold increased risk for hospitalization for heart failure and a tenfold increased risk if patients had underlying heart disease *(114)*.

10. CONSENSUS STATEMENTS

The recently published AHA/ACC guidelines (Table 10) provide a framework for the treatment of patients with hitherto asymptomatic LV systolic dysfunction (Stage B HF) and patients with LV dysfunction and current or

Table 10
AHA/ACC guidelines for the pharmacotherapy of chronic heart failure

Class of recommendation	Stage B heart failure	Stage C heart failure		
		NYHA I	NYHA II	NYHA III–IV
Class I	ACEi Beta-blockers	ACEi Beta-blockers ARB[a]	ACEi Beta-blockers ARB[a]	ACEi Beta-blockers ARB[a] Aldosterone antagonists[b]
Class IIa	ARB[a]	ARB	ARB	ARB Digoxin Hyd-Iso[c]
Class IIb		Hyd-Iso[d]	Hyd-Iso[d]	Hyd-Iso[d]
Class III	Digoxin CCB	NSAIDs Most antiarrhythmics CCB The combined use of ACEi, ARB, and aldosterone antagonists.		

Stage B: Asymptomatic left ventricular (LV) dysfunction.

Stage C: LV dysfunction with any history of heart failure symptoms.

Class I recommendation: Conditions for which there is evidence and/or general agreement that a given treatment is beneficial, useful, and effective.

Class IIa: Weight of evidence/opinion is in favor of usefulness/efficacy.

Class IIb: Usefulness/efficacy less well established by evidence/opinion.

Class III: Conditions for which there is general agreement that a treatment is not useful/effective and in some cases may be harmful.

[a]An ARB can be substituted for patients with intolerance to ACEi.

[b]The use of aldosterone antagonists is limited to patients without severe renal insufficiency and requires the ability to carefully follow serum potassium levels.

[c]In addition to ACEi and beta-blockers.

[d]In patients not able to tolerate an ACEi or an ARB. Hyd-Iso = hydralazine and isosorbide dinitrate

prior symptomatic heart failure (Stage C HF). Beta-blockers and ACEi are indicated across this spectrum of illness and unless they are not tolerated, all patients with LV dysfunction should be treated with these two agents. If patients do not tolerate an ACEi due to cough, an ARB should be used in their place. An ARB can be combined with ACEi and beta-blocker but should not be added to patients already receiving an aldosterone antagonist. For patients with persistent symptoms (NYHA class III and IV), an aldosterone antagonist is indicated and therapy with digoxin is generally recommended. Hyd-Iso is an option for patients who do not tolerate therapy with either an ACEi or ARB and can be an add-on to ACEi in patients with persistent symptoms. In spite of a wealth of clinical trial data and the reminder provided by consensus guidelines, these medications remained underprescribed in community studies and registry data. Moreover, patients with more advanced disease are incrementally less likely to receive evidence-proven, life-saving therapies such as beta-blockers and ACEi *(115)*.

REFERENCES

1. Eichhorn EJ, Gheorghiade M. Digoxin – new perspective on an old drug. N Engl J Med 2002;347:1394–1395.
2. Bristow MR, Linas S, Port JD. Drugs in the treatment of heart failure. In: Braunwald's Heart Disease: A Textbook of Cardiovascular Medicine, 7th ed., vol. 1. Philadelphia: Elsevier Saunders, 2005:569–602.
3. Smith TW. Digoxin in heart failure. N Engl J Med 1993;329:51–53.
4. Packer M, Gheorghiade M, Young JB, Costantini PJ, Adams KF, Cody RJ, Smith LK, Van Voorhees L, Gourley LA, Jolly MK. Withdrawl of digoxin from patients with chronic heart failure treated with angiotensin-converting-enzyme inhibitors. N Engl J Med 1993;329:1–7.
5. Garg R, Gorlin R, Smith T, Yusuf S. The effect of digoxin on mortality and morbidity in patients with heart failure. N Engl J Med 1997;336:525–533.
6. Rathore SS, Curtis JP, Wang Y, Bristow MR, Krumholz HM. Association of serum digoxin concentration and outcomes in patients with heart failure. JAMA 2003;289:871–878.
7. Rathore SS, Wang Y, Krumholz HM. Sex-based differences in the effect of digoxin for the treatment of heart failure. N Engl J Med 2002;347:1403–1411.
8. Adams KF, Patterson H, Gattis WA, O'Connor CM, Lee CR, Schwartz TA, Gheorghiade M. Relationship of serum digoxin concentration to mortality and morbidity in women in the Digitalis Investigation Group trial. J Am Coll Cardiol 2005;46:497–504.
9. Slatton ML, Irani WN, Hall SA, Marcoux LG, Page RL, Grayburn PA, Eichhorn EJ. Does digoxin provide additional hemodynamic and autonomic benefit at higher doses in patients with mild to moderate heart failure and normal sinus rhythm? J Am Coll Cardiol 1997;29:1206–1213.
10. Adams KF, Gheorghiade M, Uretsky BF, Young JB, Ahmed S, Tomasko L, Packer M. Patients with mild heart failure worsen during withdrawal from digoxin therapy. J Am Coll Cardiol 1997;30:42–48.
11. Hunt S, Abraham W, Chin M, et al., ACC/AHA 2005 guideline update for the diagnosis and management of chronic heart failure in the adult: A report of the American College of Cardiology/American Heart Association task force on practice guidelines. Circulation 2005;112:154–235.
12. Greger R. New insights into the molecular mechanisms of the action of diuretics. Nephrol Dial Transplant 1999;14:536–540.

13. Brater DC. Diuretic therapy. N Engl J Med 1998;339:387–395.
14. Pickkers P, Dormans TP, Russel FG, Hughes AD, Thien T, Schaper N, Smits P. Direct vascular effects of furosemide in humans. Circulation 1997;96:1847–52.
15. Eshaghian S, Horwich TB, Fonarow GC. Relation of loop diuretic dose to mortality in advanced heart failure. Am J Cardiol 2006;97:1759–1764.
16. Neuberg GW, Miller AB, O'Connor CM, Belkin RN, Carson PE, Cropp AB, Frid DJ, Nye RG, Pressler ML, Wertheimer JH, Packer M; PRAISE Investigators. Prospective randomized amlodipine survival evaluation. Diuretic resistance predicts mortality in patients with advanced heart failure. Am Heart J 2002;144:31–38.
17. Cosin J, Diez J; TORIC investigators. Torsemide in chronic heart failure: results of the TORIC study. Eur J Heart Fail 2002;4:507–13.
18. Costanzo M, Guglin M, Saltzberg M, Jessup M, Bart B, Teerlink J, Jaski B, Fang J, Feller E, Haas G, Anderson A, Schollmeyer M, Sobotka P; UNLOAD Investigators. Ultrafiltration versus intravenous diuretics for patients hospitalized for acute decompensated heart failure. J Am Coll Cardiol 2007 Feb 13;49:675–83.
19. Colucci WS, Elkayam U, Horton DP, Abraham WT, Bourge RC, Johnson AD, Wagnoner LE, Givertz MM, Liang CS, Neibaur M, Haught WH, LeJemtel TH; Nesiritide Study Group. Intravenous nesiritide, a natriuretic peptide, in the treatment of decompensated congestive heart failure. N Engl J Med 2000 Jul 27;343(4):246–53.
20. Konstam MA, Gheorghiade M, Burnett JC Jr, Grinfeld L, Maggioni AP, Swedberg K, Udelson JE, Zannad F, Cook T, Ouyang J, Zimmer C, Orlandi C. Effects of oral tolvaptan in patients hospitalized for worsening heart failure: the EVEREST outcome trial. JAMA 2007 Mar 28;297(12):1319–31.
21. Givertz MM, Massie BM, Fields TK, Pearson LL, Dittrich HC; CKI-201 and CKI-202 Investigators. The effects of KW-3902, an adenosine A1-receptor antagonist, on diuresis and renal function in patients with acute decompensated heart failure and renal impairment or diuretic resistance. J Am Coll Cardiol 2007 Oct 16;50:1551–1560.
22. Domanski M, Norman J, Pitt B, Haigney M, Hanlon S, Peyster E; Studies of Left Ventricular Dysfunction. Diuretic use, progressive heart failure, and death in patients in the Studies Of Left Ventricular Dysfunction (SOLVD). J Am Coll Cardiol 2003 Aug 20;42:705–8.
23. Juurlink DN, Mamdani MM, Lee DS, Kopp A, Austin PC, Laupacis A, Redelmeier DA. Rates of hyperkalemia after publication of the randomized aldactone evaluation study. N Engl J Med 2004;351:543–551.
24. Janssens HJ, van de Lisdonk EH, Janssen M, van den Hoogen HJ, Verbeek AL. Gout, not induced by diuretics? A case-control study from primary care. Ann Rheum Dis 2006;65:1080–3.
25. Hunter DJ, York M, Chaisson CE, Woods R, Niu J, Zhang Y. Recent diuretic use and the risk of recurrent gout attacks: The online case-crossover gout study. J Rheumatol 2006;33:1341–5.
26. Braunwald E. ACE Inhibitors – A cornerstone of the treatment of heart failure. N Engl J Med 1991;325:351–353.
27. The SOLVD Investigators. Effect of enalapril on survival in patients with reduced left ventricular ejection fractions and congestive heart failure. N Engl J Med 1991;325:293–302.
28. Swedberg K for The CONSENSUS trial Study Group. Effects of enalapril on mortality in severe congestive heart failure. Results of the Cooperative North Scandinavian Enalapril Survival Study (CONSENSUS). N Engl J Med 1987;23:1429–1435.
29. Pfeffer MA, Braunwald E, Moye LA, Basta L, Brown EJ, Cuddy TE, Davis BR, Geletman Em, Goldman S, Flaker GC, Klein M, Lamas GA, Packer M, Rouleau J, Rouleau JL, Rutherford J, Wertheimer JH, Hawkins CM. Effect of captopril on

mortality and morbidity in patients with left ventricular dysfunction after myocardial infarction. results of the survival and ventricular enlargement trial (SAVE). N Engl J Med 1992;327:669–677.

30. Ball SG for the AIRE investigators. Effect of ramipril on mortality and morbidity of survivors of acute myocardial infarction with clinical evidence of heart failure. The Acute Infarction Ramipril Efficacy (AIRE) Study Investigators. Lancet 1993;342:821–828.

31. Kober L, Torp-Pedersen C, Carlsen JE, Bagger H, Eliasen P, Lyngborg K, Videbaek J, Cole DS, Auclert L, Pauly NC. A clinical trial of the angiotensin-converting-enzyme inhibitor trandolapril in patients with left ventricular dysfunction after myocardial infarction. Trandolapril Cardiac Evaluation (TRACE) Study Group. N Engl J Med 1995;333:1670–6.

32. Rogers WJ, Johnstone DE, Yusuf S, Weiner DH, Gallagher P, Bittner VA, Ahn S, Schron E, Shumaker SA, Sheffield LT. Quality of life among 5,025 patients with left ventricular dysfunction randomized between placebo and enalapril: The Studies of Left Ventricular Dysfunction. The SOLVD Investigators. J Am Coll Cardiol 1994;23:393–400.

33. Flather MD, Yusuf S, Kober L, Pfeffer M, Hall A, Murray G, Torp-Pedersen C, Ball S, Pogue J, Moye L, Braunwald E. Long-term ACE-inhibitor therapy in patients with heart failure or left-ventricular dysfunction: A systematic overview of data from individual patients. ACE-Inhibitor Myocardial Infarction Collaborative Group. Lancet 2000;355:1575–81.

34. Konstam MA, Rousseau MF, Kronenberg MW, Udelson JE, Melin J, Stewart D, Dolan N, Edens TR, Ahn S, Kinan D, et al. Effects of the angiotensin converting enzyme inhibitor enalapril on the long-term progression of left ventricular dysfunction in patients with heart failure. SOLVD Investigators. Circulation 1992;86:431–438

35. Nanas JN, Alexopoulos G, Anastasiou-Nana MI, Kardis K, Tirologos A, Zobolos S, Pirgakis V, Anthopoulos L, Sideris D, Stamatelopoulos SF, Moulopoulos SD. Outcome of patients with congestive heart failure treated with standard versus high doses of enalapril: A multicenter study. high dose enalapril study group. J Am Coll Cardiol 2000;36:2090–2095.

36. Packer M, Poole-Wilson PA, Armstrong PW, Cleland JG, Horowitz JD, Massie BM, Ryden L, Thygesen K, Uretsky BF. Comparative effects of low and high doses of the angiotensin-converting enzyme inhibitor, lisinopril, on morbidity and mortality in chronic heart failure. ATLAS Study Group. Circulation 1999;100:2312–8.

37. Poole-Wilson PA for the NETWORK Investigators. Clinical outcome with enalapril in symptomatic chronic heart failure; a dose comparison. Eur Heart J 1998;19:481–9.

38. Kostis JB, Shelton B, Gosselin G, Goulet C, Hood WB Jr, Kohn RM, Kubo SH, Schron E, Weiss MB, Willis PW 3rd, Young JB, Probstfield J. Adverse effects of enalapril in the studies of left ventricular dysfunction (SOLVD). SOLVD Investigators. Am Heart J 1996;131:350–355.

39. Packer M, Medina N, Yushak M. Relation between serum sodium concentration and the hemodynamic and clinical responses to converting enzyme inhibition with captopril in severe heart failure. J Am Coll Cardiol 1984;3:1035–43.

40. Hood WB Jr, Youngblood M, Ghali JK, Reid M, Rogers WJ, Howe D, Teo KK, LeJemtel TH. Initial blood pressure response to enalapril in hospitalized patients (Studies of Left Ventricular Dysfunction [SOLVD]). Am J Cardiol 1991 Dec 1;68(15):1465–1468.

41. Swedberg K, Held P, Kjekshus J, Rasmussen K, Ryden L, Wedel H. Effects of the early administration of enalapril on mortality in patients with acute myocardial infarction. Results of the Cooperative New Scandinavian Enalapril Survival Study II (CONSENSUS II). N Engl J Med 1992;327:678–84.

42. Bart BA, Ertl G, Held P, Kuch J, Maggioni AP, McMurray J, Michelson EL, Rouleau JL, Warner Stevenson L, Swedberg K, Young JB, Yusuf S, Sellers MA, Granger CB,

Califf RM, Pfeffer MA. Contemporary management of patients with left ventricular systolic dysfunction. Results from the Study of Patients Intolerant of Converting Enzyme Inhibitors (SPICE) Registry. Eur Heart J 1999;20:1182–1190.

43. McDowell S, Coleman JJ, Ferner RE. Systematic review and meta-analysis of ethnic differences in risks of adverse reactions to drugs used in cardiovascular medicine. BMJ 2006;332:1177–1181.

44. Granger CB, McMurray JJ, Yusuf S, Held P, Michelson EL, Olofsson B, Ostergren J, Pfeffer MA, Swedberg K; CHARM Investigators and Committees. Effects of candesartan in patients with chronic heart failure and reduced left-ventricular systolic function intolerant to angiotensin-converting-enzyme inhibitors: the CHARM-Alternative trial. Lancet 2003;362:772–776.

45. Pitt B, Poole-Wilson PA, Segal R, et al. Effect of losartan compared with captopril on mortality in patients with symptomatic heart failure: randomised trial – the Losartan Heart Failure Survival Study ELITE II. Lancet 2000;355:1582–1587

46. Dickstein K, Kjekshus J for the OPTIMAAL Study group. Effects of losartan and captopril on mortality in high-risk patients after acute myocardial infarction: the OPTIMAAL randomized trial. Lancet 2002;360:752–760.

47. Pfeffer MA, McMurray JJV, Velazquez EJ, Rouleau J-L, Køber L, Maggioni AP, Solomon SD, Swedberg K, Van de Werf F, White H, Leimberger JD, Henis M, Edwards S, Zelenkofske S, Sellers MA, Califf RM, the Valsartan in Acute Myocardial Infarction Trial Investigators. Valsartan, captopril, or both in myocardial infarction complicated by heart failure, left ventricular dysfunction, or both. N Engl J Med 2003;349: 1893–1906.

48. McMurray JJ, Ostergren J, Swedberg K, Granger CB, Held P, Michelson EL, Olofsson B, Yusuf S, Pfeffer MA; CHARM Investigators and Committees. Effects of candesartan in patients with chronic heart failure and reduced left-ventricular systolic function taking angiotensin-converting-enzyme inhibitors: The CHARM-Added trial. Lancet 2003 Sep 6;362(9386):767–71.

49. Jong P, Demers C, McKelvie RS, Liu PP. Angiotensin receptor blockers in heart failure: meta-analysis of randomized controlled trials. J Am Coll Cardiol 2002;39:463–470.

50. Cohn JN, Ziesche S, Smith R, Anand I, Dunkman WB, Loeb H, Cintron G, Boden W, Baruch L, Rochin P, Loss L. Effect of the calcium antagonist felodipine as supplementary vasodilator therapy in patients with chronic heart failure treated with enalapril. V-HeFT III. Circulation 1997;96:856–863.

51. Packer M, O'Connor CM, Ghali JK, Pressler ML, Carson PE, Belkin RN, Miller AB, Neuberg GW, Frid D, Wertheimer JH, Cropp AB, DeMets DL. Effect of amlodipine on morbidity and mortality in severe chronic heart failure. N Engl J Med 1996;335: 1107–1114.

52. Cohn JN, Archibald DG, Ziesche S, Franciosa JA, Harston WE, Tristani FE, Dunkman WB, Jacobs W, Francis GS, Flohr K, Goldman S, Cobb FR, Shah PM, Saunders R, Fletcher RD, Loeb HS, Hughes VC, Baker B. Effect of vasodilator therapy on mortality in chronic congestive heart failure. N Engl J Med 1986;314:1547–1552.

53. Zimmet JM, Hare JM. Nitroso-Redox interactions in the cardiovascular system. Circulation 2006;114:1531–1544.

54. Taylor AL, Ziesche S, Yancy C, Carson P, D'Agostino R, Ferdinand K, Taylor M, Adams K, Sabolinski M, Worcel MM, Cohn JN. Combination of isosorbide dinitrate and hydralazine in blacks with heart failure (A-HeFT). N Engl J Med 2004;351:2049–2057.

55. Cohn JN, Johnson G, Ziesche S, Cobb F, Francis G, Tristani F, Smith R, Dunkman WB, Loeb H, Wong M, Bhat G, Goldman S, Fletcher R, Doherty J, Hughes CV, Carson P, Cintron G, Shabetai R, Haakenson C. A comparison of enalapril with hydralazine-isosorbide in the treatment of chronic congestive heart failure. N Engl J Med 1991;325:303–310.

56. Braunwald E. ACE Inhibitors – A cornerstone of the treatment of heart failure. N Engl J Med 1991;325:351–353.

57. Carson P, Ziesche S, Johnson G, Cohn JN. Racial differences in response to therapy for heart failure: analysis of the vasodilator-heart failure trials. J Card Fail 1999;5:178–187.

58. Moran AE, Cooper RS. Isosorbide and hydralazine in blacks with heart failure. N Engl J Med 2005;352:1041.

59. Bibbins-Domingo K, Fernandez A. BiDil for heart failure in black patients: implications of the U.S. food and drug administration approval. Ann Intern Med 2007;146:52–56.

60. Temple R, Stockbridge NL. BiDil for heart failure patients: The U.S. food and drug administration perspective. Ann Intern Med 2007;146:57–62.

61. Anand IS, Tam SW, Rector TS, Taylor AL, Sabolinski ML, Archambault WT, Adams KF, Olukotun AY, Worcel M, Cohn JN. Influence of blood pressure on the effectiveness of a fixed-dose combination of isosorbide dinitrate and hydralazine in the African-American Heart Failure Trial. J Am Coll Cardiol 2007;49:32–39.

62. Lewis GD, Shah R, Shahzad K, Camuso JM, Pappagianopoulos PP, Hung J, Tawakol A, Gerzten RE, Systrom DM, Bloch KD, Semigran MJ. Sildenafil improves exercise capacity and quality of life in patients with systolic heart failure and secondary pulmonary hypertension. Circulation 2007:116:1555–1562.

63. Behlin A, Rohde LE, Colombo FC, Goldraich LA, Stein R, Clausell N. Effects of a 5′phosphodiesterase four-week long inhibition with sildenafil in patients with chronic heart failure: a double-blind, placebo-controlled clinical trial. J Card Fail 2008 Apri;14(3):189–97.

64. Guazzi M, Smaja M, Arena R, Vicenzi M, Guazzi MD. Long-term use of sildenafil in the therapeutic management of heart failure. J Am Coll Cardiol 2007 Nov 27;50(22):2136–44.

65. Weber K. Aldosterone in congestive heart failure. N Engl J Med 2001;345:1689–1697.

66. Chhokar VS, Sun Y, Bhattacharya SK, Ashokas R, Myers LK, Xing Z, Smith RA, Gerling IC, Weber KT. Hyperparathyroidism and the calcium paradox of aldosteronism. Circulation 2005;111:871–878.

67. Struthers AD. Aldosterone escape during angiotensin-converting enzyme inhibitor therapy in chronic heart failure. J Card Fail 1996;2:47–57.

68. Pitt B, Zannad F, Remme WJ, Cody R, Castaigne A, Perez A, Palensky J, Wittes J. The effect of spironolactone on morbidity and mortality in patients with severe heart failure. N Engl J Med 1999;341:709–717.

69. Pitt, B, Remme W, Zannad F, Neaton J, Martinez F, Roniker B, Bittman R, Hurley S, Kleiman J, Gatlin M. Eplerenone, a selective aldosterone blocker, in patients with left ventricular dysfunction after myocardial infarction. N Engl J Med 2003;342:1309–1321.

70. Juurlink DN, Mamdani MM, Lee DS, Kopp A, Austin PC, Laupacis A, Redelmeier DA. Rates of hyperkalemia after publication of the randomized aldactone evaluation study. N Engl J Med 2004;351:543–551.

71. Cohn JN, TB Levine, MT Olivari, V Garberg, D Lura, GS Francis, AB Simon, and T Rector. Plasma norepinephrine as a guide to prognosis in patients with chronic congestive heart failure. N Engl J Med 1984;311:819.

72. Black JW, Crowther AF, Shanks RG, Smith LH, Dornhorst AC. A new adrenergic beta-receptor antagonist. Lancet 1964;283:1080–1081.

73. Waagstein F, Hjalmarson A, Varnauskas E, Wallentin I. Effect of chronic beta-adrenergic receptor blockade in congestive cardiomyopathy. Br Heart J 1975;37:1022–36.

74. Bristow, MR. β-Adrenergic receptor blockade in chronic heart failure. Circulation 2000;101:558–569.

75. Lowes BD, Gilbert EM, Abraham WT, Minobe WA, Larrabee P, Ferguson D, Wolfel EE, Lindenfield J, Tsvetkova T, Robertson AD, Quaife RA, Bristow MR. Myocardial gene expression in dilated cardiomyopathy treated with beta-blocking agents. N Engl J Med 2002;346:1357–1365.

76. Cohn JN, Ferrari R, Sharpe N. Cardiac remodeling – concepts and clinical implications: a consensus paper from an international forum on cardiac remodeling. J Am Coll Cardiol 2000;35:569–582

77. Colucci WS, Packer M, Bristow MR, Gilbert EM, Cohn JN, Fowler MB, Krueger SK, Hershberger R, Uretsky BF, Bowers JA, Sackner-Bernstein JD, Young ST, Holsclaw TL, Lukas MA. Carvedilol inhibits progression in patients with mild symptoms of heart failure. Circulation 1996;94:2800–2806.

78. Bristow MR, Gilbert EM, Abraham WT, Adams KF, Fowler MB, Hershberger RE, Kubo SH, Narahara KA, Ingersoll H, Krueger S, Young S, Shusterman N. Carvedilol produces dose-related improvements in left ventricular function and survival in subjects with chronic heart failure. Circulation 1996;94:2807–2816.

79. Packer M, Bristow MR, Cohn JN, Colucci WS, Fowler MB, Gilbert EM, Shusterman NH. The effect of carvedilol on morbidity and mortality in patients with chronic heart failure. N Engl J Med 1996;334:1349–1355.

80. Hjalmarson A, Goldstein S, Deedwania P et al. Effects of controlled-release metoprolol on total mortality, hospitalizations and well-being in patients with heart failure (MERIT-HF). JAMA 2000;283:1295–1302.

81. Packer M, Coats AJS, Fowler MB, Katus HA, Krum H, Mohacsi P, Rouleau J, Tendera M, Castaigne A, Roecker EB, Schultz MK, DeMets DL. Effect of carvedilol on survival in severe chronic heart failure. N Engl J Med 2001;344:1651–1658

82. Hjalmarson A, Goldstein S, Deedwania P et al. Effects of controlled-release metoprolol on total mortality, hospitalizations and well-being in patients with heart failure (MERIT-HF). JAMA 2000;283:1295–1302.

83. Packer M, Colucci W, Shusterman NH et al. Double-blind, placebo-controlled study of carvedilol in patients with moderate to severe heart failure. Circulation 1996;94:2793–2799.

84. Kowey PR. A review of carvedilol arrhythmia data in clinical trials. J Cardiovasc Phamacol Theraput 2005;10:S59-S68.

85. Fagerberg B et al. Effect of metoprolol CD/XL in chronic heart failure: Metoprolol CR/XL Randomized Intervention Trial in Congestive Heart Failure (MERIT-HF). Lancet 1999;353:2001–2007.

86. Dargie HJ, Lechat P et al. The Cardiac Insufficiency Bisoprolol Study II (CIBIS-II): a randomized trial. Lancet 1999;353:9–13.

87. Eichhorn E, Domanski M; et al for the BEST Investigators. A trial of the beta-blocker bucindolol in patients with advanced chronic heart failure. N Engl J Med 2001;344:1659–1667

88. Waagstein F, Bristow MR, Swedberg K, Camerini F, Fowler MB, Silver MA, Gilbert EM, Johnson MR, Goss FG, Hjalmarson A. Benefifial effects of metoprolol in idiopathic dilated cardiomyopathy. Lancet 1993;342:1441–1446

89. Yancy CW, Fowler MB, Colucci WS, Gilbert EM, Bristow MR, Cohn JN, Lukas MA, Young ST, Packer M. Race and the response to adrenergic blockade with carvedilol in patients with chronic heart failure. N Engl J Med 2001;344:1358–65.

90. Poole-Wilson PA, Swedberg K, Cleland JGF, Li Lenarda A, Hanrath P, Komajda M, Lubsen J, Lutiger B, Metra M, Remme WJ, Torp-Pedersen C, Scherhag A, Skene A. Comparison of carvedilol and metoprolol on clinical outcomes in patients with chromic heart failure in the carvedilol or metoprolol European trial (COMET): randomized controlled trial. Lancet 2003;362:7–13

91. Willenheimer R, van Veldhuisen DJ, Silke B, Erdmann E, Follath F, Krum H, Ponikowski P, Skene A, van de Ven L, Verkenne P, Lechat P. Effect on survival and

hospitalization of initiating treatment for chronic heart failure with bisoprolol followed by enalapril, as compared with the opposite sequence: Results of the randomized Cardiac Insufficiency Bisoprolol Study (CIBIS) III. Circulation 2005;112:2426–2435.

92. Fang J. Angiotensin-converting enzyme inhibitors or β-blockers in heart failure: Does it matter who goes first? Circulation 2005;112:2380–2382.

93. Eichhorn EJ, Bristow MR. Practical guidelines for initiation of beta-adrenergic blockade in patients with chronic heart failure. Am J Cardiol 1997;79:794–798.

94. Ko DT, Hebert PR, Coffey CS, Curtis JP, Foody JM, Sedrakyan A, Krumholz HM. Adverse effects of β-blocker therapy for patients with heart failure. A quantitative overview of randomized trials. Arch Intern Med 2004;164:1389–1394.

95. Krum H, Roecker EB, Mohacsi P, Rouleau JL, Tendra M, Coats AJS, Fowler MB, Packer M. Effects of initiating carvedilol in patients with severe chronic heart failure. results from the COPERNICUS Study. JAMA 2003;289:712–718.

96. Stevenson LW. Beta-blockers for stable heart failure. N Engl J Med 2002;346: 1346–1347.

97. Salpeter SR, Ormiston TM, Salpeter EE. Cardioselective β-Blockers in patients with reactive airway disease: A meta-analysis. Ann Intern Med 2002;137:715–725.

98. Fonarow GC, Abraham WT, Albert NM, Stough WG, Gheorghiade M, Greenberg BH, O'Connor CM, Sun JL, Yancy CW, Young JB; OPTIMIZE-HF Investigators and Coordinators. Influence of beta-blocker continuation or withdrawal on outcomes in patients hospitalized with heart failure: Findings from the OPTIMIZE-HF program. J Am Coll Cardiol 2008 Jul 15;52(3):190–9.

99. Beemath A, Stein PD, Skaf E, Al Sibae MR, Alesh I. Risk of venous thromboembolism in patients hospitalized with heart failure. Am J Cardiol 2006:98:793–795.

100. Freudenberger RS, Halperin JL. Should we use anticoagulation for patients with chronic heart failure? Nat Clin Pract Cardiovasc Med 2006;3:580–581.

101. Massie BM, Krol WF, Ammon SE, Armstrong PW, Cleland JG, Collins JF, Ezekowitz M, Jafri SM, O'Connor CM, Packer M, Schulman KA, Teo K, Warren S. The Warfarin and Antiplatelet Therapy in Heart Failure trial (WATCH): rationale, design, and baseline patient characteristics. J Card Fail 2004;10:113–4.

102. Cleland JG, Findlay I, Jafri S, Sutton G, Falk R, Bulpitt C, Prentice C, Ford I, Trainer A, Poole-Wilson PA. The Warfarin/Aspirin Study in Heart failure (WASH): a randomized trial comparing antithrombotic strategies for patients with heart failure. Am Heart J 2004;148:157–64.

103. Pullicino P, Thompson JLP, Barton B, Levin B, Graham S, Freudenberger RS. Warfarin Versus Aspirin in Patients with Reduced Cardiac Ejection Fraction (WARCEF): rationale, objectives, and design. J Card Fail 2006;12:39–46.

104. Khush KK, Waters DD, Bittner V, Deedwania PC, Kastelein JJ, Lewis SJ, Wenger NK. Effect of high-dose atorvastatin on hospitalizations for heart failure: subgroup analysis of the Treating to New Targets (TNT) study. Circulation 2007 Feb 6;115(5):576–83.

105. Domanski M, Coady S, Felg J, Tian X, Sachdev V. Effect of statin therapy on survival in patients with nonischemic dilated cardiomyopathy (from the Beta Blocker Evaluation of Survival Trial [BEST]). Am J Cardiol 2007 May 15:99(10):1448–50.

106. Kjekshus J, Apetrei E, Barrios V, Bohm M, Cleland JG, Cornel JH, Dunselman P, Fonseca C, Goudev A, Grande P, Gullestad L, Hjalmarson A, Hradec J, Janosi A, Kamensky G, Komajda M, Korewicki J, Kuusi T, Mach F, Mareev V, McMurray JJ, Ranjith N, Schaufelberger M, Vanhaecke J, van Veldhuisen DJ, Waagstein F, Wedel J, Wikstrand J. Rosuvastatin in older patients with systolic heart failure. N Engl J Med 2007 Nov 29;357(22):2248–61.

107. Nesto RW, Bell D, Bonow RO, Fonseca V, Grundy SM, Horton ES, Le Winter M, Porte D, Semenkovich CF, Smith S, Young LHM, Kahn R. Thiazolidinedione use, fluid retention, and congestive heart failure. A consensus statement from the American Heart Association and American Diabetes Association. Circulation 2003;108:2941–2948.

108. Amabile CM, Spencer AP. Keeping your patient with heart failure safe. Arch Intern Med 2004;164:709–720.
109. Kober L, Torp-Pederson C, McMurray JJ, Gotzsche O, Levy S, Crigins H, Amlie J, Carlsen J; Dronedarone Study Group. Increased mortality after dronedarone therapy for severe heart failure. N Engl J Med 2008 June 19:358(25):2678–87.
110. Goldstein RE, Boccuzzi SJ, Cruess D, Nattel S. Diltiazem increases late-onset congestive heart failure in post-infarction patients with early reduction in ejection fraction. Circulation 1991;83:52–60.
111. Elkayam U, Amin J, Mehra A, Vasquez J, Weber L, Rahimtoola S. A prospective, randomized, double-blind, cross-over study to compare the efficacy and safety of chronic nifedipine therapy with that of isosorbide dinitrate and their combination in the treatment of chronic congestive heart failure. Circulation 1990;82:1954–1961.
112. Cohn, JN, Ziesche, S, Smith, R, Anand, I, Dunkman, WB, Loeb, H, Cintron, G, Boden, W, Baruch, L, Rochin, P, Loss, L. Effect of the calcium antagonist felodipine as supplementary vasodilator therapy in patients with chronic heart failure treated with enalapril: V-HeFT III. Circulation 1997;96: 856–863.
113. Antman EM, Bennett JS, Daugherty A, Furberg C, Roberts H, Taubert KA. Use of nonsteroidal antiinflammatory drugs. An update for clinicians: A scientific statement from the American Heart Association. Circulation 2007;115:1634–1642.
114. Page J, Henry D. Consumption of NSAIDs and the development of congestive heart failure in elderly patients. Arch Intern Med 2000;160:777–784.
115. Lee DS, Tu JV, Juurlink DN, Alter DA, Ko DT, Austin PC, Chong A, Stukel TA, Levy D, Laupacis A. Risk-treatment mismatch in the pharmacotherapy of heart failure. JAMA 2005;294:1240–1247.

3 Device Trials in Chronic Heart Failure: Implications of Trial Design

Warren K. Laskey, MD and Renee Manring-Day, RN, MSN, ACNP

CONTENTS

Abstract

Device therapy in the treatment of patients with heart failure may add incremental therapeutic benefits on a background of optimal medical treatment. Improvements in quality of life and survival observed in clinical trials (efficacy) in patients with heart failure have led to increasing utilization of these devices in clinical practice (effectiveness). Clinical trials define the patient population in whom the device is likely to be effective, the magnitude of the expected degree of improvement, and the balance between risk and benefit. It is, therefore, essential that clinicians understand the basic elements of trial design and how they apply specifically to trials of device therapy in patients with heart failure.

Key Words: Heart failure; Clinical trials; Medical device; Statistics; Trial design; Pharmacologic treatment.

From: *Contemporary Cardiology: Device Therapy in Heart Failure*
Edited by: W.H. Maisel, DOI 10.1007/978-1-59745-424-7_3
© Humana Press, a part of Springer Science+Business Media, LLC 2010

1. INTRODUCTION

The clinician caring for a patient with heart failure is confronted with two fundamentally different yet inter-related challenges: the challenge of improving the chances of survival and the challenge of optimizing quality of life. Despite major advances in the pharmacologic treatment of patients with heart failure *(1, 2)*, patient survival with heart failure in the current era, on average, is only marginally improved over the original grim prognosis described in the incipient Framingham cohort *(3, 4)*. Although the prognosis of heart failure patients receiving optimal pharmacologic treatment is unquestionably improved compared to the untreated state, increasing rates of hospitalization and, ultimately, complications related to progressive heart failure suggest that we may be approaching a "ceiling" of therapeutic benefit related to neurohumoral blockade *(5)*. On this background, it is evident that demonstration of the incremental efficacy of novel pharmacologic treatments for heart failure will be increasingly difficult.

Given the significant morbidity and mortality risk that even "optimal" pharmacologically treated heart failure still confers, it is not surprising that alternative means of treating patients with persistent symptomatic heart failure have evolved. Leading the advance in this area of trans-pharmacologic treatment of heart failure is technologically sophisticated, invasively implanted devices. While the heart failure specialist requires expertise in the understanding of these devices, including their indications, contraindications, and expected benefits, the (non-specialist) clinician should also understand when to consider the feasibility of a device and how to appropriately assess such patients following receipt of a given device. Basically, this reduces to two deceptively simple questions: *does it work?* and *is it safe?* The answers are derived from the results of clinical trials performed to demonstrate, with reasonable assurance, device efficacy, and safety; these latter considerations determine whether a device receives regulatory approval *(6)*. This aspect of device development and application to patients with heart failure is discussed in a separate chapter.

For the clinician who manages heart failure patients to understand these issues and to answer the aforementioned questions with his or her particular patient in mind, an understanding (and appreciation) of heart failure device clinical trial design is a necessity. To that end, the fundamental tenets of clinical trial design will be reviewed, followed by a more detailed look at device trial designs for patients with heart failure.

2. TENETS OF GOOD CLINICAL TRIAL DESIGN

2.1. The Question

While it may seem intuitive, the question (related to, but frequently not identical with, the principal hypothesis) that a clinical trial addresses should be clinically meaningful, clearly stated and, with a high degree of certainty, likely to be answered by the trial. These objectives are generally met when the clinical trial design adheres to a number of well-defined criteria (Table 1).

Table 1
Elements of clinical trial design

General	Specific
Question/hypothesis	Clinically relevant; addresses an issue for which no consistent or convincing evidence exists
Nature of the endpoint	Must be "measurable," e.g., continuous; binary; categorical (hierarchical) outcomes; single response variable; composite of single response variables; surrogate response variable
Intended population	Trial inclusion criteria must match the target population characteristics
Comparator population	Must match the treatment group in all/most aspects except for treatment modality; ideally should be chosen at random from the same "universe" of patients as the treatment group
Elimination of bias	Randomization; blinding; choice of appropriate comparator; complete follow-up
Ability to detect treatment effect of specified size	Confidence, power, and sample size calculations; nature of endpoint (continuous vs. binary, time to event, etc.)
Ability to reject erroneous conclusions	Confidence, power, and sample size calculations; nature of endpoint
Ethics	Institutional review board (IRB), Data safety monitoring board (DSMB)
Mechanics of trial design	Parallel design; crossover design; non-inferiority design; superiority design, event driven; sample size driven
Trial conduct	Independent (from sponsor) steering committee; independent data safety monitoring board; timely recruitment; completeness of ascertainment of response variable(s)

These aspects of clinical trial design have been discussed in detail in several excellent texts *(7–9)* and review articles *(10–12)*. In the present chapter, these elements are referred to only insofar as they highlight specific aspects of a clinical trial in patients with heart failure.

The study *population* is defined as the segment of the general population with certain characteristics known as eligibility criteria. The study *sample* is that fraction of the study population who ultimately participate (enroll) and are observed. Without a clear definition of these criteria the patients likely to benefit from the specified treatment will remain poorly defined. However, the more restrictive the eligibility (and inclusion) criteria, the less generalizable the results.

The primary endpoint should, ideally, be assessed in all subjects; should be immune from bias (blinded); and should be question/hypothesis specific. The measure of the primary endpoint is reflected in the response variable which, as seen in Table 1, may assume many forms. In the case of a composite endpoint, each component should be assessable without bias (subject or observer), be responsive to the intervention, and have clinical import. Although this review will focus on the primary endpoint(s) of a given trial, secondary endpoints are, despite their appellation, often meaningful; in fact, on occasion, they are more clinically meaningful than the primary endpoint. However, it is the primary endpoint which defines the trial's null hypothesis, power, and sample size calculations. Surrogate endpoints are those measures of an outcome that, ideally, reflect the clinical condition under study. Implicit, therefore, are the assumptions that observed changes in the surrogate must (1) reliably predict changes in the specified clinical outcome and (2) respond in kind to the change observed in the clinical outcome. Often this is not the case and changes observed in the surrogate variable are not reflected in the specified clinical outcome.

An important consideration in interpreting time-dependent endpoints (time to event) is the effect of overall trial duration, event rate, and individual follow-up times on the study's conclusions. Differences between treatment arms with regard to clinically relevant outcomes may not be identified with short follow-up intervals and either surrogate endpoints or "soft" endpoints. The effect(s) of censoring may also impact a trial's conclusions if the primary endpoint occurs beyond the censoring interval. In that case, the observations will be biased in favor of the non-censored patients. This is an important consideration in the interpretation of "event-driven" trials (see discussion in Section 3 on cardiac resynchronization effects on mortality). Another consideration in time to event trials is that of competing risks within a composite outcome. In general, when a patient meets one of the prespecified endpoints of a composite outcome, that patient is removed from the pool of analyzable, at-risk patients. In the extreme instance, if a patient dies early in the course of the trial, this will impact the ability to identify a benefit on quality of life. Conversely, if a patient is hospitalized, that subject is also removed from the pool of subjects at risk of the combined endpoint. Under these circumstances, the ability to identify a benefit on mortality may be compromised (13).

This chapter will focus primarily on efficacy endpoints, recognizing that this is only half the story. Safety endpoints, including their definition, metrics, and influence on a study's ability to reliably detect important, sometimes infrequent, adverse outcomes, are also critical to interpreting the utility of a novel device designed to treat heart failure patients. In general, clinical trials are designed to demonstrate clinical efficacy with a certain degree of confidence ("p value") and precision (power). While many safety endpoints, e.g., stroke or death, may be detected with similar degrees of confidence and power for the same sample size, other more infrequent endpoints may not be detected. Under these circumstances, a much larger clinical trial with, possibly, longer follow-up would be necessary to address a primary safety hypothesis. In any event, it is the overall risk/benefit ratio which determines not only the "success" of a clinical trial but also its real-world applicability.

The measure of benefit should, ideally, be understood by clinicians as well as clinical trialists and statisticians, should not vary with baseline characteristics (confounding), and should be amenable to basic statistical analysis. Although the measure of benefit can be expressed in a number of ways (relative risk, odds ratio, risk reduction), both (relative and absolute) measures should be available for review as they connote distinct entities ("effectiveness" vs. "benefit").

The selection of a control group is fundamental to clinical trial design as this provides the only means of identifying outcomes related to the treatment from those caused by the natural history of the condition or observer and/or patient expectation. It is the latter factor which often plays an important part in identifying and quantifying the "placebo" effect in many clinical trials. The choice of a control group for a clinical trial is a critical decision, and often the subject of debate (historical, contemporaneous, placebo, active treatment, etc.); this choice has a profound impact on the degree to which bias is mitigated, the kind (and number) of endpoints that can be assessed, the credibility of the results, and, importantly, the soundness of the results to regulatory bodies ("reasonable assurance").

The importance of minimizing, or eliminating, bias in a clinical trial cannot be overstated. Common sources of bias originate in both patient and medical environments. The former include referral (pattern) bias, patient refusal, and differential eligibility criteria while the latter include bias in detection and evaluation and the data quality itself. The most reliable way to minimize bias in a clinical trial is through the process of randomization and appropriate blinding of both observer and patient. While this is not always possible, particularly in the setting of device implantation in patients with heart failure, randomization is the most reliable way to achieve (near) comparability in treatment and control groups. Ideally, in a randomized trial, the imbalances that remain are due to chance – something for which statistical modeling can typically account. Adequately "adjusting" for the many non-random sources of bias, such as those that frequent non-randomized trials, is much more difficult, and in some cases impossible.

Detailed discussions of sample size and power calculations are important to the understanding of clinical trial design, but are beyond the scope of this chapter. Other texts thoroughly cover this topic (7–9). An important distinction must be made between the "statistically significant" and the "clinically significant" trial results. Specifically, the clinician must recognize the clinical trial designed to detect a small, clinically irrelevant difference between treatment and control and understand how confidence intervals may be used to interpret the result (14). When outcomes are infrequent, combining events of similar pathophysiologic consequence increases the study's power and allows for a greater likelihood of observing true differences between treatment and control arms. As will be seen in subsequent examples, composite endpoints comprise a significant proportion of the response variables in current device trials. The trade-off is clear – for similar levels of precision and confidence, low-frequency (singular) outcomes require larger sample sizes to detect a treatment effect while higher-frequency (composite) outcomes require smaller sample sizes to detect a treatment effect *(12)*, albeit at the risk of increased difficulty in interpreting the clinical relevance of the endpoint.

Finally, the clinical trial must be carried out in compliance with contemporary ethical mandates. Ethical challenges include ensuring that patients receive necessary medical care (i.e., for sick patients randomized to placebo or "control" arms), and that the clinical trial is conducted without bias, conflict of interest, or intellectual dishonesty. A system of checks and balances has evolved, particularly for the conduct of large-scale, multi-center trials, to address these crucial elements *(11)*. Nevertheless, particularly in the case of severely ill heart failure patients awaiting transplantation, inability to blind subjects or observers to treatment poses substantial challenges to the interpretation of subjective endpoints.

The following overview is not intended to be comprehensive but rather to highlight important similarities and differences in clinical trial designs categorized by the nature of the endpoint. Although the review is focused on the various trials' measures of treatment efficacy, the same principles apply to measures of safety.

3. CURRENT TRIAL DESIGNS IN HEART FAILURE POPULATIONS

3.1. The Endpoint: Symptom Relief in Acute Decompensated Heart Failure

Patients with chronic heart failure frequently exhibit acute exacerbations necessitating hospitalization. Traditional therapy has relied heavily on the use of parenteral loop diuretics albeit with diminishing effectiveness as repeated treatment becomes necessary. The UNLOAD trial *(15)* examined the utility of ultrafiltration vs. intravenous diuretic therapy in hospitalized patients with volume overload superimposed on chronic heart failure (Table 2). In this multi-center, randomized controlled trial, one co-primary endpoint (weight loss) met statistical significance, while the other (dyspnea grade) did not. Neither observers nor patients were blinded to treatment assignment, and the endpoint is comprised of an ordinal variable and a continuous variable. The trial also demonstrates the dichotomy of a clinically relevant endpoint (dyspnea grade) not captured by a potential surrogate endpoint (weight loss).

Table 2
Device therapy for the improvement in symptoms in patients with decompensated heart failure

Patient population	Trial design	Primary efficacy endpoint(s)	Outcome I Weight loss (kg)		Outcome II Dyspnea grade	
			Treatment	Control	Treatment	Control
Hospitalized with clinical volume overload	Randomized within 24 h of admission; parallel design; no blinding	Weight loss and dyspnea at 48 h	5.0 ± 3.1	3.1 ± 3.5^a	6.4	6.1^b

[a] $p = 0.001$ (treatment vs. control).
[b] $p = 0.35$ (treatment vs. control).

3.2. The Endpoint: Functional Improvement and Quality of Life

The use of implantable devices for the treatment of patients with heart failure essentially began with cardiac resynchronization therapy (CRT) (16–18). The early trials were designed to establish improvements in subjective (quality of life score based on a standardized questionnaire and New York Heart Association Class) and objective (6-min walk test) measures of heart failure severity and were focused in scope in order to gain FDA approval (Table 3). Notably, all trials were performed on a background of "optimal medical therapy" appropriate to the time of the study. Patients in the control arms received optimal medical therapy alone while patients receiving devices were also maintained on optimal medical therapy. Selected published clinical trial experience with these same endpoints is summarized in Table 4. Differences between the premarket approval (PMA) submissions and the published studies reflect somewhat different patient populations, differences in the timing of acquisition of baseline data in relationship to the time of randomization, and varying degrees of ascertainment of follow-up data. Examination of the trial designs for these "pivotal" studies highlights the concepts articulated earlier. The "success" of the trial hinges on the nature of the endpoint and whether the response variable is viewed as separate co-primary endpoints (InSynch ICD) or one composite endpoint in which a statistically significant result in any one of the components would be sufficient to reject the null hypothesis. These specific endpoints are subject to both patient and observer bias and, thus, the matter of blinding (and its assurance) is crucial. The importance of a separate control group is demonstrated by the magnitude and direction of responses observed in the non-treated population. Finally, the interpretation of composite endpoints and

Table 3

Cardiac resynchronization therapy pivotal trials for the assessment of functional improvement and quality of life: pre-market applications (PMA) to FDA

Study/year (PMA #)	Patient population	Trial design	Primary efficacy endpoint(s)		Outcomes	
					Treatment	Control
InSynch ICD/2002 (P010031)	NYHA Class III/IV; ICD required; LVEF ≤0.35; QRS ≥130 ms	Randomized (0–7 days after implant), double-blind, parallel design	Median NYHA class	Base	3	3
				6 months	2	3[a]
			Median QOL score	Base	55	57
				6 months	33	44[b]
			6-min walk (m)	Base	260	275
				6 months	342	333[c]
InSynch atrial synchronous biventricular pacing device 2002 (P010015)	NYHA Class III/IV; ICD not required; LVEF≤0.35; QRS≥130 ms	Randomized (0–3 days after implant), double-blind, parallel design	Median NYHA class @ 6 months		2	3[d]
			Median QOL score @ 6 months		40.5	46.0[e]
			6-min walk (m) @6 months		371	321[e]

				Change from baseline @ 6 months	95% LCB
CONTAK-CD – focused confirmatory study 2002 (PO10012)	NYHA Class III/IV; met indication for ICD; LVEF≤0.35; QRS≥120 ms (127)	Single arm, unblinded, "optimal performance criteria" design	Peak VO$_2$	0.94 ± 0.3	0.45
			6-min walk (m)	50.9 ± 10.4	37.6
			QOL score	23.9 ± 2.6	19.7
			Percent with one-grade improvement in NYHA class	60.4%	N/A

[a] $p = 0.027$ (treatment vs. control @ 6 months).
[b] $p = 0.009$ (treatment vs. control @ 6 months).
[c] $p = 0.407$ (treatment vs. control @ 6 months).
[d] $p < 0.001$ (treatment vs. control @ 6 months).
[e] $p = 0.003$ (treatment vs. control @ 6 months).
LCB, lower confidence bound; N/A, not available.

Table 4

Cardiac resynchronization therapy trials for the assessment of functional improvement and quality of life: published clinical trials

Study/year	Patient population	Trial design	Primary efficacy endpoint(s)	Outcomes Treatment	Outcomes Control
MUSTIC-SR/2001	NYHA Class III; LVEF <0.35; QRS>150 ms	Randomized (0–14 d after implant); single-blind; crossover design	Active–inactive group ($n = 29$)	6-min walk (m) @ 3 months 384 ± 79	336 ± 128[a]
			Inactive–active group ($n = 29$)	413 ± 117	316 ± 142[a]
			Combined groups	399 ± 100	326 ± 134[b]
MIRACLE/2002	NYHA Class III/IV; LVEF ≤0.35; QRS ≥130 ms	Randomized (1–14 d after implant); double-blind; parallel control design		Change @ 6 months in: NYHA Class	
			% Improved ≥2 grades	16%	6%[b]
			% Improved 1 grade	52%	32%
			% No change	30%	59%
			Median QOL score	–18	–9[c]
			6-min walk (m)	+39	+10[d]
MIRACLE-ICD/2003	NYHA Class III/IV; LVEF ≤0.35; QRS ≥130 ms and candidate for ICD	Randomized (1–14 d); double-blind; parallel control design		Change @ 6 months	
			Median NYHA class	–1	0[e]
			Median QOL score	–17.5	–11[f]
			6-min walk (m)	55	53[a]

[a] p = ns (treatment vs. control).
[b] $p < 0.001$ (treatment vs. control).
[c] $p = 0.001$.
[d] $p = 0.005$.
[e] $p = 0.007$.
[f] $p = 0.02$.

the translation to a measure of clinical benefit, particularly when some components fail to change or respond in a discordant fashion, are conceptually difficult for the clinician to grasp. The CONTAK-CD Focused Confirmatory Study design represents a compromise between the rigor of obtaining "valid scientific evidence" and pragmatic and regulatory considerations *(19)*. Specifically, the use of optimum performance criteria for comparator arms is, in general, fraught with limitations. However, where extensive, albeit noncontemporaneous data from similar patient populations and device experience exist, such a trial design may be used for specific purposes.

The endpoints in the above trials are assessed after relatively short treatment intervals (3–6 months) and continuing optimal medical therapy. Conclusions from such studies cannot, therefore, be extrapolated to long-term efficacy, survival beyond these intervals, or patient tolerability. Conversely, while the "placebo" response observed in the control group might mitigate the measure of short-term efficacy, no such conclusions can be extrapolated to potential longer-term benefit. In addition to the potential for bias in the assessment of functional classification (observer unblinding, observer and patient motivation) the scatter in the 6-min walk data highlights the need for adequate power to support statistical significance. While crossover design trials have the advantage of requiring a smaller sample size (in comparison to parallel design trial) to demonstrate an effect, the patient groups must be well matched at baseline and the risk of "carry over" effect (real or placebo) must be minimal *(20)* in order to assess the true treatment effect. The difficulty of obtaining clinically meaningful and objective measures of functional improvement and quality of life in patients with heart failure can be appreciated in all these trials. Treatment effects remain difficult to interpret, particularly in the case of composite endpoints of "soft" response variables. While trial design cannot consistently address these issues (of "soft" endpoints and bias), use of a less subjective endpoint with unquestioned clinical relevance allows for clinical trial design consistent with the above-discussed tenets.

Taking the lead from pharmacologic trials, an endpoint of mortality and/or hospitalization, combined (composite) or separate, meets the criteria for objectivity and clinical relevance. Pre-market clinical trials sponsored by commercial manufacturers of implantable cardiac devices and utilized to obtain device approval (Table 5) as well as clinical trial data reported in the literature (Table 6) provide insight into the strengths and limitations of trial designs using these specific endpoints in heart failure patients.

As noted in the opening section of this chapter, the composite endpoints chosen reflect a balance between pragmatism (trial expense and completion) and clinical relevance. Composite endpoints allow for greater statistical power and smaller sample sizes. Despite the relatively short-term outcome assessments, the use of clear-cut measures of disease severity/progression ("hard endpoints") allows for meaningful interpretation of the observed event rates in treated patients and controls. Such "hard" endpoints also lessen

Table 5

Clinical trials designed to assess changes in risk of mortality and/or repeat hospitalization following device implantation in patients with heart failure: Pre-market applications (PMA) to the US Food and Drug Administration

Study/year (PMA#)	Patient population	Trial design	Primary efficacy endpoint(s)	Outcomes	
				Treatment	Control
CONTAK-CD-ICD/2002 (P010012)	NYHA Class III/IV; ICD indication; QRS ≥120 ms; LVEF ≤0.35	Randomized (by 30 days after implant); double-blind; parallel control (OMT)	At 6 months: Composite of All-cause mortality (%) or Hospitalization (%) or VT/VF (%)	4.5 / 12.0 / 13.5	6.5[a] / 5.1[a] / 15.1[a]
CRT-D/2004 (P010012 suppl 26) (COMPANION)	NYHA Class III/IV; ICD indication; QRS ≥120 ms; LVEF ≤0.35	Randomized (before implant); double-blind; parallel control (OMT)	All-cause mortality or hospitalization (%); All-cause mortality (%)	At 12 months 56 / 12	58[b] / 19[c]
ACORN CorCap®/2001 (P040049)	Dilated cardiomyopathy (30 mm/m² < EDDi<40 mm/m²); LVEF ≤0.35 (≤0.45 with MR); symptomatic despite optimal medical therapy	Randomized (1:1), paralleled design, stratified on mitral valve surgery; single blind	1° endpoint at >12 months[d,e]; Improved (%); Same (%); Worsened (%)	37.7 / 25.1 / 37.2	27.3 / 27.7 / 45.1

[a] $p = 0.21$ (for combined endpoint).

[b] $p = 0.011$ (treatment vs. control).

[c] $p = 0.004$ (treatment vs. control).

[d] Composite endpoint of all-cause mortality, change in NYHA class, requirement for major cardiac procedure.

[e] Summary odds ratio (T/C) = 1.73 (95% CI: 1.07–2.79), $p = 0.024$.

EDDi, left ventricular end-diastolic dimension index; OMT, optimal medical treatment.

Table 6

Clinical trials designed to assess changes in risk of mortality and/or repeat hospitalization following device implantation in patients with heart failure: published clinical trials

Study/year	Patient population	Trial design	Primary efficacy endpoint(s)	Outcome Treatment		Control
				CRT	CRT-D	
COMPANION/2004	NYHA Class III/IV; QRS ≥120 ms; LVEF <0.35; no clinical indication for ICD	1:2:2 parallel design randomization (OMT, OMT+CRT, OMT+CRT-D) prior to implant; blinded adjudication	Composite: All-cause mortality or All-cause hosp. @ 12 months (%)	56[a]	56[b]	68
CARE-HF/2005	NYHA Class III/IV; LVEF ≤0.35; EDDi ≥30 mm; QRS ≥120 ms*; no clinical indication for ICD	1:1 parallel design randomization stratified on NYHA class prior to implant; blinded adjudication	Composite: All-cause mortality or Unplanned CV-related hosp. @ 1100+ days (%)	39[c]		55
SCD-HeFT/2005	NYHA Class II/III; LVEF ≤0.35	1:1:1 parallel design randomization (placebo, amiodarone, ICD)	All-cause mortality @ 5 years (%)	ICD 22[d]	Amio 28[e]	Placebo 29

* For QRS of 120–149 ms there was an additional requirement for evidence of dyssynchrony; ICD, implantable cardiac defibrillator; OMT, optimal medical therapy.

[a] p = 0.015 (CRT vs. OMT).
[b] p = 0.011 (CRT-D vs. OMT).
[c] p < 0.001 (treatment vs. control).
[d] p = 0.007 (ICD vs. placebo).
[e] p = 0.53.

concerns regarding bias as may often be seen with the use of "softer" composite endpoints of equivocal clinical relevance. It is notable that both the COMPANION *(21)* and CARE-HF *(22)* trials designated all-cause mortality as a secondary endpoint. In the COMPANION trial, there was no significant difference in all-cause mortality between CRT and optimal medical therapy (OMT) at the conclusion of the trial (hazard ratio, 0.76; 95% confidence interval, 0.58–1.01; $p = 0.06$) whereas in the CARE-HF trial the difference in mortality between CRT and OMT at the conclusion of the trial was statistically significant (hazard ratio, 0.64; 95% confidence interval, 0.48–0.85; $p < 0.002$). Differences in trial duration and absolute numbers of events may explain the discordance.

The use, and hazard, of surrogate endpoints is noted in the ACORN trial *(23)*. While "proof of principle" was verified in the observed changes in ventricular size and shape (all secondary endpoints) in patients receiving the device, limitations in the conduct of the study, incomplete primary endpoint ascertainment, and an inability to demonstrate a decreased risk of mortality or repeat hospitalizations led the FDA to deny approval of this PMA *(23)*. This may be a critical point in other device trials seeking to use markers of ventricular remodeling as surrogates for the "hard" clinical outcomes of death and repeat hospitalization.

In contrast to the COMPANION PMA, in which CRT with a defibrillator (CRT-D) was compared to medical therapy alone, the published trial *(21)* was a three-way comparison of optimal medical therapy, CRT alone (CRT-P), and CRT-D. Notably, both trial designs specified a composite primary endpoint of mortality or hospitalization as the outcome of interest. The COMPANION trial did not possess adequate power to identify differences in the secondary endpoint (mortality) between the medical treatment alone, CRT-P, and CRT-D arms while the CARE-HF trial *(22)* was able to demonstrate a difference in this important secondary endpoint. The use of event-driven trials may preclude identifying differences in modes of event-free survival, or even all-cause mortality between treatment arms if the trials are terminated prior to the time when such differences may have been detectable (COMPANION and CARE-HF had different trial durations). The SCD-HeFT trial *(24)* was of sufficient duration and power to establish the role of ICD therapy in improving the survival of patients with heart failure, irrespective of etiology.

The discussion to this point has followed a sequence of increasingly relevant, i.e., "hard," primary outcomes and correspondingly rigorous trial design. Unfortunately, a sizeable proportion of patients with heart failure progress to a truly dire state in which all treatment modalities have failed, quality of life is dismal, and the risk of mortality approaches 100% without further intervention. Until recently, the only viable option for these patients was cardiac transplantation. However, device technology has evolved to the point where implantable devices may now serve as a "bridge to transplantation" or as "destination therapy." When serving as a bridge to transplantation, devices are intended to stabilize, if not improve, tenuous hemodynamic and critical overall clinical conditions thereby allowing for improved chances at transplantation *(25)*. Implicit in the term "bridge" is the concept of overall patient improvement and subsequent device removal. Pioneering work by a number of investigators has led to the concept of "destination therapy" where device utilization is "permanent." This therapy is reserved for selected patients who are deemed ineligible for transplantation *(26)*. Representative clinical trials from this dynamic area are summarized in Table 7 and are not meant to be all-inclusive.

It is apparent that the patient populations, relevant endpoints, and study designs displayed in Table 7 are markedly different from the discussion to date. Inherent conflicts between scientific rigor and ethical considerations preclude "randomization," "placebo control," and use of "traditional" response variables. It is in this arena that modifications to the "traditional" trial design are most needed. However, it is also in this arena where considerations of device safety vs. performance are essential and few trade-offs are satisfactory. Despite the astonishing mortality risk in this group of patients, device safety must be a primary consideration and may drive trial designs in the future. A reasonable composite primary safety endpoint might be the overall rate of freedom from death, repeat hospitalization, or stroke. It is essential to avoid a composite endpoint that is comprised of both safety and efficacy response variables as such a composite is statistically and clinically uninterpretable.

4. IMPACT OF TRIAL DESIGN ON OUTCOME

A successful device trial will have the following characteristics: (1) adequate statistical power to reject the null hypothesis with a high level of confidence, (2) a clearly defined endpoint and clinically acceptable metrics for the response variable, (3) consistent biologic/physiologic rationale, and (4) a clear idea of the intended patient population and the expected response rate in that population. Most importantly, the risk/benefit ratio will clearly favor treatment.

The unsuccessful device trial will fail to meet prespecified criteria for "success" for a number of reasons including (1) overly optimistic or inaccurate estimates of response in either the treatment or control arms, (2) deficient study design or conduct leading to excessive missing primary data, (3) abbreviated observation times in patients due either to (informative or noninformative) censoring leading to too few analyzable patients at the trial's conclusion, or (4) use of a surrogate variable as a primary endpoint with failure to demonstrate change in a clinically relevant secondary endpoint. Finally, a device trial must be considered unsuccessful when the risk of device implantation exceeds any possible benefit.

Table 7

Device therapy as "bridge to transplant" or "destination therapy" in patients with severe, end-stage heart failure

Study/year (PMA #)	Patient population	Trial design	Primary efficacy endpoint (s)	Outcome Treatment	Outcome Control
Novacor® left ventricular assist system/1998 (P980012)	NYHA Class IV; transplant candidates at risk of "imminent death"	Non-randomized; concurrent control (OMT)	Composite: survival 30 d post-transplant with acceptable neurologic function and at least NYHA Class III (%)	67	34[a]
CardioWest total artificial heart/2004 (P030011)	Transplant candidates at risk of "imminent death"	Non-randomized; historical, and concurrent controls (OMT)	Treatment success @ 30 days defined as: Alive; NYHA Class I/II; non-ventilator dependent; not requiring dialysis	69.1	37.1[b]
REMATCH/2001	NYHA Class IV (for 60–90 days) or NYHA Class III/IV (for 28 days); not candidate for transplant; LVEF ≤0.25; ongoing need for parenteral inotropic support	1:1 parallel design randomization to LVAD or OMT	All-cause mortality @ 1 y (%)	48	75[c]

LVAD, left ventricular assist device; OMT, optimal medical therapy.

[a]p = ns (treatment vs. control).
[b]p = 0.0019 (treatment vs. control).
[c]p = 0.002 (treatment vs. control).

5. NEWER APPROACHES TO CLINICAL TRIAL DESIGN FOR DEVICES IN PATIENTS WITH HEART FAILURE

The evidence required to show efficacy of a new device becomes more and more stringent due to overall improving outcomes as a result of advances in technology, improved medical options, and better and more consistent application of available treatment modalities. Device clinical trial design must correspondingly adjust. Not all devices may need to proceed via the traditional randomized controlled clinical trial, as demonstrated by bridge to transplant and destination therapy devices. Devices that are "substantially equivalent" to pivotal trial devices require a lesser degree of statistical rigor for evidence of efficacy (27) although no lesser degree of safety in high-risk patient populations. Clinical trial designs for new device evaluation on a background of optimal medical therapy and/or currently accepted device therapy may present ethical challenges regarding the inclusion or nature of a control population. Such a trial will face significant logistical and fiscal challenges if designed as a superiority trial with an expected small margin of benefit. Where substantial prior information is available and the patient characteristics in the new trial are similar to those of prior studies, a Bayesian trial design has been suggested as facilitating trial enrollment and completion (28). Such designs leverage prior study results to minimize the need for excessive patient enrollment. Similarly, adaptive trial designs allow for sample size modification while the trial is under way without compromising the integrity of the statistical analysis (29). Non-inferiority trial design, increasingly popular in pharmacologic clinical trials, poses important limitations (30) not the least of which is related to type I errors. Acceptance of a device (with its accompanying risks) as not inferior to a related device runs the risk of implanting an ineffective device in these already-compromised patients. The choice of comparator is critical and the efficacy of that comparator in the actual trial undertaken must be carefully reviewed before any conclusions regarding non-inferiority can be drawn.

6. CONCLUSIONS

The use of devices in the treatment of patients with heart failure adds a new dimension to the spectrum of treatment modalities for this increasingly prevalent disease. Device therapy may provide incremental benefits for selected patients already receiving optimal pharmacological therapy. Improvements in quality of life and survival observed in clinical trials of heart failure patients have led to increasing utilization of these devices in clinical practice. Clinical trials define the patient population in whom the device is likely to be effective, define the magnitude of the expected clinical improvement, and define the balance between benefit and risk. It is essential to understand the strengths and limitations of various clinical trial designs in order to best interpret the available data regarding management of these complex patients.

REFERENCES

1. Braunwald E, Bristow MR. Congestive heart failure: fifty years of progress. *Circulation* 2000; 102(suppl 4):IV14–23
2. Hunt SA, Abraham WT, Chin MH, Feldman AM, Francis GS, Ganiats TG, Jessup M, Konstam MA, Mancini DM, Michl K, Oates JA, Rahko PS, Silver MA, Stevenson LW, Yancy CW. ACC/AHA 2005 Guideline Update for the Diagnosis and Management of Chronic Heart Failure in the Adult: A Report of the American College of Cardiology/American Heart Association Task Force on Practice Guidelines (Writing Committee to Update the 2001 Guidelines for the Evaluation and Management of Heart Failure). Available at: http://www.acc.org/qualityandscience/clinical/guidelines/failure/update/index.pdf2005 (accessed March 1, 2007)
3. Levy D, Kenchaiah S, Larson MG, Benjamin EJ, Kupka MJ, Ho KKL, Murabito JM, Vasan RS. Long-term trends in the incidence of and survival with heart failure. *N Engl J Med* 2002; 347:1397–402
4. Roger V, Weston SA, Redfield MM, Hellermann-Homan JP, Killian J, Yawn BP, Jacobsen SJ. Trends in heart failure incidence and survival in a community-based population. *JAMA* 2004; 292:344–50
5. Cohn J, Tognoni G. A randomized trial of the angiotensin-receptor blocker valsartan in chronic heart failure. *N Engl J Med* 2001; 345:1667–75
6. Maisel WH. Medical device regulation: an introduction for the practicing physician. *Ann Int Med* 2004; 140:296–302
7. Hill AB. *A Short Textbook of Medical Statistics*. 11th ed., London: Hodder and Stoughton, 1984
8. Pocock SJ. *Clinical Trials: A Practical Approach*. Chichester: Wiley, 1983
9. Friedman LM, Furberg C, DeMets DL. *Fundamentals of Clinical Trials*. 3rd ed., St Louis, MO: Mosby-Year Book, 1996
10. DeMets DL, Califf RM. Lessons learned from recent cardiovascular clinical trials: Part I. *Circulation* 2002; 106:746–51
11. DeMets DL, Califf RM. Lessons learned from recent cardiovascular clinical trials: Part II. *Circulation* 2002; 106:880–6
12. Yusuf S, Collins R, Peto R. Why do we need some large, simple randomized trials? *Stat Med* 1984; 3:409–22
13. Freemantle N, Calvert M, Wood J, Eastaugh J, Griffin C. Composite outcomes in randomized trials: greater precision but with greater uncertainty? *JAMA* 2003; 289:2554–9
14. Braitman LE. Confidence intervals assess both clinical significance and statistical significance. *Ann Int Med* 1991; 114:515–7
15. Costanzo MR, Guglin ME, Saltzberg MT, Jessup ML, Bart BA, Teerlink JR, Jaski BE, Fang JC, Feller ED, Haas GJ, Anderson AS, Schollmeyer MP, Sobotka PA. Ultrafiltration versus intravenous diuretics for patients hospitalized for acute decompensated heart failure. *J Am Coll Cardiol* 2007; 49:675–83
16. Saxon LA, Kerwin WF, Cahalan MK, Kalman JM, Olgin JE, Foster E, Schiller NB, Shinbane JS, Lesh MD, Merrick SH. Acute effects of intraoperative multisite ventricular pacing on left ventricular function and activation/contraction sequence in patients with depressed ventricular function. *J Cardiovasc Electrophysiol* 1998; 9:13–21
17. Kass DA, Chen CH, Curry C, Talbot M, Berger R, Fetics B, Nevo E. Improved left ventricular mechanics from acute VDD pacing in patients with dilated cardiomyopathy and ventricular conduction delay. *Circulation* 1999; 99:1567–73
18. Abraham WT, Hayes DL. Cardiac resynchronization therapy for heart failure. *Circulation*. 2003; 108:2596–603
19. http://www.fda.gov/cdrh/pdf/P010012b.pdf (accessed February 1, 2007)

20. Hills M, Armitage P. The two-period cross-over clinical trial. *Br J Clin Pharmacol* 1979; 8:7–20
21. Bristow MR, Saxon LA, Boehmer J, Krueger S, Kass DA, DeMarco T, Carson P, DiCarlo L, DeMets D, White BG, DeVries DW, Feldman AM. Cardiac-resynchronization therapy with or without an implantable defibrillator in advanced chronic heart failure. *N Engl J Med* 2004; 350:2140–50
22. Cleland JGF, Daubert J-C, Erdmann E, Freemantle N, Gras D, Kappenberger L, Tavazzi L. The effect of cardiac resynchronization on morbidity and mortality in heart failure. *N Engl J Med* 2005; 352:1539–49
23. http://www.fda.gov/ohrms/dockets/ac/05/briefing/2005-4149b1_3_Draft%20SSED.pdf (accessed February 1, 2007)
24. Bardy GH, Lee KL, Mark DB, Poole JE, Packer DL, Boineau R, Domanski M, Troutman C, Anderson J, Johnson G, McNulty SE, Clapp-Channing N, Davidson-Ray LD, Fraulo ES, Fishbein DP, Luceri RM, Ip JH. Amiodarone or an implantable cardioverter-defibrillator for congestive heart failure. *N Engl J Med* 2005; 352:225–37
25. Mancini D, Burkhoff D. Mechanical device-based methods of managing and treating heart failure. *Circulation* 2005; 112:438–48
26. Rose EA, Gelijns AC, Moskowitz AJ, Heitjan DF, Stevenson LW, Dembitsky W, Long JW, Ascheim DD, Tierney AR, Levitan RG, Watson JT, Meier P. Long-term use of a left ventricular assist device for end-stage heart failure. *N Engl J Med* 2001; 345:1435–43
27. Monsein LH. Primer on medical device regulation. Part II. Regulation of medical devices by the U.S. Food and Drug Administration. *Radiology* 1997; 205:10–8
28. http://www.fda.gov/cdrh/osb/guidance/a601.pdf (accessed February 1, 2007)
29. Proschan MA, Liu Q, Hunsberger S. Practical midcourse sample size modification in clinical trials. *Con Clin Trials* 2003; 24:4–15
30. Pocock SJ. The pros and cons of noninferiority trials. *Fund Clin Pharmacol* 2003; 17:483–90

4

The FDA Perspective on Heart Failure Devices

Matthew G. Hillebrenner, MSE, Eric A. Chen, MSE, Owen P. Faris, PhD, and Kathryn M. O'Callaghan

Contents

Abstract

The Food and Drug Administration's Center for Devices and Radiological Health (CDRH) is charged with ensuring that manufacturers of new medical devices demonstrate a reasonable assurance that their devices are safe and effective prior to approval for commercial distribution in the United States.

From: *Contemporary Cardiology: Device Therapy in Heart Failure*
Edited by: W.H. Maisel, DOI 10.1007/978-1-59745-424-7_4
© Humana Press, a part of Springer Science+Business Media, LLC 2010

CDRH also monitors the performance of medical devices once approved for distribution and introduced into commerce to evaluate the ongoing risk–benefit profile in the interest of protecting the public health. This chapter reviews regulatory terminology, submission types, clinical trial design, product labeling, recalls, and other issues related to the regulation of heart failure devices.

Key Words: Regulatory; Heart failure; FDA; Premarket; Postmarket.

1. INTRODUCTION

The Food and Drug Administration's Center for Devices and Radiological Health (CDRH) is charged with ensuring that manufacturers of new medical devices demonstrate a reasonable assurance that their devices are safe and effective prior to approval for commercial distribution in the United States. CDRH also monitors the performance of medical devices once approved for distribution and introduced into commerce to evaluate the ongoing risk–benefit profile in the interest of protecting the public health.

The modern era of the Food and Drug Administration (FDA, also referred to as "the Agency") began with the passage of the Food and Drugs Act of 1906. Regulatory oversight was first extended to medical devices in 1938, when the Federal Food, Drug, and Cosmetic Act (FFDCA) was passed into law. Under this legislation, it was illegal to sell therapeutic devices that were dangerous or being marketed with false claims. In the years between 1938 and 1969, the primary focus of medical device regulation was on radiation-emitting devices such as x-ray machines. In 1969, Congress was called upon to set minimum performance standards and establish premarket clearance procedures for certain medical devices. The ground-breaking legislation that precipitated the creation of CDRH was the Medical Device Amendments of 1976 ("the Amendments"). The Amendments mandated that all medical devices be classified based on risks to patients (Class I, II, or III, see below) and stipulated that all devices be subject to regulation by the federal government. Since that time, FDA has gradually developed and refined the regulations to reflect the law enacted in the Amendments and in subsequent federal legislation such as the Medical Device User Fee and Modernization Act (MDUFMA) of 2002.

The mission of CDRH is to promote and protect the public health by ensuring the safety and effectiveness of medical devices and the safety of radiological products. Accomplishing these objectives requires a commitment to its vision of ensuring the health of the public throughout the Total Product Life Cycle (TPLC). The Total Product Life Cycle (Fig. 1) paradigm incorporates resources throughout CDRH to guide the medical device development process from the early design concept stage through preclinical testing, clinical trials, marketing application, postmarket monitoring of device performance, and ultimately market withdrawal due to obsolescence. Information learned throughout these many phases can also be used to improve devices in future design iterations. By utilizing appropriate risk management

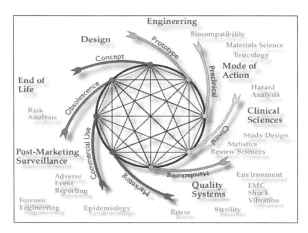

Fig. 1. The Total Product Life Cycle is shown. Medical devices typically pass through several stages of development moving from concept and prototype to pre-clinical and clinical testing before being approved for marketing and commercial use.

strategies at each stage of the product life cycle, CDRH is able to promote innovative methods for evaluating safety and effectiveness while ensuring the protection of public health. This "least burdensome" approach to medical device regulation *(1)* allows CDRH to maintain the necessary equilibrium between a comprehensive review of device performance and the timely approval of safe and effective medical devices, especially when a substantial treatment benefit is expected or there is an unmet and critical patient need. Further information about the history, organization, and mission of CDRH can be found on the Center's web site *(2)*.

2. DEVICE DEVELOPMENT, EVALUATION, APPROVAL, AND POSTMARKET SURVEILLANCE

2.1. Regulatory Terminology and Submission Types

As a manufacturer (i.e., sponsor, company, distributor, or other responsible party) begins the process of device design, produces a prototype, and initiates preclinical testing, numerous regulations are applicable. For instance, manufacturers comply with design controls, an interrelated set of practices and procedures that are incorporated throughout the device design and development process. In general, design controls make systematic assessment of the design an integral part of device development, which ideally increases the chances that the design can translate into a device appropriate for its intended use. This is addressed in Good Manufacturing Practice (GMP) requirements (outlined in 21 CFR Part 820), which require manufacturers to have a quality system for the design, manufacture, packaging, labeling, storage, installation, and servicing (where applicable) of finished medical devices intended for commercial distribution in the United States. The quality system includes such aspects as manufacturing standard operating procedures, quality controls, complaint handling procedures, and clearly defined roles for company management to ensure appropriate employee training and accountability. Each device manufacturer undergoes routine FDA inspections to evaluate compliance with the regulations. The manufacturer's design control procedures and quality system (reviewed by CDRH's Office of Compliance) are considered essential components of GMPs to guarantee that safe and effective devices can be reproducibly manufactured. The FDA's guidance document, "Design Control Guidance For Medical Device Manufacturers," is a valuable resource for additional information on this topic *(3)*.

Nonclinical testing of medical devices, typically done to assess device safety, should be conducted in compliance with Good Laboratory Practices (GLP, see 21 CFR 58). If clinical testing is conducted in humans, sponsors and investigators should take note of the relevant regulations intended to protect the welfare of those subjects, including the requirements for informed consent and Institutional Review Board (IRB) approval. If the study presents a significant risk to patients and is to be conducted in the United States, an FDA-approved Investigational Device Exemption (IDE, see 21 CFR Parts 50, 56, and 812) is required.

FDA regulates the marketing of medical devices using a risk-based classification system, assigning device types into one of three categories based on the level of control necessary to assure the safety and effectiveness of the device. Class I devices are the lowest risk devices, and are only subject to "General Controls," the minimum requirements of the Food, Drug, and Cosmetic Act (as amended) that apply to all medical devices. They consist of establishment registration and listing requirements, Good Manufacturing Practices, labeling requirements, banning provisions, medical device reporting (MDR) requirements, and submission of a premarket notification (called a 510(k) after the section of the Act in which it is described). It should be noted, however, that the vast majority of Class I devices are exempt from the requirement to submit a 510(k) prior to marketing. Elastic bandages and certain manual hand-held surgical instruments are examples of Class I devices.

Moderate risk devices are termed Class II, and most require the submission and clearance of a 510(k) application before the device can be legally marketed. In addition to General Controls, Class II devices must also comply with Special Controls, which may consist of device-specific labeling requirements, mandatory performance standards, and postmarket surveillance. Examples of Class II devices indicated for patients with heart failure are cardiopulmonary bypass systems (approved for up to 6 h of use), intra-aortic balloon pumps, and external counterpulsation devices.

For those devices that require a 510(k) submission prior to marketing, the manufacturer must demonstrate that the new device is "substantially equivalent" to one or more legally marketed devices. A legally marketed device is: (1) a device that was legally marketed prior to May 28, 1976 and does not require PMA approval; (2) a device which has been reclassified from Class III to Class II or I; (3) a device which has been found to be substantially equivalent to a marketed device through the 510(k) process; or (4) one established through Evaluation of Automatic Class III Designation. The legally marketed device(s) to which equivalence is drawn is known as the "predicate" device(s). To make a claim of substantial equivalence to a predicate device, the manufacturer must show that the new device has the same intended use and that the technological characteristics of the new device and predicate device are the same or similar. If the new device has different technological characteristics, the differences must not raise new safety and effectiveness questions, and the manufacturer must demonstrate that the new device is at least as safe and effective as the predicate. This is typically accomplished through a comparison of device descriptive characteristics, proposed labeling, and performance data, which may include bench, animal, and/or clinical testing.

The highest risk devices are categorized as Class III and include those devices for which General Controls and Special Controls are insufficient to provide reasonable assurance of safety and effectiveness. In addition, Class III devices are typically those that support or sustain human life, are of substantial importance in preventing impairment of human health, or present a potential unreasonable risk of illness or injury. An Investigational Device exemption (IDE) application is required to conduct clinical studies when the device: (1) is intended as an implant and presents a potential for serious risk to the health, safety, or welfare of a subject; (2) is for use in supporting or sustaining human life and represents a potential for serious risk to the health, safety, or welfare of a subject; (3) is for a use of substantial importance in diagnosing, curing, mitigating, or treating disease or otherwise preventing impairment of human health and presents a potential for serious risk to the health, safety, or welfare of a subject; or (4) otherwise presents a potential for serious risk to a subject [21 CFR 812.3(m)]. FDA's review of an IDE application focuses on the description of the device and its operating principles, the proposed indications for use, any prior investigations including all nonclinical studies (bench and animal), previous clinical experience, a summary of the manufacturing process and quality systems, the proposed investigational plan, and proposed labeling and informed consent documents to be used in the study (See 21 CFR 812 for full requirements). FDA's perspective regarding several critical aspects of the investigational plan for heart failure trials is discussed later in this chapter. In most cases, marketing of Class III devices requires the submission and approval of a Premarket Approval (PMA) application prior to marketing. Class III heart failure devices include cardiac resynchronization therapy pacemakers and defibrillators, implantable hemodynamic monitors, cardiac constraint devices, ventricular assist devices (bridge-to-transplant and destination therapy), and total artificial hearts.

PMA approval of Class III devices is based on valid scientific evidence that demonstrates a reasonable assurance that the device is both safe [21 CFR 860.7(d)] and effective [21 CFR 860.7(e)] for its intended use(s). Valid scientific evidence is defined in the regulations [21 CFR 860.7(c)(2)] as evidence from well-controlled investigations, partially controlled studies, studies and objective trials without matched controls, well-documented case histories conducted by qualified experts, and reports of significant human experience with a marketed device, from which it can fairly and responsibly be concluded by qualified experts that there is reasonable assurance of the safety and effectiveness of a device under its conditions of use. Isolated case reports, random experience, reports lacking sufficient details to permit scientific evaluation, and unsubstantiated opinions are not regarded as valid scientific evidence to show safety or effectiveness.

When reviewing a PMA application, FDA evaluates all information about the device and its intended use, including a complete and detailed description of the device, its components and principles of operation; the proposed indications for use; technical sections describing nonclinical studies; the results of all human clinical investigations (e.g., studies conducted under an IDE and any other clinical studies of the device); a description of the methods, facilities, and controls used in the manufacture, processing, packaging, storage, and, where appropriate, installation of the device; marketing history (if the device has been previously marketed either within the United States under a previous marketing approval or clearance, or outside of the United States); a bibliography of any relevant published information; proposed labeling; and a Summary of Safety and Effectiveness Data (SSED), which summarizes the device, studies conducted on the device, and conclusions drawn from those studies (See 21 CFR 814 for full application requirements). Specific examples of the type of information reviewed in approved PMA applications for cardiac resynchronization therapy devices and ventricular assist devices are provided below.

Some heart failure devices may be approved as a Humanitarian Use Device (HUD). This would apply to a device that is intended to benefit patients by treating or diagnosing a disease or condition that affects or is manifested in fewer than 4000 individuals in the United States per year. A device manufacturer's research and development costs could exceed its market returns in such small patient populations; therefore, the HUD provision of the regulation [21 CFR 814 Subpart H] provides an incentive for the development of devices for use in the treatment or diagnosis of diseases affecting these populations. The initial step in this process includes a review by FDA's Office of Orphan Products Development (4) to determine whether or not the device should be designated as an HUD. Once this designation has been made, a humanitarian device exemption (HDE) application can be submitted to obtain FDA approval.

An HDE is similar in both form and content to a premarket approval (PMA) application, but is exempt from the effectiveness requirements of a PMA. However, the FDA must be able to determine, during the course of their review, that the device does not pose an unreasonable or significant risk of illness or injury and that the probable benefit to health outweighs the risk of injury or illness from its use, taking into account the probable risks and benefits of currently available devices or alternative forms of treatment. More information on HUDs can be found on the FDA web site *(5)*.

The Office of Device Evaluation (ODE) comprises five system-specific divisions, including the Division of Cardiovascular Devices (DCD), each further subdivided into more specialized branches. FDA encourages sponsors to contact the specific branch responsible for review of a particular device for guidance during all stages of the device regulatory process. Device manufacturers often introduce new devices to FDA via the pre-IDE process, a method by which they can receive informal feedback within approximately 60 days, whether in the form of a teleconference, fax, email, or face-to-face meeting. Pre-IDE submissions typically contain a description of the device, its intended use, and an analysis of the risks associated with use of the device. Sponsors can also submit their proposed regulatory strategy for comment by FDA review staff, as well as specific questions for which they are seeking FDA feedback. Such an approach could include proposed test protocols for preclinical (bench and/or animal testing) or clinical evaluations of the new device. This process can be used more than once during the development of various test protocols. For example, it may be helpful to have FDA provide initial informal comments on animal studies to be conducted, then to have a subsequent meeting to discuss planned clinical studies once some preclinical testing on the device has been completed. More details on the pre-IDE process can be found in "Guidance on IDE Policies and Procedures," available on the FDA web site *(6)*.

2.2. Device Labeling

In Section 201 of the FFDCA, labeling is defined as a "display of written, printed, or graphic matter upon the immediate container of any article..." and "all labels and other written, printed, or graphic matter." As part of the approval process, sponsors must generate labeling for their device that contains a description of the device and appropriately characterizes its intended use, the patient population in whom it has been found to be safe and effective, adequate instructions for use, a summary of the safety and effectiveness outcomes demonstrated in any clinical studies, and any situations or patients in whom the device should explicitly not be used. Labeling is directed toward device users, including physicians, patients, and caregivers, and essentially tells the story of how the device was determined to be safe and effective both by the sponsor and by the FDA. The "indications for use" statement identifies the target population in a significant portion of which sufficient valid scientific evidence has demonstrated that the device as labeled will provide clinically effective results and at the same time does not present an unreasonable risk of illness or injury associated with the use of the device. When a device is used in a manner inconsistent with that described in its approved labeling, this is considered off-label use. The FDA does not regulate the practice of medicine (Section 906 of FFDCA), acknowledging that individual physicians may use legally marketed devices according to their best clinical judgment to optimize treatment for specific patients. However, in many cases data from well-designed clinical trials have not been collected to establish a reasonable assurance of safety and effectiveness for these off-label uses and there are multiple off-label use issues that may potentially compromise optimal evidence-based medical care.

2.3. Product Recalls

Medical device recalls are handled by CDRH's Office of Compliance. A recall is an action taken to address a problem with a medical device that violates FDA law. Recalls occur when a medical device is defective, when it could be a risk to health, or both. A medical device recall does not always imply that one must stop using the product or return it to the company. A recall sometimes means that the medical device needs to be checked, adjusted, or fixed. If an implanted device is recalled, it does not always have to be removed. When an implanted device has the potential to fail unexpectedly, companies often tell doctors to contact their patients to discuss the risk of removing the device compared to the risk of leaving it in place.

In most cases, a company recalls a medical device on its own (voluntarily). When a company learns that it has a product that violates FDA law, it recalls the device and notifies FDA. When a company recalls a medical device, it contacts the customers who received the product from them, and takes steps to reach others who need to be notified (e.g., by issuing press releases or providing detailed instructions), supplies information to help users identify the product and take steps to minimize health consequences, and takes action to prevent the problem from happening again. All of these actions are done with FDA oversight to ensure that the actions are adequate to protect the public health.

FDA classifies medical device recalls into three categories, reflecting the potential risk to public health and the measures that must be taken in order to ensure the effectiveness of the recall action. A Class I recall is appropriate when there is a reasonable chance that the product will cause serious health problems or death. At the other end of the spectrum, a Class III recall is necessary when a product violates FDA law, which in and of itself needs to be addressed, but there is little chance that using or being exposed to the device will cause health problems. Throughout the recall process, FDA and the company work together to take necessary actions to protect the public health. More information on medical device recalls can be found on the FDA web site *(7)*.

2.4. Premarket vs. Postmarket Review

CDRH places a significant emphasis on data collection in the postmarket setting. Review teams for original premarket approval applications typically include an epidemiologist from the Office of Surveillance and Biometrics, who works together with the review team to determine whether or not a post-approval study will be necessary if the device is ultimately approved. It should be noted there are several goals when conducting a post-approval study, namely to assess the generalizability of a new device or technology, continue long-term follow-up to ensure reasonable assurance of continued safety and effectiveness, evaluate the effectiveness of training programs, identify and assess rare events, and gather data on real-world usage. The information obtained from the post-approval study can also be used to provide information for updates to the device labeling. While the information gained from a post-approval study is a critical piece of the TPLC puzzle, it is important to remember that the promise of collecting postmarket data cannot serve as a substitute for demonstrating a reasonable assurance of safety and effectiveness prior to approval.

The above paragraphs provide a general overview of medical device regulation and the various applications that may be submitted to the Agency for review. Further information can be found on the FDA's Device Advice webpage for additional resources pertaining to medical devices *(8)*.

3. CONSIDERATIONS IN CLINICAL TRIAL DESIGN

When designing a clinical trial to support a marketing application, there are many critical aspects that require special attention. It is important for the FDA and medical device sponsors to minimize any possible bias of patients, observers, and analysts of the data. This can be a challenge in comparison to double-blinded, placebo-controlled drug trials. There are, however, several measures that can be taken to minimize bias in device trials. This section will elaborate on the FDA's perspective regarding the choice of control population, study endpoints, quality control measures, methods for handling missing data, and gender bias.

3.1. Choosing a Control Group

As discussed in a previous section, the FDA bases its determinations of safety and effectiveness on valid scientific evidence. Medical device regulations [21 CFR 860.7(e)(2)] stipulate that, when possible, such evidence shall consist of well-controlled investigations. Furthermore, the scientific community recognizes certain principles as the essentials of a well-controlled clinical investigation [21 CFR 860.7(f)]. Among them is a comparison of the results of treatment or diagnosis with a control in such a fashion as to permit quantitative evaluation. When selecting a control population for a clinical study, FDA recommends considering what therapy the patients would most likely receive if they were not enrolled in the trial. In addition, the use of risk stratification tools may also be helpful in determining the appropriate control group *(9–11)*. Referring back to the medical device regulations, four types of comparisons are generally recognized [21 CFR 860.7(f)(1)(iv)(a–d)].

(a) No treatments. Where objective measurements of effectiveness are available and placebo effect is negligible, comparison of the objective results in comparable groups of treated and untreated patients. This scenario does not occur often in heart failure device trials, primarily because most of these devices are permanent implants and the placebo effect is rarely negligible. However, this type of study could be appropriate for add-on features to already-approved device therapies. For example, after cardiac resynchronization therapy (CRT) devices were approved in the early 2000s, device manufacturers expressed an interest in adding certain features to the devices' capabilities. While these features may not imply new claims of effectiveness, the FDA wanted to ensure that they did not negatively impact the beneficial effects of CRT. Patients enrolled in this type of study could be randomized to one of two groups: CRT with the new feature ON or CRT with the new feature OFF. Because the primary therapy in this case would be CRT, it would not be unethical to deny control patients the new feature. In addition, since all patients have a device implanted and receive CRT, the placebo effect could be considered negligible.

(b) Placebo control. Where there may be a placebo effect with the use of a device, comparison of the results of use of the device with an ineffective device used under conditions designed to resemble the conditions of use under investigation as far as possible. The original cardiac resynchronization therapy trials were conducted using this paradigm. Patients who were randomized to the treatment group received a functioning CRT device in addition to the stable, optimal medical therapy that was already part of their treatment regimen. Those assigned to the control group received a CRT device that was not turned on. Therefore, those patients were only on medical therapy during the first 6 months of follow-up. At the 6-month visit, patients were unblinded to their randomization status and control patients' devices were turned on. This study design allowed for a blinded assessment of device effectiveness and the collection of more safety data associated with the new implant procedure for CRT devices. In addition, the device could be activated in the control group at 6 months, which limited the perceived negative impact of not receiving the therapy from the outset.

(c) Active treatment control. Where an effective regimen of therapy may be used for comparison, e.g., the condition being treated is such that the use of a placebo or the withholding of treatment would be inappropriate or contrary to the interest of the patient. For example, consider a ventricular assist device approved for use as "destination therapy." This device was studied in a randomized controlled trial vs. optimal medical management in an extremely sick New York Heart Association (NYHA) Class IV heart failure population. Trials designed to evaluate the safety and effectiveness of new

destination therapy devices have the opportunity to randomize patients to "standard optimal therapy," which would include any FDA-approved drugs and/or medical devices for that patient population. This allows clinicians to use any FDA-approved means available to them to treat control patients, qualifying as an active treatment option.

(d) Historical control. In certain circumstances, such as those involving diseases with high and predictable mortality or signs and symptoms of predictable duration or severity, the results of use of the device may be compared quantitatively with prior experience historically derived from the adequately documented natural history of the disease or condition in comparable patients or populations who received no treatment or who followed an established effective regimen. This situation applies to several ongoing studies, which have been discussed at recent heart failure conferences, for ventricular assist devices that are being used as a bridge to transplant (BTT). These devices are only implanted in patients who have advanced heart failure (NYHA Class IV), defined as having symptoms at rest or with little exertion, and do not have long life expectancy. In addition, these patients must be on the United Network for Organ Sharing (UNOS) cardiac transplant list (Status 1A or 1B). In such a patient population, it would be unethical to mandate that patients be randomized to only medical therapy. Therefore, a historical control is used as the basis for comparison. This has been accomplished using a performance goal that was established through a literature review of the survival to cardiac transplantation rates of approved BTT devices *(12–17)*. Based on the data in these publications, a BTT study would be considered a success if the sponsor is able to demonstrate that the lower 95% confidence limit for the rate of survival to cardiac transplantation is at least 65%. The FDA has used this performance goal as the framework for designing various ongoing BTT studies.

The examples listed above provide an overview of the issues that a sponsor must consider when choosing a control group. This decision will likely have a direct influence on other aspects of the trial, such as endpoints.

3.2. Selecting the Appropriate Endpoints

When working with sponsors in the clinical study design stage, FDA focuses on endpoints that reflect the intended use of the device and represent a clinically meaningful outcome for patients. Patients with heart failure experience a decline in quality of life as their condition worsens, ultimately resulting in a premature death in many cases. As such, the fundamental goal of heart failure device therapy is to extend the lives of patients while also improving, or at least maintaining, their health status. Unlike Phase III studies investigating the safety and efficacy of new drug therapies, heart failure device trials are often limited by a relatively small sample size and not powered to definitively examine objective, clinically meaningful endpoints such as mortality. Therefore, device trials often rely on alternative endpoints in order to maintain a least burdensome approach. Under this paradigm, secondary endpoint data are important to consider when determining the risk–benefit profile of the device being evaluated; the totality of the data is used by FDA to make decisions regarding device approvability. Due to the issues of bias mentioned earlier, it is recommended that sponsors choose the most objective endpoints possible when studying their device. In addition, while some endpoints can be used in all heart failure trials, the specific device technology and patient population involved in each study should also factor into the decision. The ensuing section provides a discussion of various endpoints that have been used in heart failure device trials, highlighting some of the advantages and disadvantages associated with them from a regulatory point of view.

All-cause mortality is the most objective and clinically meaningful endpoint that can be used in heart failure trials. However, as mentioned above, device trials do not typically involve large sample sizes, and it can be impractical to require manufacturers to demonstrate a statistically significant benefit in mortality. Alternatively, there are patient populations, such as those receiving ventricular assist devices, where survival is a realistic and appropriate primary endpoint. This is due to the severity of illness in these patients and the high mortality rate that would be expected if they did not receive a device. Furthermore, in bridge-to-transplant trials, the primary goal of the therapy is to keep the patient alive until they receive a cardiac transplant.

Heart failure-related hospitalization serves as another objective endpoint that captures the effect of device therapy on the morbidity a patient experiences as well as their quality of life. Due to the increased quality of care in heart failure programs/clinics throughout the country, the Agency prefers an expanded hospitalization definition, which includes hospitalizations ≥ 24 h or with a change in calendar date, emergency department visits, and unplanned clinic visits that are determined to be heart failure-related. Sponsors may encounter some of the same obstacles with hospitalization as with mortality, specifically that the event rate is not high enough to power the trial appropriately with a reasonable sample size. One potential solution is to combine these two endpoints and evaluate them as a composite.

Cardiopulmonary exercise (CPX) testing is conducted using a treadmill or bicycle; in this test, expired gases are collected and the oxygen uptake of the patient is measured. Oxygen uptake, VO_2, is a measure of central cardiac output and peripheral O_2 extraction and is an objective measure of functional capacity. To guarantee a valid and interpretable test result, patients must reach a recommended minimum respiratory exchange ratio (RER) of 1.10. When well-executed and interpreted, VO_2 is a powerful predictor of outcome and commonly used to list patients for transplantation *(18)*. Peak VO_2 values < 14 ml/min/kg or $< 50\%$ of predicted value by age, gender, and physical conditioning are considered markers of poor outcomes *(19, 20)*. Ventilatory threshold, occasionally referred to as anaerobic threshold, is also obtained via CPX testing and is viewed as an even more objective assessment of patient functional status since the value is reproducible regardless of testing protocol *(21, 22)*. Challenges associated with the use of cardiopulmonary exercise testing in clinical trials include the cost of the testing, expertise of administering and interpreting the test, difficulty in ensuring valid results, and the fact that sicker patients may be unable to perform the test, leading to the undesirable outcome of missing data points. Appropriate training, standardized protocols for administering and interpreting the test *(23)*, trial conduct behavior, serial testing, the use of experienced core laboratories, and a greater commitment to collecting the data provide various mechanisms for combating these impediments.

The 6-Minute Walk (6MW) test is a submaximal exercise test that is widely used as a measure of functional capacity for lower-level activity in heart failure clinical trials. It distinguishes the moderately sick from the very sick *(24, 25)*. During the test, patients walk a premeasured 20-m hall back and forth, at their own pace, for 6 min. The test is intended to measure a patient's ability to perform regular daily activities, and its correlation with mortality has varied among trials *(24, 26)*. The 6MW test is easier to conduct than cardiopulmonary exercise testing and is typically associated with fewer missing data points. However, 6MW test results are usually subject to large standard deviations, making it difficult to power statistical analyses, and can be influenced by the level of "coaching" provided by hospital staff. Serial testing, standardized protocols *(27)* adhered to by blinded test administrators, and a dedication to data collection offer several ways to minimize these concerns.

In October 2003, the Heart Failure Society of America and members of the Division of Cardiovascular Devices held a joint workshop that resulted in the formation of a working group tasked with exploring several regulatory issues associated with health status measurements in clinical trials. The findings of this working group were later published in the *Journal of Cardiac Failure (28)*, and a high-level summary of this manuscript is offered here. As mentioned previously, improving patient health status is one of the primary goals of medical therapy; therefore, the working group recommended that health status be measured in all clinical trials, regardless of how vital these assessments are to the overall approval decision. The authors also summarized five basic attributes of health status measures that are necessary to develop confidence in clinical trial results: validity, reliability, responsiveness to change, interpretability, and availability of translations in other languages *(29)*. A third key message put forth by Normand et al. was that no one assessment of health status can serve as the single determinant of overall effectiveness, a concept consistent with FDA's approach of evaluating the totality of the data. With that in mind, below is a discussion of the various health status assessment tools that have been developed and used in heart failure clinical trials.

The Minnesota Living with Heart Failure (MLHF) questionnaire has been widely used in heart failure clinical trials *(30, 31)*. In device trials, it has most often been chosen as a secondary endpoint or part of a composite primary endpoint. This quality-of-life survey measures four dimensions – physical, emotional, social, and mental. A review of drug trial literature suggests that a five-point change is viewed as the minimal clinically meaningful difference; it is unclear whether the threshold should be higher in unblinded device trials. The Kansas City Cardiomyopathy Questionnaire (KCCQ) is another heart failure-specific assessment tool that has been developed in recent years *(32)*. The KCCQ instrument rates patient responses in five distinct domains – physical function, symptoms, social function, self-efficacy/knowledge, and quality of life – with an overall summary score obtained by totaling all but the self-efficacy/knowledge domain. Similar to the MLHF questionnaire, a five-point change in the KCCQ summary score is considered a clinically significant change based on existing data. Again, most of these data are taken from blinded drug studies, making it difficult to interpret what results would need to be achieved in an unblinded device trial in order to be considered a success. The KCCQ is currently a secondary endpoint in several heart failure device studies (e.g., ventricular assist devices), which is a critical step in the validation process for any health status endpoint.

The New York Heart Association (NYHA) functional classification system provides another method for describing the severity of a patient's heart failure and is also used to specify the patient population indicated for most approved heart failure devices. This system relates symptoms to everyday activities and the patient's quality of life. A general description of each classification is supplied here:

- Class I: patients with no limitation of activities; they suffer no symptoms from ordinary activities.
- Class II: patients with slight, mild limitation of activity; they are comfortable with rest or with mild exertion.
- Class III: patients with marked limitation of activity; they are comfortable only at rest.
- Class IV: patients who should be at complete rest, confined to bed or chair; any physical activity brings on discomfort and symptoms occur at rest.

NYHA Class has been utilized as a secondary endpoint and part of composite primary endpoints in device trials. Given its categorical nature, however, it can be difficult to determine what would be a clinically meaningful change in an individual patient. In addition, there is significant variability in the way different physicians apply this measurement, making interpretation of results problematic.

The EuroQol is a self-administered, generic health status instrument meant to be easily used across a wide range of health situations and in various languages. The instrument captures physical, mental, and social functioning, and is made up of several pages. For health-related quality of life, pages 2 and 3 are primarily used. On page 2, the patient reports on five dimensions of health state including pain, self-care, and mobility.

Page 3 is perhaps the best known of the entire instrument and is called the "thermometer" where the patient marks their own level of health state from 0 (worst) to 100 (best imaginable) *(33, 34)*. The EuroQol instrument has been used in ventricular assist device trials.

All of the health status measurements described above provide a challenge when it comes to data interpretation in unblinded device trials. For each of these assessments, the patient and physicians have a considerable influence over the process. When blinding is not possible, there are several ways to minimize the potential bias associated with these types of endpoints. For example, sponsors are encouraged to use independent, blinded test administrators whenever feasible. During the time it takes to conduct a clinical trial, it is likely that some of the personnel responsible for overseeing the completion of these tests will change; therefore, study centers should consider developing a plan to re-train both new and old key personnel throughout the investigation. As with any experiment, it would be ideal to keep as many potential covariates constant as possible. Examples of factors that could impact test results include the time of day the test is administered, the format for completing the surveys (i.e., electronic, paper, telephone), whether the instruments are filled out by the patient or a health-care professional, etc. Similar to exercise testing discussed previously, it would be helpful to obtain multiple measurements from patients prior to randomization.

The clinical evaluation of cardiovascular devices that may have a direct impact on brain function should include means for testing the neurocognitive and neurological function and status of affected patients. There are several broad areas of brain function and behavior that should be assessed, including clinical stroke, mood and affect, neurological quality of life, and cognitive function. Cognitive function should evaluate the following eight domains: executive function, memory, concentration/attention, language, visual/spatial perception, processing speed, and motor function. There are various measurement tools available for these types of tests.

3.3. Utilizing Quality Control Measures

In addition to choosing a suitable control group and endpoints for a clinical study, sponsors are encouraged to use further methods of assuring the quality of the data collected. For instance, a blinded, independent clinical events committee (CEC) is often tasked with reviewing deaths and serious adverse events that occur during the study to determine whether or not they should be considered "device-related." The CEC, which should include a heart failure cardiologist and other members with the expertise necessary for the particular trial, might also be responsible for adjudicating hospitalizations that occur during the study to decide if these events meet the definition of "heart failure-related." An independent Data and Safety Monitoring Board (DSMB), ideally consisting of members with backgrounds in cardiovascular patient management and clinical trial conduct, is typically convened to review summary data related to enrollment, data quality, safety, and effectiveness outcomes. The main function of the DSMB is usually to provide recommendations regarding study management or potential early trial termination due to safety concerns. As alluded to above, sponsors are also encouraged to use blinded core laboratories when applicable. Core labs provide another layer of quality assurance when it comes to adherence to protocols and validity of test results.

3.4. Methods for Handling Missing Data

In heart failure trials, missing data points are an unfortunate reality. This can be due to many reasons, from patients dying during the course of the trial to not showing up for their follow-up visits. While we recommend that sponsors, first and foremost, increase their commitment to collecting all the data required under their investigational protocol, there are a few additional measures that can be taken to minimize the impact of missing data when it is unavoidable. First, sponsors are encouraged to prespecify a plan for handling missing data. In some instances, the missing at random assumption could apply; however, that is not always the case. When data are missing for cause, sponsors will be asked to apply a conservative model to account for the missingness. Such models would likely involve various sensitivity analyses, including worst case, available data only, and multiple imputation. FDA review staff members are available to assist device sponsors during the clinical trial design stage to devise an appropriate plan for dealing with missing data.

3.5. Gender Bias

Despite the fact that heart disease kills more women than men every year, women are still less likely to be referred for appropriate diagnosis and treatment procedures (35). For heart failure specifically, women constitute 50% of the disease population (36). However, data from the United Network for Organ Sharing (UNOS) indicate that only 26% of 2192 heart transplants performed in 2006 were in women. Similarly, the national Interagency Registry for Mechanically Assisted Circulatory Support (INTERMACS) registry database, designed to capture data on US patients receiving mechanical circulatory support devices to treat advanced heart failure, showed that only 34% of the devices implanted between March 2006 and March 2007 were used to treat women.

Statistics such as these emphasize the fundamental knowledge gap that exists when it comes to diagnosing, treating, and preventing heart disease in women. From the product development perspective, sex-based differences would ideally be taken into consideration at every stage, from drawing board to benchtop to bedside. More work needs to be done to elucidate the sex-based biological differences that relate to heart failure and other diseases, but in the meantime, researchers and those that evaluate research proposals should consider what can be done today to answer questions regarding the applicability of existing technologies that may have been studied exclusively (or predominantly) in men. The need for conclusive clinical trial data with specific relevance to women is clearly a piece of the puzzle.

It is the responsibility of health-care professionals, medical product manufacturers, research institutions, and regulatory agencies alike to pursue and promote clinical trials that produce scientific evidence that is applicable to both sexes. For example, investigational clinical studies of new medical products should strive to include a study sample group that is representative of the disease prevalence in the overall US population. Studies conducted entirely in women would provide the opportunity for obtaining much needed statistically significant information which can be used to support clinical decision-making. Examination of study entry criteria may reveal that women are unintentionally being excluded from participation. Study sponsors should make an effort to determine whether inherent referral biases exist at their investigational sites, and develop strategies for minimizing such bias. Tailored patient-informed consent processes may be needed. These measures are examples of steps that can and should be taken immediately, to bridge the existing gap in the treatment, diagnosis, and prevention of heart disease in women.

4. REVIEW PARADIGMS FOR HEART FAILURE DEVICES

As evidenced by the remaining chapters in this book, there are a myriad of devices available for the treatment of heart failure. This section will step through the FDA review process for three device areas in particular. For cardiac resynchronization therapy and ventricular assist devices, examples of the preclinical and clinical testing used to support approved marketing applications are provided, similar to the work previously published by Faris et al. *(37)*. In the case of hemodynamic monitoring technology, the discussion focuses on several factors that FDA uses to determine the level of data necessary to perform an adequate assessment of new devices in this intriguing field. Despite all being used for the treatment of heart failure, there are considerable technological differences between these three device areas, leading to various methods by which they are evaluated for safety and effectiveness.

4.1. Cardiac Resynchronization Therapy

Cardiac resynchronization therapy (CRT) devices are a relatively recent addition to the available medical therapy for heart failure patients, representing an advance in the technology used in pacemakers and defibrillators. Through the use of an additional pacing lead, placed on the outside of the left ventricle in the coronary sinus, CRT device systems are capable of coordinating the beating of the right and left ventricles to improve the heart's blood pumping efficiency. As sponsors developed this new technology, they applied many of the same principles of preclinical testing that were utilized for pacemakers and defibrillators. This included performance testing for major components of the device, such as the battery, capacitors, and connector module. When marketing applications also included novel leads for pacing the left ventricle, further testing specific to the leads was required, such as electrical resistance, pacing impedance, and flex fatigue testing. In addition, the devices underwent qualification testing to demonstrate that they would perform adequately in expected shipping, handling, and operating conditions. This set of tests included various environmental, electromagnetic compatibility, and design verification testing. Given the significant role of software in these devices, extensive verification and validation testing was conducted for both the software and firmware as well. Then the system components (i.e., implantable device, software, and device programmer) were combined and tested to ensure that they all worked together appropriately under simulated clinical conditions. Additional preclinical testing included biocompatibility, sterilization, shelf life, packaging, and animal testing. Since these devices were similar to previously reviewed and approved devices, the primary focus of the preclinical testing and review was on the incremental changes, such as validating the functionality of the biventricular pacing feature, its interaction with the existing features of the device, and new risks associated with the left ventricular lead.

The clinical studies conducted in support of CRT devices have gradually changed as the therapy has been embraced by the clinical community. As illustrated in Table 1, the initial clinical studies were randomized, double-blinded, placebo-controlled trials, focused on demonstrating a benefit in a patient's ability to exercise as well as their quality of life. For the patient population being studied, predominantly NYHA Class III, improvements in these measures were clinically meaningful. These early studies, conducted by several different manufacturers, showed a consistent and significant benefit in these parameters. Using alternative endpoints to support the original approval of these devices offers a realistic example of the least burdensome model. After receiving approval, sponsors were then able to conduct further investigations to evaluate the impact of CRT on mortality and hospitalizations in this population. In addition, due to the rapid adoption of CRT as part of standard heart failure care, a subsequent study designed to support initial device approval randomized patients to approved CRT devices as the control group as opposed to medical therapy. Please see the Summaries of Safety and Effectiveness Data (SSEDs) referenced in Table 1 for more information on the testing conducted in support of the various CRT marketing applications. As for ongoing and future clinical trials for CRT, the focus seems to be on the addition of new features to existing devices as well as investigating the safety and effectiveness in new patient populations.

4.2. Ventricular Assist Devices and Total Artificial Hearts

Ventricular assist devices (VADs) and total artificial hearts (TAHs) have been in development for several decades. Over the years, much has been

Table 1
Examples of cardiac resynchronization therapy clinical trial designs

Study design	MIRACLE (38)	MIRACLE (39) ICD	CONTAK (40) CD	RHYTHM ICD (41)	OPTION CRT/ATx (42)	COMPANION (43)	CARE-HF (44)
Year study began	1998	1999	1998	2002	2003	2000	2001
Year approved	2001	2002	2002	2004	2006	2004	2006
Type of device	CRT pacing	CRT defibrillator	CRT defibrillator	CRT defibrillator	CRT defibrillator	CRT defibrillator	CRT pacing
Comparison	On vs. Off	On vs. Off	On vs. Off	On vs. Off	Any approved CRT-D	Medical therapy	Medical therapy
Follow-up (months)	1, 3, 6	1, 3, 6	0, 3, 6	1, 3, 6	1, 6	0, 3, 6, 12	1, 3, 6, 9, 12, 18
Blinding	Double	Double	Double	Double	None	None	None
Primary effectiveness endpoint(s)	NYHA Class, 6 MW, QOL	NYHA Class, 6 MW, QOL	Mortality, heart failure hospitalizations, therapy for VT/VF	Peak VO$_2$, VF detection/redetection	6 MW, QOL	All-cause mortality or first hospitalization (time to first event)	All-cause mortality
Additional endpoints	Mortality, peak VO$_2$, QRS, hospitalization, Echo measures, neurohormones	Mortality, peak VO$_2$, QRS, hospitalization, echo measures, neurohormones	Peak VO$_2$, QOL, 6 MW, NYHA, echo measures, norepinephrine, heart rate	NYHA, QOL, 6 MW	Peak VO$_2$, NYHA, hospitalization	All-cause mortality, cardiac morbidity	NYHA, QOL, LVEF, LVESF, HF hospitalization
N (total randomized)	532	555	490	179	200	903	813

learned about the performance of these devices and then applied to the methods used to design and test them. Recent advances in technology have led to the development of continuous flow pumps, which are substantially smaller than the previous iterations of pulsatile pumps. The device design, intended clinical application (supporting the left ventricle, right ventricle, or both), as well as expected duration of use (bridge-to-transplant or destination therapy) will typically determine the conditions under which the device should be tested for reliability and durability, two critical aspects of the preclinical evaluation.

Preclinical testing for these devices also includes electrical safety, electromagnetic compatibility, battery longevity, software verification and validation, hermeticity, biocompatibility, sterilization, and packaging. In addition, individual system components such as the percutaneous leads, performance alarms, and valved conduits must be tested under simulated use conditions.

Animal studies have contributed to the safety assessment of these devices too by evaluating hemodynamic stability, end organ function, infection, pathology, and other important data. For more information on the type of preclinical testing necessary for these devices, see the SSEDs referenced in Table 2.

Also included in Table 2 are some of the basic parameters of the clinical studies conducted in support of currently approved mechanical circulatory support devices. For bridge-to-transplant (BTT) studies, the principal focus has been on the percentage of patients who survive to cardiac transplant, as well as capturing the incidence of adverse events such as bleeding, stroke, and infection. It is important to note that no randomized, prospective studies have been done comparing mechanical circulatory support devices to optimal medical therapy for the BTT patient population, due in large part to the severity of heart failure in these patients. Instead, various different control groups have been used, including historical control data from previously approved devices and non-randomized patients who were concurrently receiving medical therapy and enrolled in the trial. In 2003, the Agency combined data from several publications (12–17) to arrive at a performance goal for BTT studies, as discussed earlier in this chapter, which is used as the basis for choosing a comparator for ongoing trials of devices seeking this indication. Currently, there is only one FDA-approved ventricular assist device indicated for destination therapy (DT), which was evaluated in a randomized, controlled trial vs. medical therapy (51). While the trial was successful in demonstrating a significant difference in 2-year survival in favor of the device, there were a number of early and unexpected device failures. Present studies for the destination therapy indication are also randomized, with control patients receiving either an FDA-approved device or "standard of care," which includes any FDA-approved drug or device therapy available to this patient population. The future of this field may hinge on the success of INTERMACS, a national registry for circulatory support devices (discussed in more detail below). For example, data obtained from

Table 2
Examples of bridge-to-transplant and destination therapy clinical trial designs

Study design	Thoratec VAD (45)	HeartMate VE (46)	Novacor LVAS (47)	REMATCH (48)	Syncardia TAH-T (49)	Abiocor (50)
Year study began	1984	1996	1996	1998	1993	2001
Year approved	1995	1998	1998	2002	2004	2006
Type of device	BTT VAD	BTT VAD	BTT VAD	DT VAD	BT TAH	DT TAH
Comparison	Historical control	Historical control	Open-label medical therapy	Medical therapy	Historical control	None
Follow-up (months)	1, 6, 12	1, 3, 6, 12	1, 3, 6, 12	1, 3, 6, 12, 24	1, 3, 6, 12, 24	Monthly, post-discharge
Blinding	None	None	None	None	None	None
Primary effectiveness endpoint(s)	Survival to cardiac transplant	Survival to cardiac transplant	Survival to cardiac transplant	All-cause mortality	Survival to 30-day post-cardiac transplant	Safety and probable benefit assessment at 60-day post-implantation
Additional endpoints	Hemodynamics, adverse events, survival to 30-day post-transplant	NYHA, neurologic function, adverse events, survival to 30-day post-transplant	NYHA, neurologic function, adverse events, survival to 30-day post-transplant	NYHA, neurologic function, adverse events, device malfunctions and failures, QOL	NYHA, overall survival, adverse events, end organ function, hemodynamics	Hemodynamics, adverse events, QOL
N (total enrolled)	71	86	191	129 (Randomized)	95	14 (Feasibility study)
Regulatory pathway	PMA	PMA	PMA	PMA	PMA	HDE

INTERMACS could be used as a concurrent control group for VAD trials. Device manufacturers have also expressed an interest in conducting trials in less sick patients, an effort that would require avid participation by referring heart failure cardiologists. Similarly, if trials include less sick patients, one must identify the appropriate control patient population and clinically meaningful endpoints.

4.3. Hemodynamic Monitoring Technologies

Hemodynamic monitoring techniques have long been used to improve treatment strategies for heart failure patients. Recent advances in technology have produced several heart failure devices and features specifically designed to provide additional information to clinicians to assist them in their practice. FDA reviews these monitoring devices within the context of the entire treatment strategy with which they are associated. When evaluating the risks and benefits, there are several considerations that can help determine the type of data that are needed to provide a reasonable assurance of safety and effectiveness.

For example, FDA is interested in identifying the kind of information being presented. There is a different threshold associated with basic physiologic measurements, such as heart rate, temperature, weight, or intracardiac pressure, which are fairly well understood, as compared to novel parameters such as intrathoracic impedance or indices mathematically derived from other physiologic measurements. Furthermore, it is critical to determine whether the monitoring parameter is one that physicians are experienced in interpreting and acting upon. If that is the case, establishing the accuracy of the measurement may be acceptable. For parameters whose value is not so implicit, the clinical utility of the information will likely need to be demonstrated.

Another point to consider is to whom and where is the information being communicated. There are different concerns associated with the data being available to physicians during in-clinic follow-up vs. having access to the data via a remote monitoring network. Additional risks may be encountered when patients have direct access to the data. FDA is also interested in what triggers the presentation of data. This may be initiated by the physician or patient, as well as periodic reports based on a prespecified transmission schedule. There is an increased concern when the device includes audible or visible alarms based on the data obtained. In all situations, FDA pays particular attention to whether the data presentation implies a diagnosis and if there is a response expected by the user; therefore, sponsors are also asked to gather enough information to develop adequate instructions for use, for both physicians and patients.

When the device includes an alarm, FDA's evaluation focuses on whether the sensitivity and false alarm rate are acceptable. If the sensitivity is too low, patients may have a misplaced sense of security or ignore critical symptoms.

In contrast, if the false alarm rate is high, patients may be inappropriately treated (e.g., diuresis leading to hypovolemia) or users may choose to ignore alarms, removing any potential benefit associated with the feature.

As with all medical devices, FDA makes approval decisions by evaluating the risk–benefit profile of implantable monitoring devices. If the new technology is a monitoring feature coupled to a therapeutic device being used in a patient indicated for the therapy, the focus will be on comparing the additional risks associated with this new feature (e.g., additional or modified device hardware, longer or more difficult implant procedure, etc.) with the benefits attributable to its use. In the event that sponsors are seeking approval for a stand-alone monitoring device, the clinical benefit must outweigh all of the acute and chronic risks associated with the implant. In either instance, these risks include the possible misuse or misinterpretation of the data being captured, as well as the potential for device error. In conclusion, it is important to remember that FDA's review of heart failure monitoring devices focuses on the risks and benefits of the entire treatment strategy.

5. ROLE OF THE CIRCULATORY SYSTEM DEVICES ADVISORY PANEL

The FDA review process for heart failure device marketing applications may include a review by the Circulatory System Devices Advisory Panel at a public meeting *(52)*. This is typically the case when the device under review is the first of its kind or if additional expertise is needed based on initial evaluation of the data. The advisory panel consists of a chairperson, approximately six voting members who can serve up to two consecutive 2-year terms, and several temporary voting members who are usually recruited based on their particular expertise as it applies to the device being discussed, including heart failure cardiology, electrophysiology, cardiothoracic surgery, interventional cardiology, pediatrics, neurology, or ethics. As well, at least one statistician sits on the panel. The panel also includes two non-voting members who serve as industry and consumer representatives. All members must pass rigorous conflict of interest screening prior to being approved to sit on a particular panel.

Once decided upon, the date and location of the advisory panel meeting are publicly announced in the Federal Register. The sponsor and the FDA work together to provide a package of the pertinent information to the panel members in advance of the meeting. After all proprietary information has been redacted, the materials included in this panel package are posted on the Internet prior to the meeting. During the meeting, the sponsor typically provides an overview of their device and the results of their clinical trial. The FDA also presents a summary of their review, highlighting the particular areas in which the review team is looking for panelist input. There are also opportunities for the public to speak during the open public hearing sessions. At the conclusion of the meeting, the panel is asked to make a recommendation regarding the approvability of the marketing application that has been reviewed. The panel has the option of recommending approval, not approvable, or approval with conditions. Each voting member has the opportunity to cast their vote or abstain. The panel chair votes only in the event of a tie. If a majority votes in favor of a particular motion, that is the overall recommendation of the panel. FDA review staff will then take this recommendation, as well as the deliberations of the panel, into consideration as they make their final decision. It should be noted that while FDA typically reaches the same conclusion as the advisory panel, this is not a requirement. A transcript of the entire meeting is later published on the FDA web site and serves as the official public record of the meeting. Examples of web sites for recent panel meetings where heart failure device applications were reviewed are included in the references section (53–56).

It should be mentioned that advisory panel meetings may also be held for the discussion of general issues not necessarily associated with a particular marketing application. For meetings such as this, several companies in the device field affected by the issue are usually invited to make short presentations (often including proprietary information) during a session that is closed to the public and the other companies. A majority of the proceedings take place during the open public session, during which the panelists provide guidance to the FDA on how to handle the challenging issue. One major difference between this and a typical panel meeting is that there is no vote held at its conclusion. A recent example of this type of panel meeting was held on December 7 and 8, 2006, to discuss issues related to stent thrombosis following coronary drug-eluting stent placement (57).

6. INTERACTIONS WITH EXTERNAL STAKEHOLDERS AND GOVERNMENT PARTNERS

CDRH believes that in order to accomplish its mission, it must strive to foster collaborative relationships with our many stakeholders. On a daily basis, medical device reviewers interact with members of the industry to provide feedback on preclinical testing protocols as well as clinical trial designs. This partnership forms the basis by which safe and effective devices are made available to patients who need them. In addition to communication during the premarket review of medical devices, there are other venues by which the Agency has developed its relationship with device sponsors. For example, ODE has formed the Site Visit Program, providing an educational activity during which medical device reviewers can visit manufacturing firms, hospitals, and clinics to observe the design and manufacturing process, or application, of the medical devices the Agency reviews (58). The FDA also works together with various industry trade groups to identify needs such as guidance document development for a particular device area or topic.

Similarly, the Agency maintains close ties with the medical community in an effort to align regulatory practices and policies with standard clinical practice. In the heart failure arena, there have been several recent interactions with the Heart Failure Society of America (HFSA). This has been accomplished through workshops held between members of HFSA and FDA review staff who work together in small groups to address current challenging topics. FDA also held other workshops with HFSA where device companies are invited to attend and share their experiences on similar thought-provoking issues. Additionally, FDA interacts with various other professional societies that have an interest in heart failure, such as the Heart Rhythm Society, American College of Cardiology, American Heart Association, and International Society of Heart & Lung Transplantation. FDA reviewers frequently attend the annual scientific sessions held by each of these groups and are often invited to participate as presenters, panelists, or session moderators.

CDRH has also developed a working relationship with other entities that are part of the Department of Health and Human Services (DHHS), such as the Centers for Medicare & Medicaid Services (CMS) and the National Institutes of Health (NIH). For example, members of all three agencies have teamed up with various clinicians, scientists, industry representatives, the University of Alabama at Birmingham, and the United Network for Organ Sharing to create the Interagency Registry for Mechanically Assisted Circulatory Support (INTERMACS) *(59)*. INTERMACS is a national registry for all patients who receive FDA-approved mechanical circulatory support device therapy to treat advanced heart failure. Reviewers from the Division of Cardiovascular Devices (DCD) are part of the INTERMACS Operations Committee, working together with other participants to provide direction, oversight, and approval for the major design features of the registry, as well as other functional components. For instance, members of DCD have helped develop standardized adverse event definitions for ventricular assist devices, which will aid in our ability to interpret the data collected. It is the hope of everyone involved with this major enterprise that eventually propensity score analysis can be used to compare investigational device patients to similarly matched control patients who are enrolled in the INTERMACS registry.

The National Heart, Lung, and Blood Institute (NHLBI) recently undertook another key project to fund the development of new devices in the field of pediatric mechanical circulatory support devices, having recognized the need for improved technology in this area. In 2004, NHLBI awarded five contracts to applicants based on the proposals submitted and several assessment criteria *(60)*. CDRH has also been involved with this project, sponsoring a workshop in January 2006 to describe the regulatory process for pediatric ventricular assist device approval as well as indicate to the community that effective pediatric device development is an important issue for FDA *(61)*. The examples cited in the above section illustrate just a few ways in which CDRH works together with its many stakeholders to accomplish its mission.

7. CONCLUSIONS

CDRH views itself as a collaborative organization, working within its own boundaries to achieve effective results under the Total Product Life Cycle paradigm and through its relationship with various external stakeholders. Specifically, DCD would like to remind device manufacturers that interaction with the Agency is encouraged early in the device development process. As discussed, there are many challenges involved with designing clinical trials for heart failure devices. However, the Agency is always willing to work with sponsors to overcome these obstacles, as evidenced by the successful clinical trials that have been conducted in both the CRT and VAD arenas.

REFERENCES

1. The Least Burdensome Provisions of the FDA Modernization Act of 1997: Concept and Principles; Final Guidance for FDA and Industry. Available at: http:// www.fda.gov/ cdrh/ode/guidance/1332.pdf. Accessed November 29, 2007.
2. US Food and Drug Administration – Center for Devices and Radiological Health. Available at: http://www.fda.gov/cdrh/. Accessed November 29, 2007.
3. Design Control Guidance for Medical Device Manufacturers. Available at: http://www.fda.gov/ cdrh/comp/designgd.pdf. Accessed November 29, 2007.
4. Office of Orphan Products Development. Available at: http://www.fda.gov/orphan/. Accessed November 29, 2007.
5. Humanitarian Use Devices. Available at: http://www.fda.gov/cdrh/ode/hdeinfo.html. Accessed November 29, 2007.
6. Guidance on IDE Policies and Procedures. Available at: http://www.fda.gov/cdrh/ode/ idepolcy.pdf. Accessed November 29, 2007.
7. Medical Device Recalls. Available at: http://www.accessdata.fda.gov/scripts/cdrh/ cfdocs/cfTopic/medicaldevicesafety/recalls.cfm. Accessed November 29, 2007.
8. Device Advice. Available at: http://www.fda.gov/cdrh/devadvice. Accessed November 29, 2007.
9. Aaronson KD, Schwartz JS, Chen TM, Wong KL, Goin JE, Mancini DM. Development and prospective validation of a clinical index to predict survival in ambulatory patients referred for cardiac transplant evaluation. Circulation 1997 Jun; 95(12): 2597–9.
10. Levy WC, Mazaffarian D, Linker DT, Sutradhar SC, Anker SD, Cropp AB, et al. The Seattle Heart Failure Model: Prediction of survival in heart failure. Circulation 2006 Mar; 113(11): 1424–33.
11. Frankel DS, Piette JD, Jessup M, Craig K, Pickering F, Goldberg LR. Validation of prognostic models among patients with advanced heart failure. J Card Fail 2006 Aug; 12(6): 430–8.
12. Farrar DJ, Hill JD, Pennington DG, McBride LR, Holman WL, Kormos RL, et al. Preoperative and postoperative comparison of patients with univentricular and biventricular support with the Thoratec ventricular assist device as a bridge to cardiac transplantation. J Thorac Cardiovasc Surg 1997 Jan; 113(1): 202–9.
13. El-Banayosy A, Arusoglu L, Kizner L, Tenderich G, Minami K, Inoue K, et al. Novacor left ventricular assist system versus Heartmate vented electric left ventricular assist

system as a long-term mechanical circulatory support device in bridging patients: a prospective study. J Thorac Cardiovasc Surg 2000 Mar; 119(3): 581–7.

14. Minami K, El-Banayosy A, Sezai A, Arusoglu L, Sarnowsky P, Fey O, et al. Morbidity and outcome after mechanical ventricular support using Thoratec, Novacor, and Heart-Mate for bridging to heart transplantation. Artif Organs 2000 Jun; 24(6): 421–6.

15. Di Bella I, Pagani F, Banfi C, Ardemagni E, Capo A, Klersy C, et al. Results with the Novacor assist system and evaluation of long-term assistance. Eur J Cardiothorac Surg 2000 Jul; 18(1): 112–6.

16. El-Banayosy A, Korfer R, Arusoglu L, Kizner L, Morshuis M, Milting H, et al. Device and patient management in a bridge-to-transplant setting. Ann Thorac Surg 2001 Mar; 71(3 Suppl): S98–102.

17. Frazier OH, Rose EA, Oz MC, Dembitsky W, McCarthy P, Radovancevic B, et al. Multi-center clinical evaluation of the HeartMate vented electric left ventricular assist system in patients awaiting heart transplantation. J Thorac Cardiovasc Surg 2001 Dec; 122(6): 1186–95.

18. Mancini DM, Eisen H, Kussmaul W, Mull R, Edmunds LH, Wilson JR. Value of peak exercise oxygen consumption for optimal timing of cardiac transplantation in ambulatory patients with heart failure. Circulation 1991 Mar; 83(3): 778–86.

19. Stelken AM, Younis LT, Jennison SH, Miller DD, Miller LW, Shaw LJ, et al. Prognostic value of cardiopulmonary exercise testing using percent achieved of predicted peak oxygen uptake for patients with ischemic and dilated cardiomyopathy. J Am Coll Cardiol 1996 Feb; 27(2): 345–52.

20. Lund LH, Aaronson KD, Mancini DM. Validation of peak exercise oxygen consumption and the Heart Failure Survival Score for serial risk stratification in advanced heart failure. Am J Cardiol 2005 Mar; 95(6): 734–41.

21. Pina IL, Karalis DG. Comparison of four exercise protocols using anaerobic threshold measurement of functional capacity in congestive heart failure. Am J Cardiol 1990 May; 65(18): 1269–71.

22. Chua TP, Ponikowski P, Harrington D, Anker SD, Webb-Peploe K, Clark AL, et al. Clinical correlates and prognostic significance of the ventilatory response to exercise in chronic heart failure. J Am Coll Cardiol 1997 Jun; 29(7): 1585–90.

23. Whellan DJ, O'Connor CM, Lee KL, Keteyian SJ, Cooper LS, Ellis SJ, et al. Heart failure and a controlled trial investigating outcomes of exercise training (HF-ACTION): design and rationale. Am Heart J 2007 Feb; 153(2): 201–11.

24. Lipkin DP, Scriven AJ, Crake T, Poole-Wilson PA. Six minute walking test for assessing exercise capacity in chronic heart failure. Br Med J (Clin Res Ed) 1986 Mar; 292(6521): 653–55.

25. Lipkin DP, Canepa-Anson R, Stephens MR, Poole-Wilson PA. Factors determining symptoms in heart failure: comparison of fast and slow exercise tests. Br Heart J 1986 May; 55(5): 439–45.

26. Bittner V, Weiner DH, Yusuf S, Rogers WJ, McIntyer KM, Bangdiwala, SI, et al. Prediction of mortality and morbidity with a 6-minute walk test in patients with left ventricular dysfunction. SOLVD Investigators. JAMA 1993; 270(14): 1702–07.

27. ATS Committee on Proficiency Standards for Clinical Pulmonary Function Laboratories. ATS Statement: Guidelines for the six-minute walk test. Am J Respir Crit Care Med 2002 Jul; 166(1): 111–7.

28. Normand SL, Rector TS, Neaton JD, Pina IL, Lazar RM, Proestel SE, et al. Clinical and analytical considerations in the study of health status in device trials for heart failure. J Card Fail 2005 Jun; 11(5): 396–403.

29. Guyatt GH, Kirshner B, Jaeschke R. Measuring health status: what are the necessary measurement properties? J Clin Epidemiol 1992 Dec; 45(12): 1341–5.

30. Rector TS, Cohn JN. Assessment of patient outcome with the Minnesota Living with Heart Failure questionnaire: reliability and validity during a randomized, double-blind,

placebo-controlled trial of pimobendan. Pimobendan Multicenter Research Group. Am Heart J 1992 Oct; 124: 1017–25.

31. Rector TS, Kubo SH, Cohn JN. Validity of the Minnesota Living with Heart Failure questionnaire as a measure of therapeutic response to enalapril or placebo. Am J Cardiol 1993 May;71: 1106–10.

32. Green CP, Porter CB, Bresnahan DR, Spertus JA. Development and evaluation of the Kansas City Cardiomyopathy Questionnaire: a new health status measure for heart failure. J Am Coll Cardiol 2000 Apr; 35: 1245–55.

33. Brooks, RG, Jendteg S, Lindgren B, Persson U, Bjork S. EuroQol: health-related quality of life measurement. Results of the Swedish questionnaire exercise. Health Policy 1991; 18(1): 37–48.

34. Brooks RG. EuroQol: the current state of play. Health Policy 1996; 37(1): 53–72.

35. Mosca L, Merz NB, Blumenthal RS, Cziraky MJ, Fabunmi RP, Sarawate C, et al. Opportunity for intervention to achieve American Heart Association guidelines for optimal lipid levels in high-risk women in a managed care setting. Circulation 2005 Feb; 111(4): 488–93.

36. Rosamond W, Flegal K, Friday G, Furie K, Go A, Greenlund K, et al. Heart disease and stroke statistics—2007 update: a report from the American Heart Association Statistics Committee and Stroke Statistics Subcommittee. Circulation 2007 Feb; 115(5): e69–171.

37. Faris O, Chen E, Berman M, Moynahan M, Zuckerman B. A US Food and Drug Administration perspective on cardiac resynchronization and ventricular assist device trials. Congest Heart Fail 2005 Jul–Aug; 11(4): 207–11.

38. Summary of safety and effectiveness. Medtronic InSync. Available at: http://www.fda.gov/cdrh/pdf/P010015b.pdf. Accessed November 29, 2007.

39. Summary of safety and effectiveness. Medtronic InSync ICD. Available at: http://www.fda.gov/cdrh/pdf/P010031b.pdf. Accessed November 29, 2007.

40. Summary of safety and effectiveness. Guidant CONTAK CD. Available at: http://www.fda.gov/cdrh/pdf/P010012b.pdf. Accessed November 29, 2007.

41. Summary of safety and effectiveness. St. Jude Epic and Atlas CRT-D. Available at: http://www.fda.gov/cdrh/pdf/P010012b.pdf. Accessed November 29, 2007.

42. Summary of safety and effectiveness. Biotronik Tupos and Kronos CRT-D. Available at: http://www.fda.gov/cdrh/pdf5/p050023b.pdf. Accessed November 29, 2007.

43. Summary of safety and effectiveness. Guidant COMPANION Trial. Available at: http://www.fda.gov/cdrh/pdf/P010012S026b.pdf. Accessed November 29, 2007.

44. Cleland JG, Daubert JC, Erdmann E, Freemantle N, Gras D, Kappenberger L, et al. The effect of cardiac resynchronization on morbidity and mortality in heart failure. Cardiac Resynchronization-Heart Failure (CARE-HF) Study Investigators. N Engl J Med 2005 Apr; 352(15): 1539–49.

45. Premarket Approval (PMA) Database. Thoratec Ventricular Assist Device (VAD) System. Available at http://www.accessdata.fda.gov/scripts/cdrh/cfdocs/cfPMA/PMA.cfm?ID=13935. Accessed November 29, 2007.

46. Summary of safety and effectiveness. Thoratec HeartMate VE VAD. Available at: http://www.fda.gov/cdrh/pdf/p920014s007b.pdf. Accessed November 29, 2007.

47. Summary of safety and effectiveness. WorldHeart Novacor Left Ventricular Assist System. Available at http://www.fda.gov/cdrh/pdf/P980012b.pdf. Accessed November 29, 2007.

48. Premarket Approval (PMA) Database. Thoratec HeartMate Left Ventricular Assist System (SNAP-VE LVAS). Available at: http://www.accessdata.fda.gov/scripts/cdrh/cfdocs/cfPMA/PMA.cfm?ID=13924. Accessed November 29, 2007.

49. Summary of safety and effectiveness. Syncardia temporary Total Artificial Heart (TAH-T). Available at http://www.fda.gov/cdrh/PDF3/p030011b.pdf. Accessed November 29, 2007.

50. Summary of safety and probable benefit. Abiomed Abiocar Replacement Heart. Available at http://www.fda.gov/cdrh/pdf4/H040006b.pdf. Accessed November 29, 2007.

51. Rose EA, Gelijns AC, Moskowitz AJ, Heitjan DF, Stevenson LW, Dembitsky W, et al. Long-term mechanical left ventricular assistance for end-stage heart failure. Randomized Evaluation of Mechanical Assistance for the Treatment of Congestive Heart Failure (REMATCH) Study Group. N Engl J Med 2001 Nov; 345(20): 1435–43.

52. CDRH Advisory Committees. Available at: http://www.fda.gov/cdrh/panel/. Accessed November 29, 2007.

53. Thoratec REMATCH and Medtronic InSync ICD Advisory Meetings. Available at: http://www.accessdata.fda.gov/scripts/cdrh/cfdocs/cfAdvisory/details.cfm?mtg=281. Accessed November 29, 2007.

54. Guidant COMPANION Advisory Meeting. Available at: http://www.accessdata.fda.gov/scripts/cdrh/cfdocs/cfAdvisory/details.cfm?mtg=514. Accessed November 29, 2007.

55. Acorn CorCap Cardiac Support Device and Abiomed Abiocor Total Artificial Heart Advisory Meetings. Available at: http://www.accessdata.fda.gov/scripts/cdrh/cfdocs/cfAdvisory/details.cfm?mtg=596. Accessed November 29, 2007.

56. Medtronic Chronicle Implantable Hemodynamic Monitoring System Advisory Meeting. Available at: http://www.accessdata.fda.gov/scripts/cdrh/cfdocs/cfAdvisory/details.cfm?mtg=677. Accessed November 29, 2007.

57. Stent Thrombosis in Coronary Drug-Eluting Stents Advisory Meeting. Available at: http://www.accessdata.fda.gov/scripts/cdrh/cfdocs/cfAdvisory/details.cfm?mtg=672. Accessed November 29, 2007.

58. ODE Site Visit Program. Available at: http://www.fda.gov/cdrh/ode/ode-sitevisit.html. Accessed November 29, 2007.

59. Interagency Registry for Mechanically Assisted Circulatory Support. Available at: http://www.intermacs.org/. Accessed November 29, 2007.

60. Baldwin JT, Borovetz HS, Duncan BW, Gartner MJ, Jarvik RK, Weiss WJ, et al. The national heart, lung, and blood institute pediatric circulatory support program. Circulation 2006 Jan; 113: 147–55.

61. FDA Workshop on Regulatory Process for Pediatric Mechanical Circulatory Support Devices (Ventricular Assist Devices), January 20, 2006. Available at: http://www.fda.gov/cdrh/meetings/012006workshop/index.html. Accessed November 29, 2007.

5 Hemodynamic Monitoring in Heart Failure

Anju Nohria, MD and Ami Bhatt, MD

CONTENTS

Abstract

Symptoms of pulmonary congestion, resulting from elevated left atrial and left ventricular filling pressures, are the most common cause of heart failure hospitalization. The basic goals of HF therapy are therefore grounded in improving congestion, thereby decreasing hospitalizations and improving outcomes and quality of life in patients with HF. Ongoing evaluation of the patient's volume status is vital for appropriate selection and monitoring of therapy and prevention of recurrent hospitalizations. This chapter discusses the clinical, laboratory, invasive, and non-invasive tools available for hemodynamic assessment of the heart failure patient.

Key Words: Heart failure; Hemodynamics; Pulmonary edema; Implantable monitors.

From: *Contemporary Cardiology: Device Therapy in Heart Failure*
Edited by: W.H. Maisel, DOI 10.1007/978-1-59745-424-7_5
© Humana Press, a part of Springer Science+Business Media, LLC 2010

1. INTRODUCTION

Heart failure (HF) affects five million adults in the United States and results in approximately one million hospitalizations per year *(1)*. New developments in HF treatment continue to improve patients' quality of life as well as reduce morbidity and mortality. Despite these advances, HF remains a progressive disease. Hospitalization for HF is associated with a poor prognosis with 1-year mortality estimates ranging from 25 to 40% *(2–4)*. Symptoms of pulmonary congestion, resulting from elevated left atrial and left ventricular (LV) filling pressures, are the most common cause of HF hospitalization *(3–6)*. The basic goals of HF therapy are therefore grounded in improving congestion, thereby decreasing hospitalizations and improving outcomes and quality of life in patients with HF.

Several studies of patients undergoing evaluation for cardiac transplantation demonstrate that elevated filling pressures are associated with adverse outcomes *(7, 8)*. Furthermore, inadequate reduction of filling pressures with therapy *(9)*, or persistent symptoms of congestion 4–6 weeks after hospital discharge, results in significantly reduced survival in patients admitted with New York Heart Association (NYHA) Class IV symptoms of HF *(10)*. Although it is a compensatory mechanism to maintain stroke volume, elevated filling pressures compromise coronary venous drainage and result in increased myocardial turgor and stiffening of the LV wall. This impairs LV function by increasing oxygen demand while reducing subendocardial perfusion *(11)*. Moreover, high filling pressures exacerbate dynamic mitral regurgitation, which can consume up to 50% of total stroke volume during decompensation *(12)*. Therapy aimed at lowering filling pressures improves LV diastolic distensibility *(11)* and reduces regurgitant volumes by decreasing LV end-diastolic dimensions and mitral orifice area *(12)*. Reduction of filling pressures thus improves LV function and forward cardiac output (CO), while relieving symptoms of congestion. Therefore, once the diagnosis of HF has been established, ongoing evaluation of the patient's volume status is vital for appropriate selection and monitoring of therapy and prevention of recurrent hospitalizations.

2. CLINICAL ASSESSMENT OF HEMODYNAMIC PROFILES

2.1. Symptoms

Many physicians rely on the symptom history to assess a change in volume status. Symptoms of congestion may be related to increased left or right ventricular filling pressures. Dyspnea on minimal exertion, orthopnea, and paroxysmal nocturnal dyspnea may indicate elevated left-sided filling pressures. Abdominal discomfort, early satiety, nausea, and vomiting may be due to right-sided volume overload. Of these, orthopnea correlates best with elevated pulmonary capillary wedge pressure (PCWP) with a sensitivity approaching 90% *(13)*. The remaining symptoms are relatively non-specific and less helpful in diagnosing volume overload. Unfortunately, chronic symptoms blunt patient expectations and symptoms severe enough to require HF hospitalization often occur late in the course of decompensation *(5)*. Furthermore, diuretic therapy improves symptoms substantially in approximately 66% of patients by 24 h and over 80% of patients by 3 days of discharge *(13)*. Patients frequently feel "back to normal" early during therapy when they remain decompensated by other measures. Thus, although symptoms are useful indicators of elevated filling pressures, they cannot be used to judge the adequacy of HF treatment.

Symptoms of depressed CO are less specific than those associated with congestion. Patients often complain of fatigue, which may also be a manifestation of exertional dyspnea, disordered sleep patterns, peripheral deconditioning, anemia, and depression related to HF. Complaints of feeling cold do not necessarily reflect low CO. Altered mentation is occasionally described by patients as difficulty in concentrating while reading or doing routine tasks, but is more often noted by the family.

2.2. Physical Examination

Several physical exam findings are reliable indicators of elevated filling pressures in patients with HF. Jugular venous pressure remains the most reliable and commonly used test for evaluating elevated right-sided filling pressures (sensitivity = 70% and specificity = 79%) *(14)*. Rondot's sign, or the presence of abdominojugular reflux, can be used to enhance both the sensitivity and the specificity of jugular venous distention to greater than 80% *(15)*. Right-sided pressures reliably reflect left-sided pressures in about 80% of patients (right atrial pressure (RAP) > or < 10 with PCWP > or < 22 mmHg; $r = 0.64$, $p < 0.001$) *(14)*. Furthermore, a change in RAP usually parallels a change in PCWP during ongoing therapy. Although infrequently utilized by clinicians, an abnormal blood pressure response (square wave) to the Valsalva maneuver can also be used to directly assess elevated left-sided filling pressures with a positive predictive value of 82% *(16)*. Unfortunately, this test is highly dependent on clinician experience and patient effort and may not be possible in patients with significant dyspnea or arrhythmias. The absence of other commonly evaluated signs such as rales and peripheral edema does not exclude volume overload since these are only present in one-third to one-half of patients with elevated intra-cardiac filling pressures *(13)*. Rales can be absent in patients with chronic systolic HF due to increased lymphatic drainage and chronic perivascular compensation. Leg edema is rarely seen in children and young adults with HF, but is more common in older individuals. The third heart sound (S3) is useful to diagnose LV dysfunction and can vary in intensity with fluid overload. Thus, on serial examinations, the S3 may be a helpful indicator of volume status. Increased intensity of the pulmonary component of the second heart sound (P2) indicates elevated pulmonary artery pressures. A P2 that can be heard to the left of the lower sternal border usually indicates elevated PCWP *(13)*. Data from the Evaluation Study of Congestive Heart Failure and Pulmonary Artery Catheterization (ESCAPE) trial demonstrate that even though clinicians specializing in HF can qualitatively identify jugular venous distention in majority of patients, there is significant inter-observer variability regarding the extent of elevation *(17)*. Thus, while the clinical examination may be sufficient to determine the presence or absence of congestion in many patients, its accuracy depends on patient habitus and physician experience.

Compromised perfusion is much harder to assess on physical examination and is only seen in approximately 20% of patients presenting to a specialized HF center *(18)*. Particular attention should be given to the auscultation of blood pressure as an indicator of compromised perfusion. In general, the detection of pulsus alternans indicates more severe compromise than otherwise suspected. A decrement in the proportional pulse pressure (pulse pressure/systolic blood pressure) to less than 25% has previously been suggested to reflect a cardiac index ≤ 2.2 ml/kg/min^2 *(13)*. However, analysis from the ESCAPE trial suggests that although physicians are good at judging volume overload, their assessment of perfusion does not correlate well with invasive measures of cardiac index *(17)*.

Despite its shortcomings, the history and physical examination remain the primary tool for adjusting medical therapy in patients with HF. The signs and symptoms described above can be successfully used to categorize patients into four hemodynamic profiles based on the absence or presence of congestion and adequacy of perfusion (Fig. 1). These hemodynamic profiles have prognostic value with a 2-fold greater risk of death in "wet and warm" (Profile B) patients and a 2.5-fold increased risk in "wet and cold" (Profile C) patients compared to "dry and warm" (Profile A) patients at 1 year *(18)*. These bedside hemodynamic profiles can be used to guide and monitor therapy non-invasively in patients with chronic HF with the clinical goals of attaining a jugular venous pressure < 8 cm while maintaining a systolic blood pressure of at least 80 mmHg and resolving the symptoms of congestion and fatigue.

3. LABORATORY EVALUATION OF ELEVATED FILLING PRESSURES

Biomarkers such as the natriuretic peptides have been shown to be useful in the diagnosis of HF in patients presenting to the emergency department with dyspnea of unclear etiology *(19, 20)*. A brain natriuretic peptide (BNP) cut-off value of 100 pg/ml has a 96% negative predictive value for HF *(19)*. Similarly, an N-terminal proBNP (NT-proBNP) cut-off value of < 125 pg/ml for patients < 75 years of age and < 450 pg/ml for patients ≥ 75 years of age has a negative predictive value approaching 100% for the diagnosis of HF *(20)*. While elevations in natriuretic peptide levels have been shown to correlate with left-sided filling pressures in the individual patient

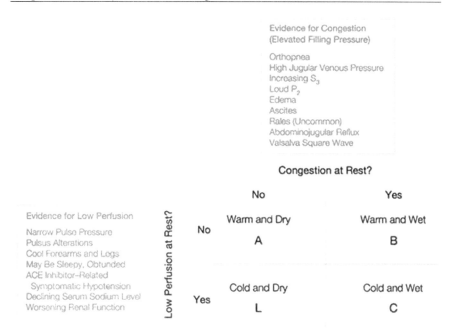

Fig. 1. Bedside assessment of hemodynamic profiles. A careful history and physical examination can be used to create a 2 × 2 grid that allows classification of patients into four hemodynamic profiles based on the absence or presence of congestion and adequacy of perfusion. These hemodynamic profiles can then be used to guide and monitor therapy. See test for details. (Reprinted with permission from Nohria et al.) *(77).*

(21, 22), there is significant variation between individuals based on the etiology of HF *(23),* LV dimensions *(24),* age *(19),* renal function *(25),* and body mass index *(26).* Thus it has been suggested that serial measurements of natriuretic peptides in a given patient can be used to detect a change in filling pressures *(27, 28)* and may be of potential value in monitoring volume status and guiding therapy. Several trials have attempted to address this question and have shown that using BNP levels to guide HF therapy results in greater utilization of evidence-based drugs (i.e., angiotensin-converting enzyme inhibitors and beta-blockers) rather than increased diuresis *(29–31).* Not surprisingly, these trials demonstrated an improvement in cardiovascular *(29)* and HF-related events *(30)* with BNP-guided therapy. However, the utility of serial natriuretic peptide measurements to monitor HF and guide therapies is limited by the large intra-individual variability seen in patients with stable HF. Taking both analytic precision and biological variation into account, intra-individual variation over a 1-week interval is approximately 66% for BNP and 50% for NT-proBNP, respectively *(32).* Thus, although it is clear that variation in natriuretic peptides reflects active physiologic processes, the percent change that should trigger a clinical response remains unclear.

Given the limitations of bedside and laboratory evaluations described above, an accurate and reliable means of monitoring fluid status in chronic HF patients is needed to adequately diurese patients during hospitalization such that outpatient diuretic regimens are successful at maintaining optimal volume status. Similarly, and perhaps more importantly, methods to detect early decompensation and affect early intervention in the ambulatory setting are needed to prevent recurrent hospitalizations. Currently, patients followed in comprehensive HF disease management programs require frequent interventions including phone calls, clinic visits, and diuretic adjustments in order to maintain clinical stability (33). While effective at reducing hospitalizations, these interventions are costly and inefficient. New and established device-based hemodynamic monitoring techniques for HF may allow repeated assessment of filling pressures and impending decompensation thereby improving survival and reducing hospitalization rates while decreasing the rising costs of health care for this population.

4. MODALITIES OF HEMODYNAMIC MONITORING

Multiple modalities are available to determine hemodynamics in patients with HF. These include non-invasive measurements such as the clinical examination (described above), echocardiography, and impedance cardiography as well as invasive techniques including the pulmonary artery (PA) catheter and novel implantable hemodynamic monitors. The following sections will focus on device-based methods of evaluating hemodynamic indices, in particular filling pressures, and their utility in the inpatient and ambulatory settings. PA catheters will be discussed first, as these represent the gold standard for measuring hemodynamics, and the accuracy of all other device-based modalities is determined relative to measurements derived from the PA catheter.

5. INVASIVE MODALITIES OF HEMODYNAMIC MONITORING

5.1. The Pulmonary Artery Catheter

In 1929, Werner Forssmann demonstrated that a catheter could be advanced safely into the human heart and that it allowed measurements of right heart pressures to be performed urgently at the bedside of critically ill patients. Dr. H.J. Swan improved this catheter by attaching a sail-like device for easier manipulation, and from that concept, the balloon-tipped catheter was fabricated. William Ganz then developed the thermodilution method of measuring cardiac output (CO) that was incorporated into the version of the pulmonary artery (PA) catheter that is still in use today.

The PA catheter is a multi-lumen catheter with a 1.5-cc balloon located just proximal to the tip. Approximately 4 cm proximal to the balloon is the thermistor used to measure temperature changes for calculation of CO. In

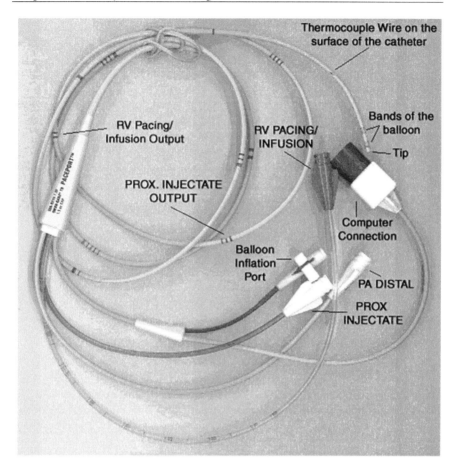

Fig. 2. Swan-Ganz pulmonary artery catheter.

addition to a distal lumen, there are two additional lumens present 19 cm and 30 cm from the distal tip (Fig. 2). Generally, the distal tip resides in the PA, and the additional lumens reside in the right ventricle (RV), right atrium, or superior vena cava (depending on right heart size). A semirigid noncompliant tubing filled with isotonic saline connects the catheter to a fluid-filled pressure transducer. This system transmits intra-cardiac pressures to the transducer, causing deformation of the transducer membrane leading to a proportional electric current that is amplified and transmitted to the monitor (Fig. 3).

5.1.1. INDICATIONS FOR THE USE OF THE PULMONARY ARTERY CATHETER

The invasive PA catheter is an important tool in the management of patients with cardiogenic shock or other life-threatening circulatory

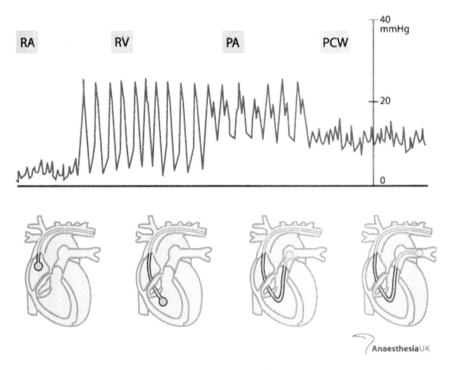

Fig. 3. Characteristic intra-cardiac pressure waveforms derived from the pulmonary artery catheter. The diagram below shows the characteristic cardiac waveforms as the pulmonary artery catheter is advanced through different chambers of the heart. RA = right atrial pressure; RV = right ventricular pressure; PA = pulmonary artery pressure; and PCW = pulmonary capillary wedge pressure.

compromise. In patients with symptoms of dyspnea whose initial clinical hemodynamic profile is unclear, the PA catheter has often been used to determine the contribution of HF relative to other concomitant conditions such as pulmonary disease or active ischemia. Furthermore, in patients with established HF and an inadequate response to empiric treatment, the PA catheter has been used to examine the relationship between right- and left-sided filling pressures to help guide future therapy. Additionally, during evaluation for cardiac transplantation, the use of PA catheters is routine to determine the presence and reversibility of secondary pulmonary hypertension.

5.1.2. USE OF THE PULMONARY ARTERY CATHETER TO "TAILOR THERAPY" IN HEART FAILURE

In addition to the above-mentioned indications, PA catheters have been used to optimize therapy for chronic decompensated HF. In the late 1970s, several investigators demonstrated that acute intravenous vasodilator therapy lowered filling pressures and improved CO by lowering systemic vascular resistance (SVR) *(34, 35)*. Importantly, in patients who were responsive to acute intravenous vasodilator therapy, the hemodynamic effects persisted after transitioning to oral vasodilator therapy *(36, 37)*. This led to the concept of using the PA catheter to "tailor therapy" in patients refractory to empiric HF treatment. For patients with the usual ratio of RAP to PCWP of 0.5, the recommended hemodynamic goals of tailored therapy are to reduce filling pressures to a PCWP≤16 mmHg and RAP≤8 mmHg. SVR is a target of therapy only as necessary to reduce filling pressures, with a goal being 1000–1200 dyne/s per cm^5 in individuals in whom the PCWP is still high. (Further reduction of SVR in patients with a normal PCWP can cause hypotension.) CO and mixed venous saturation are useful for trending circulatory status and usually improve with effective reduction of filling pressures *(38)*. Beyond that, however, therapy targeted specifically to improve CO has not proven beneficial in the management of chronic HF *(39)*.

5.1.3. CONTROVERSY SURROUNDING THE USE OF PULMONARY ARTERY CATHETERS

There has been considerable controversy surrounding the use of PA catheters in critically ill patients. The Study to Understand Prognoses and Preferences for Outcomes and Risks of Treatments (SUPPORT) trial was a propensity score, case-matched analysis of 5735 patients receiving care in an intensive care unit (ICU) with or without the aid of a PA catheter in the first 24 h *(40)*. The study evaluated the association between PA catheter use and subsequent survival, length of stay, intensity, and cost of care. In this observational study, PA catheter use was associated with increased mortality (odds ratio (OR), 1.24; 95% confidence interval (CI), 1.03–1.49) and increased utilization of resources (median cost $30,500 vs $20,600). The mean length of stay in the ICU was not significantly altered with PA catheter use (14.8 vs 13 days). These adverse results spurred several subsequent randomized controlled trials of PA catheter-guided therapy that failed to show any evidence of harm or benefit in a variety of patient populations including high-risk surgical patients *(41)*, patients with shock and acute respiratory distress syndrome *(42, 43)*, as well as a heterogeneous ICU population (Table 1) *(44)*. These results have led to a recommendation against the routine use of PA catheters for hemodynamic monitoring in patients in shock *(45)* with a resultant decline in PA catheter use from 5.66 per 1000 medical admissions in 1993 to 1.99 per 1000 medical admissions in 2004 *(46)*. However, specific data pertaining to the utility of PA catheter-guided therapy in patients with chronic decompensated HF have only recently been studied in the Evaluation Study of Congestive Heart Failure and Pulmonary Catheter Effectiveness (ESCAPE) trial *(38)*.

Table 1
Overview of the major randomized trials evaluating the safety and efficacy of pulmonary artery catheters (Modified from Shah et al.) (47)

Source	PAC vs no PAC	Population	Design	Hemodynamic targets	Treatment strategy	Results
Harvey et al. (44)	519/522	ICU	PAC vs no PAC	No	No	Death: HR 1.09 (0.94–1.27)
Schultz et al. (78)	35/35	Hip fracture	PAC vs no PAC	No	No	Death: 2.9%/29%
Shoemaker et al. (79)	30/28/30	High-risk general surgery	Grp 1: PAC w/ normal goals; Grp 2: PAC w/ supranormal goals; Grp 3: no PAC	Yes Grp 1: CI 2.8–3.5, O$_2$ delivery 400–550, VO$_2$ 120–140 Grp2: CI >4.5, O$_2$ delivery >600, VO$_2$ >170	No	Death: 10/1/7 Days hospitalized: 25.2/19.3/22.2
Isaacson et al. (80)	49/53	Abdominal aortic surgery	PAC vs no PAC	No	No	Death: 1/0 Days hospitalized: 10.2/9.4

Berlauk et al. (81)	45/23/21	Limb salvage arterial surgery	Grp1: PAC 12 h pre-op; Grp 2: PAC 3 h pre-op; Grp 3: no PAC	Yes PCWP < 15; CI ≥ 2.8; SVR ≤1100	Yes SVR >1100 & SBP >100 (vasodilator); SVR ≤1100 (inotrope); PCWP < 15 (crystalloid); CI < 2.8 (inotrope)	Death: 1/0/1 Days hospitalized: 19.4/18.0/15.4
Guyatt et al. (82)	16/17	ICU	PAC vs no PAC	No	No	Death: 10/9 Days hospitalized: 10.3/8.1
Bender et al. (83)	51/53	Elective vascular surgery	PAC vs no PAC	Yes PCWP ≤14; CI >2.8; SVR ≤1100	Yes PCWP < 14 (crystalloid); CI < 2.8 (inotrope); SVR >(vasodilator)	Death: 1/1 Days hospitalized: 12.5/12

(Continued)

Table 1
(Continued)

Source	PAC vs no PAC	Population	Design	Hemodynamic targets	Treatment strategy	Results
Valentine et al. (84)	60/60	Aortic surgery	PAC vs no PAC	Yes PCWP < 15; CI >2.8; SVR < 1000	Yes PCWP < 15 (crystalloid); CI < 2.8 (inotrope); SVR >1000 (vasodilator)	Death: 3/1 Days hospitalized: 13/13
Bonazzi et al. (85)	50/50	Aortic surgery	PAC vs no PAC	Yes PCWP ≤18; CI ≥ 3.0; SVR < 1450; O_2 delivery >600	Yes PCWP < 18 (crystalloid); CI, 3.0 (inotrope); SVR >1450 (vasodilator)	Death: 0/0 Days hospitalized: 12/11
Rhodes et al. (86)	96/105	ICU	PAC vs no PAC	No	No	Death: 46/50 Days hospitalized: 13/14

Study	n	Condition	Comparison	Protocol target	Intervention	Outcome
Sandham et al. (41)	997/997	High-risk major surgery	PAC vs no PAC	Yes PCWP ≤18; CI ≥ 3.5; O_2 delivery >600; MAP ≥ 70; bpm < 120, Hct ≥ 27%	Yes In order: Crystalloid; inotropes; vasodilators; vasopressors; blood transfusion	Death: 78/77 Days hospitalized: 10/10
Richard et al. (42)	335/341	ICU w/ ARDS, sepsis, or both	PAC vs no PAC	No	No	Death: 199/208 Days hospitalized: 14/14
Binanay et al. (38)	215/218	NYHA IV heart failure	PAC vs no PAC	Yes PCWP ≤15; RA ≤8	No	Days alive and out of hospital: HR 1.0 (0.8–1.2)

bpm = heart rate; CI = cardiac index; HR =hazard ratio; Hct = hematocrit; MAP = mean arterial pressure; O_2 = oxygen delivery; PAC = pulmonary artery catheter; PCWP = pulmonary capillary wedge pressure; RA = right atrial pressure; SVR = systemic vascular index; VO_2 = oxygen consumption.

5.1.4. SAFETY AND EFFICACY OF THE PULMONARY ARTERY CATHETER IN ADVANCED DECOMPENSATED HEART FAILURE: THE ESCAPE TRIAL

The ESCAPE trial was a randomized study designed to evaluate whether therapy guided by PA catheter monitoring and clinical assessment would improve 6-month outcomes compared to therapy based on clinical assessment alone in patients admitted with advanced decompensated HF *(38)*. This study enrolled 433 patients at 26 experienced HF centers in the United States and Canada. Patients with a left ventricular ejection fraction (LVEF) $\leq$30%, recent hospitalization or escalation of outpatient diuretic therapy, and systolic blood pressure $\leq$125 mmHg who were admitted to the hospital with at least one sign and one symptom of HF, despite adequate treatment with angiotensin-converting enzyme inhibitors and diuretics, were included. Important exclusion criteria included a creatinine >3.5 mg/dl, the use of dobutamine/dopamine >3 μg/kg/min, or milrinone prior to randomization, and requirement for early right heart catheterization (RHC). The treatment goal in the clinical arm was resolution of clinical signs and symptoms of congestion and that in the PA catheter arm was similar with the addition of PCWP $\leq$15 mmHg and RAP $\leq$8 mmHg. The protocol did not specify drug selection but the routine use of inotropic agents was discouraged. The primary end-point of the ESCAPE trial was days alive and out of the hospital for 6 months after randomization. Secondary end-points included mitral regurgitation, natriuretic peptides, functional capacity, and quality of life.

In the ESCAPE trial, both treatment strategy groups experienced a substantial reduction in symptoms, jugular venous pressure, and edema. Use of the PA catheter in addition to clinical assessment significantly improved measured hemodynamics (RAP, PCWP, SVR, and cardiac index), but did not affect the primary end point of days alive and out of the hospital during the first 6 months (hazard ratio (HR), 1.00; 95% CI, 0.82–1.21) (Fig. 4). Secondary end-points including mortality (OR = 1.26; 95% CI, 0.78–2.03) and the number of days hospitalized (HR = 1.04; 95% CI, 0.86–1.27) also did not differ between the two groups. In-hospital adverse events were more common among patients in the PA catheter group (21.9% vs 11.5%, p = 0.04); however, there were no deaths related to its use and no difference in in-hospital plus 30-day mortality *(38)*.

There was a consistent trend for better functional capacity and quality of life in patients whose therapy was adjusted with the PA catheter (Fig. 4). The ESCAPE trial utilized a time trade-off assessment representing survival months to be traded for better health. Use of the PA catheter resulted in a greater improvement in time trade-off despite a non-significant, although greater, improvement in the Minnesota Living with Heart Failure Questionnaire as an assessment of quality of life. The extent of reduction in PCWP correlated with greater improvement in functional status, and the final PCWP was a strong predictor for the primary end-point demonstrating

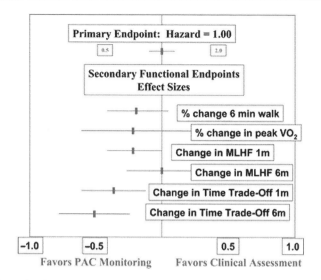

Fig. 4. Selected primary and secondary end-points from the ESCAPE trial. The ESCAPE trial randomized 433 patients admitted with advanced decompensated HF to therapy guided by a PA catheter in addition to clinical assessment ($N = 215$) vs therapy guided by clinical assessment alone ($N = 218$). The figure shows the hazard ratios for selected primary and secondary end-points. PA-catheter-guided therapy was not associated with an improvement in the primary end-point of days alive and out of hospital in the first 6 months. There was a trend toward benefit in the secondary functional end-points measured by the 6-minute walk distance and peak oxygen consumption (VO_2). Secondary end-points related to quality of life measured by the Minnesota Living with Heart Failure score (MLHF) and time trade-off instrument were also improved with PA catheter use. (Reprinted with permission from Stevenson.) *(76)*.

the importance of lowering filling pressures to the maximum extent possible (Fig. 5) *(38)*.

The findings of the ESCAPE trial were confirmed by a subsequent meta-analysis of 13 randomized controlled trials of 5051 patients treated with PA catheters in diverse clinical settings (Table 1). The combined odds ratio for mortality was 1.04 ($p = 0.59$) and there was no significant difference in the mean number of days hospitalized ($p = 0.73$) *(47)*.

5.1.5. RECOMMENDATIONS FOR THE USE OF PULMONARY ARTERY CATHETERS IN HEART FAILURE

Based on the largely neutral findings with PA catheter-guided therapy, the routine use of invasive hemodynamic monitoring in patients with advanced decompensated HF is not recommended *(48)*. Instead, PA catheter-based hemodynamic monitoring should only be considered in those patients who (1) have an unclear volume status on clinical examination, (2) have

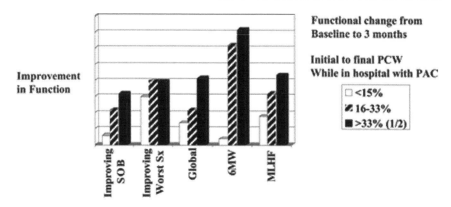

Fig. 5. Relationship between reduction in pulmonary capillary wedge pressure during hospitalization and improvement in symptoms and functional capacity at 3 months in the ESCAPE trial. The mean pulmonary capillary wedge pressure (PCW) fell from 25 ± 9 mmHg at baseline to 17 ± 7 mmHg after a median of 1.9 days of pulmonary catheter-guided therapy. Patients who experienced the largest percentage change in PCW pressure during hospitalization had the greatest improvement in symptoms and indices of functional capacity (6 MW) and quality of life (MLHF) at 3 months after discharge. SOB = shortness of breath; 6 MW = 6-min walk distance; MLHF = Minnesota Living with Heart Failure score. (Reprinted with permission from Stevenson.) *(76)*.

recurrent or refractory symptoms despite standard therapy adjusted according to clinical assessment, (3) have significant hypotension or renal failure during therapy and might benefit from delineation of the relationship between right- and left-sided filling pressures, (4) require documentation of an adequate hemodynamic response to an inotropic agent, if chronic outpatient infusion is being considered *(48)*, or (5) prior to consideration of advanced therapies such as transplantation. It is important to note that in the ESCAPE trial there was a trend toward better outcomes with PA catheters in centers with high-volume enrollment *(38)*. Perhaps it is not the inadequacy of the PA catheter as a diagnostic tool, but rather our inability to utilize the hemodynamic information appropriately, that resulted in a lack of benefit in the above-mentioned studies. Therefore, it is recommended that PA catheter use be minimized and restricted to those clinicians with adequate experience in the acquisition and interpretation of hemodynamic data *(49)*.

5.2. Implantable Hemodynamic Monitors (IHM)

One of the criticisms of the ESCAPE trial has been that it is difficult to judge the value of a diagnostic tool on long-term outcomes if the tool itself is only utilized for a short duration (i.e., during the initial hospitalization). It has been argued that since patients have fluctuating volume status after hospital discharge and require multiple medication changes based on clinical assessment *(33)*, the initial benefits of hemodynamic monitoring might have been negated by these subsequent interventions. Therefore, it has been postulated that continuous hemodynamic monitoring with an implantable device might allow early detection and optimization of filling pressures in the ambulatory setting, leading to a more sustained improvement in symptoms, decreased hospitalizations, and better outcomes. Additionally, continuous hemodynamic monitoring might provide a unique opportunity to better understand the pathophysiology of chronic HF and the response to different treatment modalities.

Several implantable hemodynamic monitoring (IHM) devices are currently under development and investigation for the frequent and long-term monitoring of hemodynamic parameters in patients with chronic HF. The IHM devices that have been investigated most extensively to date have relied on using the pulmonary artery diastolic pressure (PAD) as a surrogate for PCWP. Some of the earlier devices consisted of a transvenous lead positioned directly in the pulmonary artery with a direct pressure sensor for measuring pulmonary artery pressures *(50)*. Subsequent models have utilized an RV lead with a pressure sensor capable of measuring RV pulse pressure and the maximum derivative of RV pressure (dP/dt_{max}). These later devices rely on the concept that the pulmonic valve opens at the time of maximum rate of positive pressure development (dP/dt_{max}) in the RV when RV pressure equals PAD (Fig. 6) *(51–53)*. This estimation of the pulmonary artery diastolic pressure (ePAD) from a sensor in the RV rather than in the pulmonary artery capitalizes on the extensive safety experience with transvenous RV leads in pacemakers and implantable cardioverter defibrillators (ICDs). Several models also contain a lead with a sensor capable of measuring mixed venous oxygen saturation (SvO_2), allowing estimation of CO (Fig. 7) *(50, 54, 55)*.

5.2.1. THE MEDTRONIC CHRONICLE® IMPLANTABLE HEMODYNAMIC MONITOR DESIGN

The Chronicle IHM (Medtronic, Inc., Minneapolis, Minnesota) has the largest amount of clinical data thus far; therefore, the discussion on IHMs will focus on this device. The Chronicle® IHM is a long-term implantable device designed to record ongoing RV pressures, pressure derivatives, and heart rate (HR) *(56)*. It does not contain an SvO_2 sensor due to bio-interface problems (fibrin deposition and encapsulation) with this optical sensor in earlier IHM models. It consists of a programmable memory device placed in the pectoral area and a transvenous electrode carrying a pressure sensor in the RV outflow tract. The device continuously measures RV systolic and diastolic pressures, RV dP/dt_{max}, ePAD, HR (via a unipolar electrogram recorded at the tip of the lead), patient activity, and temperature. An external device, which patients keep with them, records ambient barometric pressure

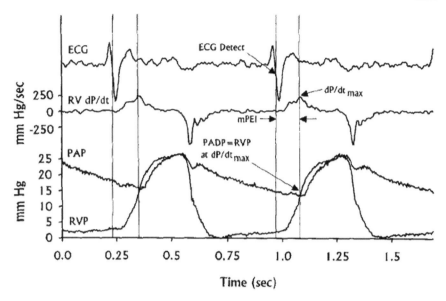

Fig. 6. Schematic illustration depicting estimation of pulmonary artery diastolic pressure from the maximal first derivative of right ventricular pressure. The computer detects each QRS complex on the electrocardiogram (ECG) to mark the onset of each beat (ECG detect) and measures right ventricular (RV) pressure signals on a beat-by-beat basis. From each cardiac cycle, it derives the value of the first derivative of the RV pressure waveform (RV dP/dt). The time from detection of the QRS complex to the occurrence of dP/dt_{max} is defined as the modified pre-ejection period (mPEI) and refers to the period of isovolumic contraction. Because pulmonary valve opening occurs at the end of isovolumic contraction, the RV pressure at the time of dP/dt_{max} is the estimate of pulmonary artery diastolic pressure (PADP). PAP = pulmonary artery pressure; RVP = right ventricular pressure. (Reprinted with permission from Reynolds et al.) *(51)*.

once per minute for calibration (similar to zeroing standard pressure transducers). When stored hemodynamic information from the device is interrogated, the barometric pressure is subtracted from the device data to provide relative pressures in the RV. Information stored in the device is transmitted via standard radio-frequency telemetry methods that have been verified for pacemakers and ICDs. Data are then available to caregivers on a secure centralized file server via an Internet web site. Thus caregivers can access relevant physiologic quantitative data as well as real-time ventricular pressure waveforms, allowing visual verification of device function (Fig. 8).

5.2.2. VALIDATION OF THE CHRONICLE® IMPLANTABLE HEMODYNAMIC MONITOR

Validation of the data obtained by the Chronicle® IHM device was performed by comparing IHM signals with hemodynamic values obtained from

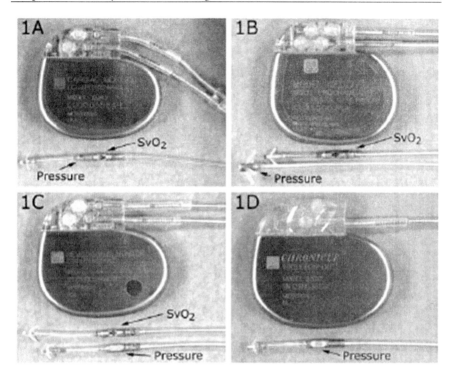

Fig. 7. Different models of implantable hemodynamic monitoring devices. All devices shown are manufactured by Medtronic, Inc. (Minneapolis, MN). (1A) Model 10040 IHM-0 with single lead for measuring right ventricular (RV) oxygen saturation (SvO_2) and pressures; (1B) Model 2507 CHF-Pacer with separate leads to measure RV SvO_2 and pulmonary artery absolute pressures; (1C) Model 10343 IHM-1 with separate leads for monitoring RV SvO_2 and RV absolute pressures, including estimated pulmonary artery diastolic pressure; (1D) Model 9520 IHM-2 (Chronicle®) with single lead for measuring RV absolute pressures, including estimated pulmonary artery diastolic pressure. (Reprinted with permission from Bennett et al.) *(6)*.

simultaneous serial RHCs. In 32 patients with chronic HF (LVEF, 29 ± 11%) the Chronicle® IHM device was implanted and pressure parameters derived from the device were correlated to measurements made with a balloon-tipped catheter at implantation, 3, 6, and 12 months *(57)*. Values were recorded during supine rest, peak response of the Valsalva maneuver, sitting, peak of a two-stage bicycle exercise test, and a recovery period. Combining all interventions, correlation coefficients (r) at implantation and at 1 year were 0.96 and 0.94 for RV systolic pressure, 0.96 and 0.83 for RV diastolic pressure, and 0.87 and 0.87 for ePAD, respectively (Fig. 9) *(57)*. Similar results have been obtained with other IHMs that contain both sensors that measure RV pressures and SvO_2 *(50, 54, 55)*. These data suggest that IHMs are accurate in a variety of physiologic conditions and over time,

A.

Mean Hemodynamic Values at Rest	This Transmission 05–Sep–2007	Previous Transmission 28–Aug–2007	Difference	
Total nights at rest (12AM to 4AM)	8 / 8	15 / 15		
Heart Rate (bpm)	66	62	4	(6.5%)
RV Diastolic Pressure (mmHg)	**12**	**1**	**11**	**(1100.0%)**
RV Systolic Pressure (mmHg)	**34**	**25**	**9**	**(36.0%)**
ePAD (mmHg)	**21**	**12**	**9**	**(75.0%)**
Mean Pulmonary Artery Pressure (mmHg)	27	17	10	(58.8%)
RV dP/dt max (mmHg/sec)	**176**	**166**	10	(6.0%)
RV Pulse Pressure (mmHg)	15	14	1	(7.1%)

Note: Out of range values highlighted in bold.

B.

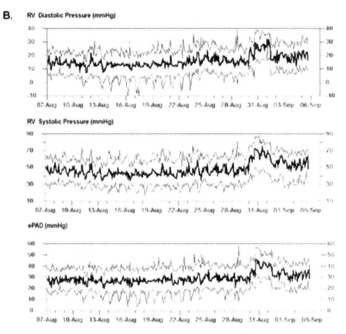

Fig. 8. Representative output from the Chronicle® implantable hemodynamic monitor. Panel A reflects the median value for the nightly (12 am to 4 am) minimum pressures over a 2-week interval. Panel B shows some of the waveform trends over a 1-month period for the same patient. RV = right ventricular; ePAD = estimated pulmonary artery diastolic pressure; dP/dt = first derivative of RV pressure waveform.

providing a potentially important tool to continuously monitor hemodynamics in ambulatory patients with chronic HF.

5.2.3. CLINICAL TRIALS WITH THE CHRONICLE® IMPLANTABLE HEMODYNAMIC MONITOR IN HEART FAILURE

Thus far, two clinical trials evaluating the impact of the Chronicle® IHM on HF hospitalizations have been completed. An initial non-randomized

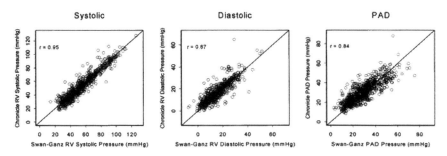

Fig. 9. Regression analyses relating pressures derived from the Chronicle® Implantable hemodynamic monitor to pressures measured by a pulmonary artery catheter. Plots are based on composite data from 32 HF patients subjected to various physiologic condition including rest, exercise, and the Valsalva maneuver at time of implantation, 3, 6, and 12 months. RV = right ventricle; PAD = pulmonary artery diastolic pressure. (Reprinted with permission from Magalski, et al.) *(57)*.

prospective study enrolled 32 patients with NYHA Class II/III HF (LVEF 29 ± 11%) *(56)*. Clinicians were blinded to information obtained from the Chronicle® IHM device for the first 9 months after implantation and were allowed to use the IHM information to make clinical decisions for the next 17 months. The effect of the Chronicle® IHM on HF hospitalization was compared to the blinded phase (9 months) plus historical information from the 12 months prior to implantation. In the 28 patients not lost to follow-up, there were 52 HF hospitalizations prior to the availability of IHM-derived hemodynamic information compared to 18 hospitalizations in the 17 months of follow-up (p <0.01). During the blinded phase, in 9/12 cases a sustained increase (>20%) in at least one pressure parameter was observed 4 ± 2 days prior to a clinical exacerbation requiring hospitalization. In all exacerbations, including those requiring hospitalization or outpatient diuretic adjustment, IHM pressures increased 24 h prior to clinical intervention. These findings supported the hypothesis that continuous, ambulatory invasive hemodynamic monitoring permits early detection of volume overload, thus allowing early intervention and a reduction in HF hospitalizations.

The encouraging preliminary experience with the Chronicle® IHM device led to a multi-center, randomized, single-blind, controlled study of 274 patients with NYHA Class III/IV HF who had at least one HF-related hospitalization, emergency room visit, or urgent care visit within the 6 months prior to enrollment. All patients enrolled in the Chronicle Offers Management to Patients with Advanced Signs and Symptoms of Heart Failure (COMPASS-HF) trial *(58, 59)* underwent placement of the Chronicle® IHM device and were randomized to optimal HF management alone ($N = $ 140) or optimal HF therapy plus IHM-guided care ($N = 134$). Patients were blinded to their treatment assignment and transmitted data remotely to their physicians on a regular basis (at least once per week). In the COMPASS-

HF trial, 99% of the devices were successfully implanted. There were fewer than 10% device complications and no sensor failures. Although, there was a 21% reduction in heart-failure-related events (hospitalizations, emergency visits, and urgent care visits) in the Chronicle® IHM group over the 6-month follow-up period, this difference was not statistically significant ($p = 0.33$) (Table 2). However, retrospective analyses revealed that the time to first HF event was delayed significantly in the Chronicle group (36% relative risk reduction, $p = 0.03$) and patients with NYHA Class III HF symptoms appeared to benefit more from the Chronicle® device than those with NYHA Class IV symptoms.

Table 2
Results of the primary end-point in the COMPASS-HF trial

	Chronicle (N = 134)	Control (N = 140)
No. of patients with events	44	60
Total HF-related events	84	113
Hospitalizations	72	99
Emergency room visits	10	11
Urgent care visits	2	3
Event rate/6 months	0.67	0.85
Percentage of reduction in event rate	21% ($p = 0.33$)	

HF = heart failure.

5.3. Other Investigational Implantable Hemodynamic Monitoring Devices

Other implantable hemodynamic monitoring devices currently under investigation in humans include left atrial pressure (LAP) sensing devices and the wireless CardioMEMS HF sensor (CardioMEMS Inc., Atlanta, Georgia). The LAP sensing devices consist of a pressure transducer implanted in the inter-atrial septum or in the left atrial appendage via a transseptal approach. The pressure transducer is connected to an electrical lead which is then connected to a device implanted in the pectoral region that processes the electrical signal. The device is interrogated with a radio-frequency hand-held wand to provide measurements of LAP. Alternatively, some of the devices are designed to interpret the LAP information to generate a signal that is communicated to the patient via a signaling device (vibration or spoken command), following which the patient administers to him/herself the therapy prescribed by the signaling device (60). A feasibility study using an implantable LAP sensor was recently conducted in nine patients with NYHA Class II–IV symptoms and evidence of recent HF decompensation. Patients were asked to interrogate the device twice daily.

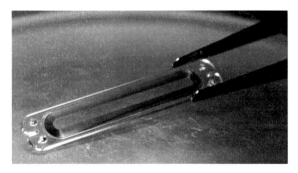

Fig. 10. CardioMEMS® wireless pulmonary artery pressure monitor.

Clinicians were blinded to device readings for the first 3 months. There-after, patients were managed dynamically based on LAP readings according to preset physician-prescribed instructions programmed into the signaling device. Dynamic therapy led to improved hemodynamics (p <0.001), fewer episodes of LAP >25 mmHg (p <0.001), better utilization of neurohormonal antagonists, and reduction in loop diuretic doses without any HF hospital-izations during this period *(60)*.

The CardioMEMS® wireless HF sensor is a proprietary miniature device, the size of a grain of rice, which is implanted in the pulmonary artery via a catheter-based procedure (Fig. 10). The device is capable of measuring pulmonary artery pressures and CO that can be interrogated with a hand-held antenna and transmitted wirelessly to a secure database that is accessible via a proprietary web site. A similar device has been extensively studied in patients who have undergone endovascular abdominal aortic aneurysm repair *(61)* and a feasibility trial of the HF device is now underway in the United States *(58)*.

Based on available clinical trial data, no IHM device has yet been approved by the Food and Drug Administration for clinical use. Future stud-ies in the field of IHM devices, either independent or combined with other modalities such as pacemakers and ICDs, will further define the role of inva-sive ambulatory monitoring in the outpatient management of patients with HF.

6. NON-INVASIVE METHODS OF HEMODYNAMIC MONITORING

It remains unclear whether the lack of benefit from invasive RHC relates to device complications or an inability to appropriately utilize hemody-namic information obtained from the catheter to improve outcomes in HF. RHC has been associated with complications including arrhythmias, RV or pulmonary artery perforation, pulmonary infarction, and infection. The fear of these potential complications has led to a shift away from the PA catheter to increasingly available non-invasive methods for the assessment of ventricular filling pressures and CO. In the section below we will discuss some of the commonly utilized non-invasive hemodynamic modalities and the clinical data supporting their use.

6.1. Non-invasive Assessment of Hemodynamics by Echocardiography

Echocardiography has long been the mainstay for assessing RV and LV functions and severity of valvular regurgitation in patients with HF. The widespread availability and versatility of echocardiography makes it an important tool in the non-invasive assessment of hemodynamics in HF. Non-invasive measurements of CO, pulmonary artery pressures, and left- and right-sided filling pressures can be obtained with reasonable accuracy and at frequent intervals to titrate and assess the response to therapy.

Doppler techniques have emerged as the modality of choice for the echocardiographic evaluation of hemodynamics. Non-invasive hemodynamic variables can be estimated as follows: CO by pulsed Doppler of the LV outflow tract, PCWP by a regression equation involving mitral and pulmonary venous flow variables, pulmonary artery pressures from tricuspid valve velocities, and pulmonary vascular resistance from the previous measurements (62). Although the feasibility and accuracy of Doppler-derived hemodynamics have been validated with simultaneous RHC by several investigators (62), the technique is criticized because of its dependence on patient habitus and operator skill for the appropriate acquisition and interpretation of data. The use of contrast-enhanced Doppler echocardiography can substantially increase the feasibility and accuracy of obtaining PCWP, mean pulmonary artery pressure, and pulmonary vascular resistance in patients with LV dysfunction (63). When compared to invasive techniques, the correlation coefficients for these variables were consistently about 0.90 (63). Newer modalities such as tissue Doppler of diastolic mitral annular velocity (Ea) combined with pulsed Doppler of transmitral flow in early diastole (E) can provide an E/Ea ratio which is also well correlated with LV filling pressures (21). An E/Ea ratio >15 can predict a PCWP >15 mmHg with a sensitivity of 86% and a specificity of 88% (21). These predictive values have been shown to be superior to those for BNP in patients with systolic HF (21).

6.2. Bioimpedance Cardiography

Bioimpedance cardiography (ICG) allows for the non-invasive measurement of hemodynamics by applying Ohm's law to assess impedance to the conduction of an alternating current applied across the thorax as a function of blood volume in the heart and great vessels (64). Because blood is a strong conductor of current compared to the surrounding thoracic tissues, the greater the blood velocity in the great vessels, the lower the impedance *(64)*. There are two basic technologies of ICG: whole-body ICG (established in 1948) and thoracic ICG (established in 1964) whereby the electrodes are applied either to the distal limbs or to the root of the neck and lower chest, respectively. The basic tool for measuring impedance in the body is the potentiometer and the two bipolar electrodes applied to the body as described in Fig. 11. Continuous electric current stimulation is transmitted across the thorax while the sensors measure the changes in electrical impedance caused by changes in the thoracic cavity. Alignment of the waveform for the first derivative of impedance (dZ/dt) with the simultaneous electrocardiogram is shown in Fig. 11. ICG distinguishes two phases of systole as follows: (1) the pre-ejection period (PEP) or isovolumic contraction which corresponds to the period from the beginning of the Q wave on the ECG to the B wave on the dZ/dt waveform and (2) the left ventricular ejection time (LVET) which corresponds to the period between the B and X waves on the impedance curve. ICG estimates stroke volume using baseline impedance (Z_0), maximum thoracic impedance (dZ/dt_{max}), and LVET *(64)*. As cardiac function deteriorates, PEP lengthens and LVET shortens. The baseline impedance (Z_0) can also be used to estimate intravascular volume status or thoracic fluid content (TFC). Increased pericardial, intra-alveolar, or pleural fluid can decrease Z_0 while normal or volume depleted states can increase Z_0 *(64)*.

Non-invasive ICG has been used to estimate CO and filling pressures in both patients with and without HF. When the CO is measured in subjects with healthy hearts, the results are usually reliable and many validation studies have been performed comparing ICG with CO determination by thermodilution or the Fick method in these relatively healthy patients. A meta-analysis of 112 studies comparing CO derived by ICG to various reference methods demonstrated an overall correlation coefficient of 0.82 (95% CI, 0.80–0.84) *(65)*. However, CO measurements taken by ICG in studies restricted to patients with cardiac diseases were not so reliable (r 0.73; 95% CI, 0.66–0.79) *(65)*. Of note, the correlation improved substantially with repeated measurements, compared to a single measurement, in the same patient *(65)*.

Since then, several studies have compared non-invasive ICG assessment of CO and TFC with CO and PCWP obtained by simultaneous RHC in patients with HF (Table 3). Three small studies of patients with systolic HF (stable and unstable) have demonstrated a significant correlation between ICG CO and that measured by thermodilution *(66–68)* and Fick methodologies *(67)*. However, there have been conflicting results regarding the correlation between TFC obtained by non-invasive ICG and PCWP *(66, 67)*. The accuracy of non-invasive ICG as a means for evaluation of hemodynamics in patients hospitalized with advanced decompensated HF was further investigated in the Bioimpedance Cardiography (BIG) substudy of the

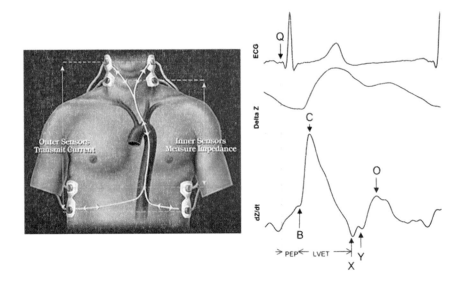

Fig. 11. Thoracic impedance cardiography. Four dual sensors with eight lead wires are placed on the neck and chest. Current transmitted by the outer sensors seeks the path of least resistance (i.e., blood-filled aorta). Baseline impedance (resistance) to the signal is measured by the inner sensors. With each heartbeat, blood volume and velocity in the aorta change and the corresponding change in impedance is measured. The first tracing is an electrocardiogram (ECG), the second represents thoracic impedance with baseline impedance (Z_0) represented by the straight line, and the third tracing depicts dZ/dt. The thoracic fluid content (TFC) is the inverse of Z_0. Q = ventricular depolarization on the ECG; PEP = pre-ejection period; LVET = left ventricular ejection time; B = opening of the aortic valve; C = maximal acceleration of blood in the aorta (dZ/dt_{max}); X = closing of the aortic valve; Y = pulmonic valve closure; O = mitral valve opening. Cardiac output is calculated from LVET $(dZ/dt)_{max}$ and Z_0.

ESCAPE trial *(69)*. In this study, 170 patients randomized to the PA catheter arm underwent simultaneous ICG and PA catheter measurements at baseline and prior to discharge. ICG-derived measures correlated modestly at baseline and after medical intervention with PA catheter-derived measures of CO and cardiac index. However, there was no correlation at baseline or after interventions between TFC and PCWP. Although, RAP at baseline was correlated with TFC, this association was no longer seen after HF therapy *(69)*. Based on these findings, it is felt that non-invasive ICG measurements do not yet provide an accurate assessment of filling pressures in patients hospitalized with decompensated HF and therefore should not be used as a surrogate for RHC, where clinically indicated.

The utility of serial non-invasive ICG monitoring to improve outcomes in ambulatory HF patients is currently being evaluated. In a study of stable

Table 3
ICG accuracy studies in heart failure

Source	Population	N	EF, %	Index	Comparison	R	P value
Woltjer et al. (66)	Stable HF	24	–	CO	ICG–TD	0.69	<0.05
				PCWP	TFC	0.92	<0.0001
Drazner et al. (67)	HF in cath lab	59	25 ± 12	CO	ICG–TD	0.76	<0.001
				PCWP	ICG–Fick	0.73	<0.001
				RA	TFC	0.05	0.71
					TFC	0.08	0.56
Albert et al. (68)	HF in ICU	29	17 ± 8	CO	ICG–TD	0.89	<0.0001
Yancy et al. (69)	Decompensated HF	170	20 ± 7	*Baseline*	ICG–TD	0.41	<0.001
				CO	TFC	0.18	0.20
				PCWP	TFC	0.40	<0.001
				RA	ICG–TD	0.62	<0.001
				Post-Rx	TFC	−0.01	0.94
				CO	TFC	−0.08	0.60
				PCWP			
				RA			

HF = heart failure; EF = ejection fraction; R = correlation coefficient; CO = cardiac output; PCWP = pulmonary capillary wedge pressure; RA = right atrial pressure; ICG = impedance cardiography; TD = thermodilution; TFC = thoracic fluid content. $P<0.05$ considered statistically significant.

patients with known HF and a recent episode of clinical decompensation, ICG measurements of stroke index and TFC, in addition to clinical variables, were used to generate a risk score to successfully identify patients at increased near-term risk of recurrent decompensation *(69)*. In this study, 212 patients underwent serial clinical evaluation and blinded ICG testing every 2 weeks for 26 weeks. Patients were followed up for the occurrence of death from any cause or worsening HF requiring hospitalization or emergent care. Multivariate analysis identified six clinical and three ICG variables that independently predicted an event within 14 days of assessment. The clinical variables included visual analog score, NYHA functional class, and systolic blood pressure. ICG parameters were velocity index, TFC index, and LVET. The three ICG parameters combined into a composite score were useful in predicting an event during the next 14 days ($p = 0.0002$). Additionally, the authors demonstrated that ICG-derived stroke index and TFC index alone could be used to construct a 2×2 table that identified low-, intermediate-, and high-risk subsets among ambulatory patients with chronic HF (Fig. 12) *(70)*. Further validation of this risk score in an independent population is required before it can be clinically applied.

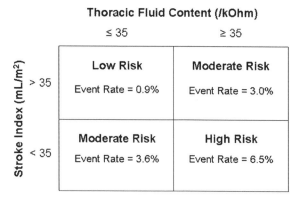

Fig. 12. Risk profiles for heart failure event within 14 days based on bioimpedance hemodynamic assessment. The PREDICT study *(69)* proposes that patients can be placed into a 2 × 2 table according to low or high thoracic fluid content and low or high stroke index to identify hemodynamic profiles that predict risk of HF event defined as death, worsening HF hospitalization, or emergency visit. The relative risk for the highest risk profile was seven times that for the lowest risk profile (95% CI, 4.7–9.9). (Modified from Packer et al.) *(70)*.

Serial monitoring for fluid overload with non-invasive ICG may not be reliable because of the variation in TFC measurements due to placement of the external electrodes, skin–electrode contact, and chest wall movement *(71)*. Moreover, non-invasive monitoring is limited since the measurements are only available at clinic visits and do not allow remote, continuous evaluation of the patient. This has led to the incorporation of thoracic impedance detection algorithms in existing devices such as ICDs or biventricular pacemakers. These devices utilize the pacemaker's activity and minute ventilation sensors and an RV lead. A constant current is sent from the device case electrode to the RV coil electrode where voltage (used to calculate impedance) is measured (Fig. 13A). The vector between these two locations encompasses a portion of the thoracic cavity. As fluid accumulates in the pulmonary vasculature, resistance across the cavity, measured as impedance, decreases. Post-surgical local edema decreases impedance in the first month after device implantation. Daily impedance measurements thereafter can be averaged to create a baseline impedance value (Z_0) specific to each patient.

A study of 33 patients with NYHA Class III/IV HF was used to define an impedance threshold that predicted clinical decompensation leading to HF hospitalization *(71)*. Intrathoracic impedance decreased before each admission by $12.3 \pm 5.3\%$ ($p < 0.001$) (Fig. 13B). Impedance reduction was observed 15 days before the onset of symptoms of HF, confirming that symptoms are a late marker of clinical decompensation. Simultaneous RHC revealed an inverse correlation between intrathoracic impedance and PCWP

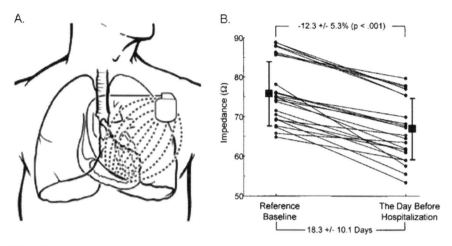

Fig. 13. Invasive assessment of filling pressures using intrathoracic impedance algorithms. (**A**) The OptiVol fluid status monitoring (Medtronic, Inc., Minneapolis, MN) measures intrathoracic impedance using the vector between the device case and the right ventricular lead. (**B**) Comparison of intrathoracic impedance at reference baseline and 1 day before admission for 24 hospitalizations resulting from worsening HF in nine patients. (Reprinted with permission from Yu et al.) *(71)*.

($r = -0.61$, $p < 0.001$) and net fluid loss ($r = -0.71$, $p < 0.001$) in hospitalized patients *(71)*. Validation of this algorithm in 26 additional patients suggested that an impedance index (absolute change in impedance from baseline × number of days) $\geq$ 60 Ohm-days has a sensitivity of 76.9% and a false positive rate of 1.5 false positives per patient-year *(71)*. This detection threshold was further validated in 115 patients with NYHA Class III/IV HF who required biventricular cardioverter defibrillators *(72)*. Out of 45 alerts in 30 patients, only 15 alerts occurred in concert with a clinical diagnosis of HF decompensation. With a threshold of 60 Ohm-days, sensitivity was excellent, but specificity was quite poor. A new optimal threshold of 120 Ohm-days demonstrated a sensitivity and specificity of 60 and 73%, respectively (Fig. 14).

6.3. Non-invasive Measurement of Left Ventricular End-Diastolic Pressure Based on the Arterial Blood Pressure Response to the Valsalva Maneuver

It is worth recalling that simple bedside measures of hemodynamic status have been established previously and continue to be valid tools. The response of the arterial blood pressure to the Valsalva maneuver is an accurate non-invasive predictor of PCWP *(16)*. In 1992, McIntyre et al.

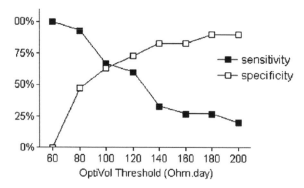

Fig. 14. Receiver-operating characteristic curve analysis on the threshold for the OptiVol® alert ($\Omega \cdot$ day) in predicting decompensated heart failure. (Reprinted with permission from Ypenburg et al.) *(72)*.

(74) demonstrated that the ratio of the final to the initial amplitude of the arterial pulse waveform during the strain phase of the Valsalva maneuver (pulse–amplitude ratio) was highly correlated with invasive PCWP in both stable ($r = 0.89$) and unstable ($r = 0.92$) catheterized cardiac patients. Moreover, the pulse–amplitude ratio was also capable of predicting changes in the PCWP after medical interventions including acute vasodilation, diuresis, and volume loading ($r = 0.89$) *(74)*. This concept has been leveraged in the VeriCor® device (CVP Diagnostics, Inc., Boston, MA) which is FDA approved for the non-invasive estimation of LV end-diastolic pressure. The VeriCor® device consists of a digital expiratory manometer coupled with a continuous arterial pressure monitor and a computer. A tonometric sensor is attached to the patient's wrist with a blood pressure cuff attached to the arm. After an 8-min calibration period, the patient is asked to perform a Valsalva maneuver by blowing into the mouthpiece of the digital manometer to produce an expiratory pressure of 20–35 mmHg for a minimum of 8 s. The arterial pressure signals are then analyzed according to algorithms designed to predict PCWP *(74)*. The accuracy of this device was validated in a study of 49 patients undergoing elective right and left heart catheterization *(75)*. VeriCor® measurements were compared to LV end-diastolic pressure measured directly and by the use of a PA catheter. The VeriCor® measurements correlated well with direct measurements of LV end-diastolic pressure ($r = 0.86$; $p < 0.001$) and outperformed the PCWP, which had a correlation coefficient of 0.81 with LV end-diastolic pressure *(75)*. Despite its accuracy and non-invasive nature, this device has not gained popularity because of practical limitations. Beat-to-beat variation in arterial pulse pressure prohibits use of this device in patients with arrhythmias. Furthermore, patients must maintain uniform strain at the desired level (20–35 mmHg) during the Valsalva maneuver as erratic strain may transiently increase arterial pressure and make results unreliable *(75)*. Greater experience with this device and

studies evaluating its impact on outcomes in patients with HF are needed before it can be widely used.

7. SUMMARY

Despite substantial therapeutic advances, patients with HF continue to experience significant morbidity and mortality. Most of the symptoms that limit daily life and routine activities result primarily from elevated filling pressures *(76, 77)*. The basic goals of therapy therefore remain grounded in improving symptoms of congestion, decreasing hospitalizations, and improving quality of life, in addition to promoting longevity. Evaluation of hemodynamic parameters is therefore necessary to guide and monitor the effect of therapies in both the inpatient and ambulatory settings.

A careful history and physical examination can successfully identify hemodynamic profiles based on the absence or presence of congestion and adequacy of perfusion in most patients with HF *(18)*. However, symptoms may resolve before optimal diuresis or persist due to concomitant conditions. The physical examination can also be limited by patient habitus and physician experience. The invasive PA catheter has long been the gold standard for evaluating hemodynamics and the adequacy of treatment in cases where the clinical profile is ambiguous, symptoms persist despite empiric therapy, treatment is thwarted by hypotension or progressive renal dysfunction, or consideration is being given to advanced modalities such as ventricular assist device placement or transplantation *(48)*. Despite its widespread use, several randomized trials *(47)*, including the ESCAPE trial in patients with advanced decompensated HF *(38)*, have failed to show significant reductions in hospitalization or mortality with PA catheter-guided therapy. However, patients randomized to PA catheter-guided therapy in the ESCAPE trial demonstrated a significant short-term improvement in quality of life measures compared to those randomized to empiric treatment *(38)*. This observation begs us to question whether the apparent failure of PA catheterization reflects risks inherent to the invasiveness of the procedure or is due to the transient nature of the intervention with empiric management thereafter. Future trials of non-invasive hemodynamic monitoring modalities and continuous implantable hemodynamic monitors will help answer this question better.

In conclusion, it is clear that hemodynamic variables can be accurately measured, but that interventions based on this information improve outcomes in patients with HF has not been established. Although available data caution against the routine use of PA catheters, it remains unclear whether alternate hemodynamic monitoring tools are any better. The trend toward benefit with PA catheter-guided therapy in high-enrollment centers also leaves open the larger question that it is not the catheter per se, but rather the ability to make medical changes based on the information derived from it, that requires further refinement.

REFERENCES

1. Rosamond W, Flegal K, Friday G, et al. Heart disease and stroke statistics – 2007 update: a report from the American Heart Association Statistics Committee and Stroke Statistics Subcommittee. *Circulation.* Feb 6 2007;115(5):e69–171.

2. Rector TS, Ringwala SN, Ringwala SN, et al. Validation of a risk score for dying within 1 year of an admission for heart failure. *J Card Fail.* May 2006;12(4):276–280.

3. Siirila-Waris K, Lassus J, Melin J, et al. Characteristics, outcomes, and predictors of 1-year mortality in patients hospitalized for acute heart failure. *Eur Heart J.* Dec 2006;27(24):3011–3017.

4. Goldberg RJ, Ciampa J, Lessard D, et al. Long-term survival after heart failure: a contemporary population-based perspective. *Arch Intern Med.* Mar 12 2007;167(5): 490–496.

5. Friedman M. Older adults' symptoms and their duration before hospitalization for heart failure. *Heart Lung.* 1997;26:169–176.

6. Bennett S, Huster G, Baker S, et al. Characterization of the precipitants of hospitalization for heart failure decompensation. *Am J Crit Care.* 1998;7:168–174.

7. Keogh AM, Baron DW, Hickie JB. Prognostic guides in patients with idiopathic or ischemic dilated cardiomyopathy assessed for cardiac transplantation. *Am J Cardiol.* Apr 1 1990;65(13):903–908.

8. Campana C, Gavazzi A, Berzuini C, et al. Predictors of prognosis in patients awaiting heart transplantation. *J Heart Lung Transplant.* Sep–Oct 1993;12(5): 756–765.

9. Stevenson LW, Tillisch JH, Hamilton M, et al. Importance of hemodynamic response to therapy in predicting survival with ejection fraction less than or equal to 20% secondary to ischemic or nonischemic dilated cardiomyopathy. *Am J Cardiol.* Dec 1 1990;66(19):1348–1354.

10. Lucas C, Johnson W, Hamilton MA, et al. Freedom from congestion predicts good survival despite previous class IV symptoms of heart failure. *Am Heart J.* 2000;140(6): 840–847.

11. Watanabe J, Levine MJ, Bellotto F, et al. Effects of coronary venous pressure on left ventricular diastolic distensibility. *Circ Res.* Oct 1990;67(4):923–932.

12. Rosario LB, Stevenson LW, Solomon SD, et al. The mechanism of decrease in dynamic mitral regurgitation during heart failure treatment: importance of reduction in the regurgitant orifice size. *J Am Coll Cardiol.* Dec 1998;32(7):1819–1824.

13. Stevenson LW, Perloff JK. The limited reliability of physical signs for estimating hemodynamics in chronic heart failure. *Jama.* Feb 10 1989;261(6):884–888.

14. Chakko S, Woska D, Martinez H, et al. Clinical, radiographic, and hemodynamic correlations in chronic congestive heart failure: conflicting results may lead to inappropriate care. *Am J Med.* Mar 1991;90(3):353–359.

15. Ewy GA. The abdominojugular test: technique and hemodynamic correlates. *Ann Intern Med.* Sep 15 1988;109(6):456–460.

16. Schmidt DE, Shah PK. Accurate detection of elevated left ventricular filling pressure by a simplified bedside application of the Valsalva maneuver. *Am J Cardiol.* Feb 15 1993;71(5):462–465.

17. Drazner MH, Yancy CW, Shah MR, et al. Utility of the history and physical examination in assessing hemodynamics in patients with advanced heart failure: the ESCAPE trial. *Circulation.* 2005;112(17):II-640.

18. Nohria A, Tsang SW, Fang JC, et al. Clinical assessment identifies hemodynamic profiles that predict outcomes in patients admitted with heart failure. *J Am Coll Cardiol.* 2003;41(10):1797–1804.

19. Maisel AS, Clopton P, Krishnaswamy P, et al. Impact of age, race, and sex on the ability of B-type natriuretic peptide to aid in the emergency diagnosis of heart failure:

results from the Breathing Not Properly (BNP) multinational study. *Am Heart J.* Jun 2004;147(6):1078–1084.

20. Januzzi JL, Jr., Camargo CA, Anwaruddin S, et al. The N-terminal Pro-BNP investigation of dyspnea in the emergency department (PRIDE) study. *Am J Cardiol.* Apr 15 2005;95(8):948–954.

21. Dokainish H, Zoghbi WA, Lakkis NM, et al. Optimal noninvasive assessment of left ventricular filling pressures: a comparison of tissue Doppler echocardiography and B-type natriuretic peptide in patients with pulmonary artery catheters. *Circulation.* May 25 2004;109(20):2432–2439.

22. Parsonage WA, Galbraith AJ, Koerbin GL, et al. Value of B-type natriuretic peptide for identifying significantly elevated pulmonary artery wedge pressure in patients treated for established chronic heart failure secondary to ischemic or idiopathic dilated cardiomyopathy. *Am J Cardiol.* Apr 1 2005;95(7):883–885.

23. O'Donoghue M, Chen A, Baggish AL, et al. The effects of ejection fraction on N-terminal ProBNP and BNP levels in patients with acute CHF: analysis from the ProBNP Investigation of Dyspnea in the Emergency Department (PRIDE) study. *J Card Fail.* Jun 2005;11(5 Suppl):S9–14.

24. Vanderheyden M, Goethals M, Verstreken S, et al. Wall stress modulates brain natriuretic peptide production in pressure overload cardiomyopathy. *J Am Coll Cardiol.* Dec 21 2004;44(12):2349–2354.

25. Tsutamoto T, Wada A, Sakai H, et al. Relationship between renal function and plasma brain natriuretic peptide in patients with heart failure. *J Am Coll Cardiol.* Feb 7 2006;47(3):582–586.

26. Krauser DG, Lloyd-Jones DM, Chae CU, et al. Effect of body mass index on natriuretic peptide levels in patients with acute congestive heart failure: a ProBNP Investigation of Dyspnea in the Emergency Department (PRIDE) substudy. *Am Heart J.* Apr 2005;149(4):744–750.

27. Kazanegra R, Cheng V, Garcia A, et al. A rapid test for B-type natriuretic peptide correlates with falling wedge pressures in patients treated for decompensated heart failure: a pilot study. *J Card Fail.* Mar 2001;7(1):21–29.

28. Bettencourt P, Azevedo A, Pimenta J, et al. N-terminal-pro-brain natriuretic peptide predicts outcome after hospital discharge in heart failure patients. *Circulation.* Oct 12 2004;110(15):2168–2174.

29. Troughton RW, Frampton CM, Yandle TG, et al. Treatment of heart failure guided by plasma aminoterminal brain natriuretic peptide (N-BNP) concentrations. *Lancet.* Apr 1 2000;355(9210):1126–1130.

30. Jourdain P, Jondeau G, Funck F, et al. Plasma brain natriuretic peptide-guided therapy to improve outcome in heart failure: the STARS-BNP Multicenter Study. *J Am Coll Cardiol.* Apr 24 2007;49(16):1733–1739.

31. Shah M, Investigators S. STARBRITE: a randomized pilot trial of BNP-guided therapy in patients with advanced heart failure. *Circulation.* Oct 31 2006;114(18): II-528.

32. O'Hanlon R, O'Shea P, Ledwidge M, et al. The biologic variability of B-type natriuretic peptide and N-terminal pro-B-type natriuretic peptide in stable heart failure patients. *J Card Fail.* Feb 2007;13(1):50–55.

33. Shah MR, Flavell CM, Weintraub JR, et al. Intensity and focus of heart failure disease management after hospital discharge. *AmHeart J.* 2005;149(4):715–721.

34. Cohn JN, Franciosa JA. Vasodilator therapy of cardiac failure (second of two parts). *N Engl J Med.* Aug 4 1977;297(5):254–258.

35. Cohn JN, Franciosa JA. Vasodilator therapy of cardiac failure: (first of two parts). *N Engl J Med.* Jul 7 1977;297(1):27–31.

36. Kovick RB, Tillisch JH, Berens SC, et al. Vasodilator therapy for chronic left ventricular failure. *Circulation.* Feb 1976;53(2):322–328.

37. Pierpont GL, Cohn JN, Franciosa JA. Combined oral hydralazine-nitrate therapy in left ventricular failure. Hemodynamic equivalency to sodium nitroprusside. *Chest*. Jan 1978;73(1):8–13.

38. Binanay C, Califf RM, Hasselblad V, et al. Evaluation study of congestive heart failure and pulmonary artery catheterization effectiveness: the ESCAPE trial. *JAMA*. Oct 5 2005;294(13):1625–1633.

39. Cuffe MS, Califf RM, Adams KF, Jr., et al. Short-term intravenous milrinone for acute exacerbation of chronic heart failure: a randomized controlled trial. *JAMA*. Mar 27 2002;287(12):1541–1547.

40. Connors AF, Jr, Speroff T, Dawson NV, et al. The effectiveness of right heart catheterization in the initial care of critically ill patients. SUPPORT Investigators. *JAMA*. 1996;276(11):889–897.

41. Sandham JD, Hull RD, Brant RF, et al. A randomized, controlled trial of the use of pulmonary-artery catheters in high-risk surgical patients. *N Engl J Med*. Jan 2 2003 348(1):5–14.

42. Richard C, Warszawski J, Anguel N, et al. Early use of the pulmonary artery catheter and outcomes in patients with shock and acute respiratory distress syndrome: a randomized controlled trial. *JAMA*. 2003;290(20):2713–2720.

43. Wheeler AP, Bernard GR, Thompson BT, et al. Pulmonary-artery versus central venous catheter to guide treatment of acute lung injury. *N Engl J Med*. May 25 2006;354(21):2213–2224.

44. Harvey S, Harrison DA, Singer M, et al. Assessment of the clinical effectiveness of pulmonary artery catheters in management of patients in intensive care (PAC-Man): a randomised controlled trial. *The Lancet*. 2005;366(9484):472–477.

45. Antonelli M, Levy M, Andrews PJ, et al. Hemodynamic monitoring in shock and implications for management. International Consensus Conference, Paris, France, April 27–28 2006. *Intensive Care Med*. Apr 2007;33(4):575–590.

46. Wiener RS, Welch HG. Trends in the use of the pulmonary artery catheter in the United States, 1993–2004. *JAMA*. Jul 25 2007;298(4):423–429.

47. Shah MR, Hasselblad V, Stevenson LW, et al. Impact of the pulmonary artery catheter in critically ill patients: meta-analysis of randomized clinical trials. *JAMA*. 2005;294(13):1664–1670.

48. Executive summary: HFSA 2006 Comprehensive Heart Failure Practice Guideline. *J Card Fail*. Feb 2006;12(1):10–38.

49. Rubenfeld GD, McNamara-Aslin E, Rubinson L. The pulmonary artery catheter, 1967–2007: rest in peace? *JAMA*. Jul 25 2007;298(4):458–461.

50. Steinhaus DM, Lemery R, Bresnahan DR, Jr., et al. Initial experience with an implantable hemodynamic monitor. *Circulation*. Feb 15 1996;93(4):745–752.

51. Reynolds DW, Bartelt N, Taepke R, et al. Measurement of pulmonary artery diastolic pressure from the right ventricle. *J Am Coll Cardiol*. Apr 1995;25(5):1176–1182.

52. Ohlsson A, Bennett T, Nordlander R, et al. Monitoring of pulmonary arterial diastolic pressure through a right ventricular pressure transducer. *J Card Fail*. Mar 1995;1(2):161–168.

53. Chuang PP, Wilson RF, Homans DC, et al. Measurement of pulmonary artery diastolic pressure from a right ventricular pressure transducer in patients with heart failure. *J Card Fail*. Mar 1996;2(1):41–46.

54. Ohlsson A, Bennett T, Ottenhoff F, et al. Long-term recording of cardiac output via an implantable haemodynamic monitoring device. *Eur Heart J*. Dec 1996;17(12):1902–1910.

55. Ohlsson A, Kubo SH, Steinhaus D, et al. Continuous ambulatory monitoring of absolute right ventricular pressure and mixed venous oxygen saturation in patients with heart failure using an implantable haemodynamic monitor: results of a 1 year multicentre feasibility study. *Eur Heart J*. Jun 2001;22(11):942–954.

56. Adamson PB, Magalski A, Braunschweig F, et al. Ongoing right ventricular hemody-namics in heart failure: clinical value of measurements derived from an implantable monitoring system. *J Am Coll Cardiol.* 2003;41(4):565–571.

57. Magalski A, Adamson P, Gadler F, et al. Continuous ambulatory right heart pressure measurements with an implantable hemodynamic monitor: a multicenter, 12-month follow-up study of patients with chronic heart failure. *Journal of Cardiac Failure.* 2002;8(2):63–70.

58. Cleland JG, Coletta AP, Freemantle N, Velavan P, Tin L, Clark AL. Clinical trials update from the American College of Cardiology meeting: CARE-HF and the remission of heart failure, Women's Health Study, TNT, COMPASS-HF, VERITAS, CANPAP, PEECH and PREMIER. *Eur J Heart Fail.* 2005; 7: 931–936.

59. Bourge RC, Abraham WT, Adamson PB, Aaron MF, Aranda JM Jr, Magalski A, Zile MR, Smith AL, Smart FW, O'Shaughnessy MA, Jessup ML, Sparks B, Naftel DL, Stevenson LW, COMPASS-HF Study Group. Randomized controlled trial of an implantable continuous hemodynamic monitor in patients with advanced heart failure: the COMPASS-HF study. J Am Coll Cardiol. Mar 18 2008;51(11):1073–1079.

60. Ritzema J, Troughton R, Melton I, et al. Medical therapy directed by a new implantable left atrial pressure sensing device reduces episodes of hemodynamic deterioration in ambulatory heart failure patients. *Circulation.* 2006;114(18):II-528.

61. Ohki T, Ouriel K, Silveira PG, et al. Initial results of wireless pressure sensing for endovascular aneurysm repair: the APEX Trial–Acute Pressure Measurement to Con-firm Aneurysm Sac EXclusion. *J Vasc Surg.* Feb 2007;45(2):236–242.

62. Nagueh SF. Noninvasive evaluation of hemodynamics by Doppler echocardiography. *Curr Opin Cardiol.* May 1999;14(3):217–224.

63. Dini FL, Traversi E, Franchini M, et al. Contrast-enhanced Doppler hemodynamics for noninvasive assessment of patients with chronic heart failure and left ventricular systolic dysfunction. *J Am Soc Echocardiogr.* Feb 2003;16(2):124–131.

64. Rosenberg P, Yancy CW. Noninvasive assessment of hemodynamics: an emphasis on bioimpedance cardiography. *Curr Opin Cardiol.* 2000;15(3):151–155.

65. Raaijmakers E, Faes TJ, Scholten RJ, et al. A meta-analysis of published stud-ies concerning the validity of thoracic impedance cardiography. *Ann NY Acad Sci.* 1999;873:121–127.

66. Woltjer HH, Bogaard HJ, Bronzwaer JG, et al. Prediction of pulmonary capillary wedge pressure and assessment of stroke volume by noninvasive impedance cardiography. *Am Heart J.* Sep 1997;134(3):450–455.

67. Drazner MH, Thompson B, Rosenberg PB, et al. Comparison of impedance cardiogra-phy with invasive hemodynamic measurements in patients with heart failure secondary to ischemic or nonischemic cardiomyopathy. *Am J Cardiol.* 2002;89(8):993–995.

68. Albert NM, Hail MD, Li J, et al. Equivalence of the bioimpedance and thermodilution methods in measuring cardiac output in hospitalized patients with advanced, decompen-sated chronic heart failure. *Am J Crit Care.* Nov 2004;13(6):469–479.

69. Yancy C, Rogers J, Pauly D, et al. Diagnostic implications of impedance cardiography in the setting of severe acute decompensated heart failure: results of the bioimpedance cardiography (BIG) substudy in the ESCAPE trial. *Circulation.* 2005;112(17):II-639.

70. Packer M, Abraham WT, Mehra MR, et al. Utility of impedance cardiography for the identification of short-term risk of clinical decompensation in stable patients with chronic heart failure. *Journal of the American College of Cardiolog* 2006;47(11): 2245–2252.

71. Yu C-M, Wang L, Chau E, et al. Intrathoracic impedance monitoring in patients with heart failure: correlation with fluid status and feasibility of early warning preceding hospitalization. *Circulation.* Aug 9 2005;112(6):841–848.

72. Ypenburg C, Bax JJ, van der Wall EE, et al. Intrathoracic impedance monitoring to predict decompensated heart failure. *Am J Cardiol.* Feb 15 2007;99(4):554–557.

73. OptiLink HF. Study: Optimization of Heart Failure Management Using Medtronic OptiVol Fluid Status Monitoring and Medtronic CareLink Network (OptiLink-HF). Accessed at http://clinicaltrials.gov/ct2/show/NCT00769457.

74. McIntyre K, Vita J, Lambrew C, et al. A noninvasive method of predicting pulmonary-capillary wedge pressure. *N Engl J Med.* Dec 10, 1992;327(24):1715–1720.

75. Sharma GVRK, Woods PA, Lambrew CT, et al. Evaluation of a noninvasive system for determining left ventricular filling pressure. *Arch Intern Med.* Oct 14 2002;162(18):2084–2088.

76. Stevenson LW, Le Jemtel TH, Alt EU. Hemodynamic goals are relevant. *Circulation.* Feb 21 2006;113(7):1020–1033.

77. Nohria A, Lewis E, Stevenson LW. Medical management of advanced heart failure. *JAMA.* Feb 6 2002;287(5):628–640.

78. Schultz RJ, Whitfield GF, LaMura JJ, Raciti A, Krishnamurthy S. The role of physiologic monitoring in patients with fractures of the hip. *J Trauma.* Apr 1985;25(4): 309–316.

79. Shoemaker WC, Appel PL, Kram HB, Waxman K, Lee TS. Prospective trial of supranormal values of survivors as therapeutic goals in high-risk surgical patients. *Chest.* Dec 1988;94(6):1176–1186.

80. Isaacson IJ, Lowdon JD, Berry AJ, et al. The value of pulmonary artery and central venous monitoring in patients undergoing abdominal aortic reconstructive surgery: a comparative study of two selected, randomized groups. *J Vasc Surg.* Dec 1990;12(6): 754–760.

81. Berlauk JF, Abrams JH, Gilmour IJ, O'Connor SR, Knighton DR, Cerra FB. Preoperative optimization of cardiovascular hemodynamics improves outcome in peripheral vascular surgery. A prospective, randomized clinical trial. *Ann Surg.* Sep 1991;214(3): 289–297; discussion 298–299.

82. Guyatt G. A randomized control trial of right-heart catheterization in critically ill patients. Ontario Intensive Care Study Group. *J Intensive Care Med.* Mar-Apr 1991; 6(2):91–95.

83. Bender JSMD, F.A.C.S.; Smith-Meek, Melissa A. B.A.; Jones, Calvin E. M.D., F.A.C.S. Routine Pulmonary Artery Catheterization Does Not Reduce Morbidity and Mortality of Elective Vascular Surgery: Results of a Prospective, Randomized Trial. *Annals of Surgery.* 1997;226(3):229–237.

84. Valentine RJ, Duke ML, Inman MH, et al. Effectiveness of pulmonary artery catheters in aortic surgery: a randomized trial. *J Vasc Surg.* Feb 1998;27(2):203–211; discussion 211–212.

85. Bonazzi M, Gentile F, Biasi GM, et al. Impact of perioperative haemodynamic monitoring on cardiac morbidity after major vascular surgery in low risk patients. A randomised pilot trial. *Eur J Vasc Endovasc Surg.* May 2002;23(5):445–451.

86. Rhodes A, Cusack RJ, Newman PJ, Grounds MR, Bennett DE. A randomised, controlled trial of the pulmonary artery catheter in critically ill patients. *Intensive Care Medicine.* 2002/03/01/ 2002;V28(3):256–264.

6 Implantable Cardioverter-Defibrillators

Rachel Lampert, MD and Zachary Goldberger, MD

CONTENTS

Abstract

Sudden cardiac death (SCD) causes 300,000–400,000 deaths annually in the United States and is responsible for nearly 50% of all cardiovascular mortality worldwide. Ventricular tachycardia (VT) degenerating into ventricular fibrillation (VF) causes two-thirds of SCD. Among patients with heart failure (HF), one-third to one-half of deaths are sudden. Because there are often no warning symptoms to identify potential victims of SCD, successful therapy has focused on identifying high-risk patients and implanting cardioverter-defibrillators (ICDs), which continuously monitor the heart rhythm and deliver therapy (a shock or an antitachycardia pacing) upon detection of a sustained ventricular arrhythmia. This chapter focuses on the clinical indications and technical aspects of ICDs for heart failure patients.

Key Words: Heart failure; Implantable defibrillator; Sudden death; Ventricular tachycardia; Ventricular fibrillation.

1. SUDDEN CARDIAC DEATH IN HEART FAILURE

Sudden cardiac death (SCD) causes 300,000–400,000 deaths annually in the United States and is responsible for nearly 50% of all cardiovascular mortality worldwide *(1–3)*. Ventricular tachycardia (VT) degenerating into

From: *Contemporary Cardiology: Device Therapy in Heart Failure*
Edited by: W.H. Maisel, DOI 10.1007/978-1-59745-424-7_6
© Humana Press, a part of Springer Science+Business Media, LLC 2010

ventricular fibrillation (VF) causes two-thirds of SCD *(4–6)*. Among patients with heart failure (HF), one-third to one-half of deaths are sudden *(7)*. While overall mortality increases as functional status worsens, the proportion of deaths which are sudden is highest in those patients with less-severe signs and symptoms *(8)*. This holds true for both ischemic and nonischemic etiologies *(7)*. While more recent pharmacological advances have improved overall mortality, the percentage of deaths which are sudden remain similar *(7, 9, 10)*. Of sudden deaths in patients with HF, about half are due to ventricular tachyarrhythmias and half due to bradycardia or electromechanical dissociation *(11)*. Because there are no warning symptoms to identify potential victims of tachyarrhythmic SCD *(4)*, successful therapy has focused on identifying high-risk patients and implanting cardioverter-defibrillators (ICDs), which continuously monitor the heart rhythm and deliver therapy (a shock or an antitachycardia pacing) upon detection of a sustained ventricular arrhythmia *(12)*.

2. INDICATIONS FOR ICD IMPLANTATION IN PATIENTS WITH HF

The introduction of the ICD into clinical practice has been a process in evolution. While secondary prophylaxis for patients surviving a life-threatening ventricular arrhythmia has long been the standard of care, more recent trials demonstrate the survival benefit of the ICD in expanding groups of patients at high risk (primary prophylaxis) for SCD as well.

2.1. Secondary Prevention Trials

Several trials have investigated the role of the ICD in secondary prevention of SCD (Table 1) *(13–17)*. The largest include the Antiarrhythmics Versus Implantable Defibrillators (AVID) trial *(13)*, the Cardiac Arrest Study – Hamburg (CASH) *(14)*, and the Canadian Implantable Defibrillator Study (CIDS) *(15)*. Each randomized patients to ICD vs pharmacologic therapy, and in each, the ICD reduced total mortality, although only AVID reached statistical significance.

AVID was also the largest and best designed, including nearly exclusive use of transvenous defibrillators and comparing the ICD against the best available antiarrhythmic drug therapy (amiodarone and sotalol) unlike CASH and CIDS. Further, a meta-analysis of AVID, CASH, and CIDS confirmed that ICD therapy resulted in significant relative reductions in total mortality (27%) and arrhythmic mortality (51%) *(18)*. The ICD improved survival regardless of beta-blockade, surgical revascularization, or presenting arrhythmia (VT or VF). There was no difference in benefit gained from ICD implantation between those patients with coronary disease and those with nonischemic cardiomyopathies *(18)*.

Table 1
Secondary prevention of sudden cardiac death – randomized trials

Study	Randomization	N	Inclusion criteria	CHF enrollment by class[a]	Mean follow-up (months)	Main findings
AVID (13)	Antiarrhythmic medications (97% amiodarone, 3% sotalol) vs ICD	1016	Survived VT/VF/cardiac arrest; VT with syncope; VT with LVEF ≤ 0.40	None 42% I/II 48% III 10%	18	27% relative risk reduction in total mortality with ICD therapy ($P < 0.02$)
CASH (14)	Antiarrhythmic medications propafenone (withdrawn early), metoprolol, or amiodarone vs ICD	288	Survived VT/VF/cardiac arrest	I 27% II 57% III 16%	57	23% relative risk reduction in total mortality with ICD therapy ($P = 0.08$)
CIDS (15)	Amiodarone vs ICD	659	Survived VT/VF/cardiac arrest; VT with syncope; VT with LVEF ≤ 0.35 and cycle length ≤ 400 ms	None 50% I/II 38% III/IV 11%	35	19.7% relative risk reduction in death from any cause with ICD therapy ($P = 0.142$); 32.8% reduction in the risk of death from arrhythmia with ICD therapy ($P = 0.094$)

Table 1
(Continued)

Study	Randomization	N	Inclusion criteria	CHF enrollment by class[a]	Mean follow-up (months)	Main findings
DEBUT (16)	Beta-blocker vs ICD	86	Survived VT/VF/cardiac arrest; no structural abnormalities	I 100%	36	Seven total deaths, all of which occurred in the beta-blocker group – (three deaths during 2-year follow-up, $P = 0.07$; four deaths during 3-year follow-up, $P = 0.02$)
MAVERIC (17)	EP-guided therapy (antiarrhythmic, revascularization, or ICD) vs amiodarone	214	Survived VT/VF/cardiac arrest	Any CHF 26%	60[b]	Lower mortality with ICD therapy compared to non-ICD therapy ($P = 0.04$). No advantage to EP testing

Abbreviations: AVID, Antiarrhythmics Versus Implantable Defibrillators; CASH, Cardiac Arrest Study – Hamburg; CIDS, Canadian Implantable Defibrillator Study; DEBUT, Defibrillator Versus beta-Blockers for Unexplained Death in Thailand; MAVERIC, The Midlands Trial of Empirical Amiodarone Versus Electrophysiologically Guided Intervention and Cardioverter Implant in Ventricular Arrhythmias; EP, electrophysiologic; ICD, implantable cardioverter-defibrillator; LVEF, left ventricular ejection fraction; VF, ventricular fibrillation; VT, ventricular tachycardia.

[a] As defined for the trial.
[b] Median follow-up.

Interestingly, the AVID registry, enrolling patients not qualifying for randomization, showed that some groups previously considered at lower risk for SCD – patients with hemodynamically stable VT or arrhythmias attributed to "reversible causes" – actually had significantly worse survival than did randomized ICD-treated patients. In particular those with lower ejection fractions fared poorly, suggesting that these groups may also benefit from ICDs *(19)*.

2.2. Primary Prevention Trials

The dismal survival rate after cardiac arrest *(20–22)* provides strong impetus to identify high-risk patients who might benefit from an ICD, before a first life-threatening arrhythmia. How best to stratify risk has been a process in evolution. Historically, patients with LV dysfunction, postmyocardial infarction, and a history of nonsustained VT underwent electrophysiology (EP) testing to identify higher risk patients with inducible, nonsuppressible, ventricular tachyarrhythmias *(23, 24)*. This population was the target for the first primary prevention trial (Table 2), the Multicenter Automatic Defibrillator Trial (MADIT) *(25)*, which compared ICDs to conventional therapy (mainly amiodarone) (ejection fraction (EF) $\leq 35\%$), and the Multicenter Unsustained Tachycardia Trial (MUSTT) *(26)*, which compared EP-guided therapy (ICDs or drug therapy) vs no EP-guided therapy (EF $\leq 40\%$).

MADIT was prematurely aborted after enrolling only 196 patients, when preliminary analysis revealed a dramatic benefit of ICD therapy in reducing overall mortality by 54% ($P = 0.009$). MADIT had no placebo group, raising the question of whether the trial proved benefit of ICD or detriment of amiodarone. Also, beta-blocker use was higher in the ICD arm. However, MUSTT, while not designed to evaluate the ICD, supported the MADIT findings. The original hypothesis of MUSTT was that EP-guided therapy, either pharmacological or device based, could reduce arrhythmic and total mortality in high-risk patients who had arrhythmias induced at EP study. In patients randomized to EP-guided therapy, antiarrhythmic drugs were tested first and, at the physician's discretion, nonresponders received ICDs. MUSTT did show a decrease in arrhythmic death/cardiac arrest with EP-guided therapy, supporting the primary hypothesis. However, subgroup analysis revealed that the benefits were due entirely to the ICD: at 5 years, there were absolute reductions in total mortality of 31% when compared to those receiving pharmacological therapy and of 24% when compared to those receiving no therapy (mortality 24% in the ICD group, 55% with pharmacological therapy, and 48% with no therapy). In MUSTT, few patients received amiodarone, and ICD use was not randomized. However, taken together, MUSTT and MADIT clearly demonstrate the benefit of the ICD in the relatively small population of patients with coronary artery disease (CAD), low LVEF, and inducible ventricular arrhythmia.

The MUSTT registry *(27)*, however, followed patients who had clinical criteria for the trial but had no inducible arrhythmias. Surprisingly,

Table 2
Primary prevention of sudden cardiac death in ischemic cardiomyopathy – randomized trials

Study	Randomization	N	Population	HF NYHA Class	Mean F/U (months)	Main findings
MADIT (25)	Antiarrhythmic therapy (74% amiodarone) vs ICD	196	Prior MI; LVEF ≤ 0.35; asymptomatic NSVT; NYHA Class I–III; inducible VT refractory to intravenous procainamide on EPS	II/III 65%	27	56% RR reduction in mortality with ICD therapy ($P = 0.009$)
MUSTT (26)	EP-guided therapy (AAD or ICD) vs conventional therapy	704	Prior MI; LVEF ≤ 0.40; CAD; NSVT; inducible VT on EPS	I 37%, II 38%, III 25%	39[a]	60% RR reduction in mortality with ICD therapy ($P < 0.001$)
MADIT II (28)	Conventional therapy vs ICD	1232	Prior MI; LVEF ≤ 0.30	I 37%, II 34%, III 24%, IV 5%	20	31% RR reduction in mortality with ICD therapy ($P = 0.016$)
SCD-HeFT (29)	Conventional therapy vs amiodarone vs ICD	2521	NYHA Class II–III CHF (ischemic and nonischemic); LVEF ≤ 0.35	II 70%, III 30%	45.5[a]	Overall: 23% RR reduction in mortality with ICD therapy ($P = 0.007$) Ischemic heart disease: 21% relative reduction in mortality with ICD therapy ($P = 0.05$)

CABG Patch (44)	CABG with an ICD vs CABG	900	Patients scheduled for CABG; LVEF ≤ 0.35; positive SAECG	II/III 72%	32	No reduction in mortality with ICD therapy ($P = 0.64$)
DINAMIT (33)	Conventional therapy vs ICD	674	Recent MI (within 4–40 days), LVEF ≤0.35; impaired cardiac autonomic modulation (HRV)	I 13%, II 59%, III 27%	39	No reduction in death with ICD therapy ($P = 0.66$); risk of arrhythmic death lower with ICD therapy ($P = 0.009$)

Abbreviations: MADIT, Multicenter Automatic Defibrillator Trial; MUSTT, Multicenter Unsustained Tachycardia Trial; SCD-HeFT, Sudden Cardiac Death in Heart Failure Trial; CABG Patch, Coronary Artery Bypass Graft Patch; DINAMIT, Defibrillator in Acute Myocardial Infarction Trial; AAD, antiarrhythmic drug; CAD, coronary artery disease; EPS, electrophysiological study; HRV, heart rate variability; ICD, implantable cardioverter-defibrillator; LVEF, left ventricular ejection fraction; MI, myocardial infarction; NSVT, nonsustained ventricular tachycardia; NYHA, New York Heart Association; RR, relative risk; SAECG, signal-averaged electrocardiogram; VF, ventricular fibrillation; VT, ventricular tachycardia.

[a]Median follow-up.

while 5-year mortality for these patients was statistically lower than that for inducible patients randomized to no therapy (44% and 48%, respectively, $P = 0.005$), it was significantly higher than that for the inducible, ICD-treated patients (24%). These data implied that noninducible patients with LV dysfunction and nonsustained ventricular tachycardia (NSVT) may also benefit from a prophylactic ICD and that EP study may be an inadequate risk stratifier.

The second MADIT trial (MADIT II) *(28)* directly addressed the value of prophylactic ICD implantation in patients with CAD and EF $\leq$30%, without EP risk stratification. The ICD showed a 31% relative reduction in mortality at any interval ($P = 0.016$). Of note, among 593 patients in the ICD arm who underwent peri-implant EP testing (not an entry criterion), inducibility did not predict later ventricular arrhythmia, supporting a low sensitivity for EP testing.

The more recently published Sudden Cardiac Death in Heart Failure Trial (SCD-HeFT) *(29)* enrolled patients with either ischemic or nonischemic cardiomyopathy, New York Heart Association (NYHA) Class II or III heart failure, and LVEF $\leq$35%. The results confirmed the benefit of ICD in ischemic patients as found in MADIT II, as well as the findings of a previous smaller study of nonischemic cardiomyopathy patients, the Prophylactic Defibrillator Implantation in Patients with Nonischemic Dilated Cardiomyopathy (DEFINITE) trial *(30)*. (Selected studies of primary prophylaxis of SCD in patients with nonischemic cardiomyopathy can be found in Table 3 *(29, 31–33)*.) In SCD-HeFT, ICD-treated patients lived longer than those treated with amiodarone (which had no benefit) or conventional medical therapy. While previous studies have shown the benefits of pharmacological therapy of HF in preventing sudden death *(9, 10)*, the majority of patients in SCD-HeFT were receiving standard HF therapies (87% receiving an ACE inhibitor or ARB, 78% receiving beta-blockers), implying an incremental benefit of the ICD even among appropriately treated HF patients. Further, while the concern has been raised that ICD benefit in MADIT II may have been skewed by the short follow-up *(34)*, SCD-HeFT showed ICD benefit extending to 5 years, independent of heart failure etiology (ischemic vs nonischemic). These studies suggest that patients with LVEF $\leq$35% and NYHA Class II or III HF are candidates for an ICD (based on SCD-HeFT) as are patients with LVEF $\leq$30% and history of MI (based on MADIT II).

However, whether ejection fraction and heart failure functional class alone should be the primary factor determining ICD eligibility remains somewhat controversial *(35–38)*. In MUSTT, left ventricular EF had poor specificity in predicting SCD *(39)*, and in other studies, combinations of factors were more predictive *(40, 41)*. Limiting both the MADIT II and SCD-HeFT study designs, neither evaluated ICD benefit in patients known to be noninducible. This may explain why the absolute reductions in all-cause mortality for MADIT II and SCD-HeFT (6% and 7%, respectively) are much smaller than that for MADIT I and MUSTT (23% and 31%, respectively), which selected

Table 3
Primary prevention of sudden cardiac death in nonischemic dilated cardiomyopathy – randomized trials

Study	Randomization	N	Population	CHF enrollment by class	Mean follow-up (months)	Main findings
CAT (31)	Conventional therapy vs ICD	104	NYHA Class II–III, NIDCM; LVEF $\leq$ 0.30; asymptomatic NSVT	II 66% III 34%	66	No reduction in total mortality with ICD therapy ($P = 0.554$)
AMIOVERT (32)	Amiodarone vs ICD	103	NYHA Class I–III, NIDCM; LVEF $\leq$ 0.35; asymptomatic NSVT	I 15% II 64% III 20%	36	No reduction in total mortality with ICD therapy ($P = 0.80$)
DEFINITE (30)	Conventional therapy vs ICD	458	NIDCM; LVEF < 0.36; NSVT or PVCs	I 22% II 57% III 21%	29	35% relative risk reduction in total mortality with ICD therapy ($P = 0.08$; 80% reduction in death from arrhythmia with ICD therapy ($P = 0.006$)

(Continued)

R. Lampert and Z. Goldberger

Table 3
(Continued)

Study	Randomization	N	Population	CHF enrollment by class	Mean follow-up (months)	Main findings
SCD-HeFT (29)	Conventional therapy vs amiodarone vs ICD	2521	NYHA class II–III CHF (ischemic and nonischemic); LVEF ≤ 0.35	See above	45.5[a]	Overall: 23% relative risk reduction in mortality with ICD therapy ($P = 0.007$). Nonischemic heart disease: 27% relative reduction in mortality with ICD therapy ($P = 0.06$)

Abbreviations: CAT, Cardiomyopathy Trial; AMIOVERT, Amiodarone Versus Implantable Defibrillator in Patients with Nonischemic Cardiomyopathy and Asymptomatic Nonsustained Ventricular Tachycardia; DEFINITE, Prophylactic Defibrillator Implantation in Patients with Nonischemic Dilated Cardiomyopathy; SCD-HeFT, Sudden Cardiac Death in Heart Failure Trial; CAD, coronary artery disease; ICD, implantable cardioverter-defibrillator; LVEF, left ventricular ejection fraction; NIDCM, nonischemic dilated cardiomyopathy; NSVT, nonsustained ventricular tachycardia; NYHA, New York Heart Association; PVC, premature ventricular contraction; VF, ventricular fibrillation; VT, ventricular tachycardia.
[a]Median follow-up.

higher risk patients using EP criteria. As a result, SCD-HeFT/MADIT II had a much higher number needed to treat than did MUSTT/MADIT (15–17 vs 3–4). Thus, the benefit of ICD therapy may be greater in patients with SCD risk beyond low LVEF (although these differences in absolute risk reduction may also be due to better medical therapy in the control groups in the later trials *(42)*. The validity of ICD implantation in all post-MI patients with reduced LVEF has been questioned *(35, 43, 44)*, suggesting that further risk stratification is still needed *(35)*. The potential role of noninvasive risk stratifiers shown to have good predictive value, such as T-wave alternans *(45, 46)*, remains undetermined.

Two studies failed to show benefit of ICD for primary prophylaxis in specific populations: the Coronary Artery Bypass Graft (CABG) Patch Trial *(47)* and the Defibrillator in Acute Myocardial Infarction Trial (DINA-MIT) *(33)*. CABG Patch randomized patients with an abnormal signal-averaged electrocardiogram undergoing CABG to treatment with an ICD, implanted during surgery, or to treatment with no ICD. The ICD showed no benefit, likely due to the lower risk profile of the patient population. While preoperative ejection fractions were low, they may improve with surgery. Also, the signal-averaged electrocardiogram may lack specificity *(23, 24)*. Revascularization itself may have protected against arrhythmia, although in AVID, the ICD offered similar survival rates independent of revascularization *(13)*.

A recent substudy of the large Valsartan in Acute Myocardial Infarction Trial (VALIANT) *(48)* demonstrated that SCD risk is highest in the first 30 days after MI complicated by reduced LVEF and/or HF, suggesting that early ICDs might save lives. However, the DINAMIT study, which randomly assigned such patients to receive an ICD or conventional medical therapy, showed no ICD benefit early after MI, possibly due to the low event rate in this small study. It is also possible that the VALIANT patients with SCD were sicker than the survivors, with competing risks. DINAMIT supports this theory, as the decrease in arrhythmic deaths in the ICD group was offset by an increase in nonarrhythmic cardiac death. Whether further risk stratification or noninvasive measures such as an external wearable vest or an automatic external defibrillator might be more beneficial and cost-effective early after MI *(49)* is unknown.

2.3. Benefit of the ICD in Patients with Advanced Heart Failure

The benefit of the ICD for primary prevention of SCD in patients with more severe HF has been mixed among the different studies. In SCD-HeFT, analysis of prespecified subgroups showed that while patients with NYHA Class II HF (70% of the study population) showed an absolute reduction of mortality of 12% at 5 years, there was no apparent reduction in risk of death with an ICD for those with Class III HF (30% of the population, hazard ratio 1.16, 97.5% CI 0.84–1.61) *(29)*. Other studies, however, have shown equal or greater benefit in patients with more advanced HF. Among the secondary prevention trials, most patients had NYHA Class I–II HF, with Class III comprising just 9% of AVID patients, 19% of CASH, and 11% of CIDS. However, meta-analysis of the three trials revealed that patients with the lowest left ventricular ejection fraction (LVEF) and more advanced HF benefited most *(18)*. In a subanalysis of the MADIT II trial, while patients with Class III HF (29% of the population) had overall higher mortality and higher risk of arrhythmic events than those with Class I–II HF, there was no interaction between functional class, ICD treatment, and mortality, implying similar benefit of ICD treatment regardless of NYHA class *(50)*. Further, in the DEFINITE trial, there was a greater benefit for those with Class III HF.

The role of the ICD for patients with Class IV HF has not been well studied, as most trials of standard defibrillators have excluded these individuals. However, the Comparison of Medical Therapy, Pacing, and Defibrillation in Heart Failure (COMPANION) trial *(51)* randomized patients with NYHA Class III or IV HF, reduced EF, and conduction delays (QRS > 120 ms) to receive conventional medical therapy alone, cardiac resynchronization therapy (CRT) alone, or CRT incorporated in an ICD. While patients in the CRT-alone arm had a 19% risk reduction in the primary end point of death or hospitalization ($P = 0.014$), patients in the CRT plus ICD arm had a significant improvement in total mortality, with a relative reduction of 36%. (A limitation of COMPANION was its lack of power to directly compare CRT with vs without defibrillation.) While the number of Class IV patients was small (14%), the mortality benefit with the combined CRT-ICD device was similar between Class III and IV patients.

Overall, these trials strongly support ICD implantation for secondary prevention in patients with prior life-threatening arrhythmia and as primary prophylaxis for many patients with a low LVEF and CAD and/or HF *(52–54)*. Current ACC/AHA/HRS guidelines reflect the inclusion and exclusion criteria from the landmark studies and are displayed in Table 4 *(53, 54)*. Importantly, the 2008 AHA/ACC/HRS guidelines note that Class IV heart failure may be a "heterogeneous and dynamic state," requiring a careful individualized approach to decisions about further invasive interventions. ICD therapy is generally not recommended, however, for patients with severe, persistent Class IV symptoms who are not candidates for CRT and are already receiving optimal medical *(54)*. The Centers for Medicare and Medicaid Services has expanded coverage for ICDs for most heart failure patients based on the results of MADIT II and SCD-HeFT and for patients with more Class IV HF meeting criteria for CRT (Table 5) *(55)*.

ICDs are also used to prevent SCD in other high-risk patient subsets, such as those with ion-channel abnormalities [i.e., Brugada syndrome, long QT syndrome (LQTS)] or other structural heart disease (i.e., RV dysplasia and hypertrophic cardiomyopathy). Although prospective randomized trials in these rare conditions are not likely to be pursued *(56)*, case series

Table 4
ACC/AHA/HRS guidelines (2008): indications for ICD therapy

Class I indications

1. ICD therapy is indicated in patients who are survivors of cardiac arrest due to VF or hemodynamically unstable sustained VT after evaluation to define the cause of the event and to exclude any completely reversible causes (*Level of Evidence: A*)

2. ICD therapy is indicated in patients with structural heart disease and spontaneous sustained VT, whether hemodynamically stable or unstable (*Level of Evidence: B*)

3. ICD therapy is indicated in patients with syncope of undetermined origin with clinically relevant, hemodynamically significant sustained VT or VF induced at electrophysiological study (*Level of Evidence: B*)

4. ICD therapy is indicated in patients with LVEF less than 35% due to prior MI who are at least 40 days post-MI and are in NYHA functional Class II or III (*Level of Evidence: A*)

5. ICD therapy is indicated in patients with nonischemic DCM who have an LVEF ≤ 35% and who are in NYHA functional Class II or III (*Level of Evidence: B*)

6. ICD therapy is indicated in patients with LV dysfunction due to prior MI who are at least 40 days post-MI, have an LVEF less than 30%, and are in NYHA functional Class I (*Level of Evidence: A*)

7. ICD therapy is indicated in patients with nonsustained VT due to prior MI, LVEF less than 40%, and inducible VF or sustained VT at electrophysiological study (*Level of Evidence: B*)

Class IIa indications

1. ICD implantation is reasonable for patients with unexplained syncope, significant LV dysfunction, and nonischemic DCM (*Level of Evidence: C*)

2. ICD implantation is reasonable for patients with sustained VT and normal or near-normal ventricular function (*Level of Evidence: C*)

3. ICD implantation is reasonable for patients with HCM who have one or more major risk factors for SCD (*Level of Evidence: C*)

4. ICD implantation is reasonable for the prevention of SCD in patients with ARVD/C who have one or more risk factors for SCD (*Level of Evidence: C*)

5. ICD implantation is reasonable to reduce SCD in patients with long QT syndrome who are experiencing syncope and/or VT while receiving beta-blockers (*Level of Evidence: B*)

(Continued)

Table 4
(Continued)

6. ICD implantation is reasonable for nonhospitalized patients awaiting transplantation (*Level of Evidence: C*)
7. ICD implantation is reasonable for patients with Brugada syndrome who have had syncope (*Level of Evidence: C*)
8. ICD implantation is reasonable for patients with Brugada syndrome who have documented VT that has not resulted in cardiac arrest (*Level of Evidence: C*)
9. ICD implantation is reasonable for patients with catecholaminergic polymorphic VT who have syncope and/or documented sustained VT while receiving beta-blockers (*Level of Evidence: C*)
10. ICD implantation is reasonable for patients with cardiac sarcoidosis, giant cell myocarditis, or Chagas disease (*Level of Evidence: C*)

Class IIb indications

1. ICD therapy may be considered in patients with nonischemic heart disease who have an LVEF $\leq$ 35% and who are in NYHA functional Class I (*Level of Evidence: C*)
2. ICD therapy may be considered for patients with long QT syndrome and risk factors for SCD (*Level of Evidence: B*)
3. ICD therapy may be considered in patients with syncope and advanced structural heart disease in whom thorough invasive and noninvasive investigations have failed to define a cause (*Level of Evidence: C*)
4. ICD therapy may be considered in patients with a familial cardiomyopathy associated with sudden death (*Level of Evidence: C*)
5. ICD therapy may be considered in patients with LV noncompaction (*Level of Evidence: C*)

Class III indications

1. ICD therapy is not indicated for patients who do not have a reasonable expectation of survival with an acceptable functional status for at least 1 year, even if they meet ICD implantation criteria specified in the Class I, IIa, and IIb recommendations above (*Level of Evidence: C*)
2. ICD therapy is not indicated for patients with incessant VT or VF (*Level of Evidence: C*)
3. ICD therapy is not indicated in patients with significant psychiatric illnesses that may be aggravated by device implantation or that may preclude systematic follow-up (*Level of Evidence: C*)
4. ICD therapy is not indicated for NYHA Class IV patients with drug-refractory congestive heart failure who are not candidates for cardiac transplantation or CRT-D (*Level of Evidence: C*)

5. ICD therapy is not indicated for syncope of undetermined cause in a patient without inducible ventricular tachyarrhythmias and without structural heart disease (*Level of Evidence: C*)

6. ICD therapy is not indicated when VF or VT is amenable to surgical or catheter ablation (e.g., atrial arrhythmias associated with the Wolff–Parkinson–White syndrome, RV or LV outflow tract VT, idiopathic VT, or fascicular VT in the absence of structural heart disease) (*Level of Evidence: C*)

7. ICD therapy is not indicated for patients with ventricular tachyarrhythmias due to a completely reversible disorder in the absence of structural heart disease (e.g., electrolyte imbalance, drugs, or trauma) (*Level of Evidence: B*)

Class I: Conditions for which there is evidence and/or general agreement that a given procedure or treatment is beneficial, useful, and effective.

Class II: Conditions for which there is conflicting evidence and/or a divergence of opinion about the usefulness/efficacy of a procedure or treatment.

Class IIa: The weight of evidence/opinion is in favor of usefulness/efficacy.

Class IIb: The usefulness/efficacy is less well established by evidence/opinion.

Class III: Conditions for which there is evidence and/or general agreement that a procedure/treatment is not useful/effective and in some cases may be harmful.

Level of Evidence A: Data derived from multiple randomized clinical trials or meta-analyses.

Level of Evidence B: Data derived from a single randomized trial or nonrandomized studies.

Level of Evidence C: Consensus opinion of experts, case studies, or standard of care in the absence of the above.

Table 5

Centers for Medicare and Medicaid Services (CMS) coverage requirements for ICD implantation (53)

---

(1) Patients with IDCM, documented prior MI, NYHA Class II and III heart failure, and measured LVEF ≤ 0.35

(2) Patients with NIDCM > 3 months, NYHA Class II or III heart failure, and measured LVEF ≤ 0.35

(3) Patients who meet all current CMS coverage requirements for a CRT device and have NYHA Class IV heart failure

For all groups, patients must not have:

Cardiogenic shock or symptomatic hypotension while in a stable baseline rhythm

A CABG or a PTCA within the past 3 months

An acute MI within the past 40 days

Clinical symptoms or findings that would make them a candidate for coronary revascularization

Irreversible brain damage from preexisting cerebral disease

Any disease, other than cardiac disease associated with a likelihood of survival less than < 1 year

---

Abbreviations: CABG, coronary artery bypass grafting; CAD, coronary artery disease; ICD, implantable cardioverter-defibrillator; IDCM, ischemic dilated cardiomyopathy; LVEF, left ventricular ejection fraction; NIDCM, nonischemic dilated cardiomyopathy; NSVT, non-sustained ventricular tachycardia; NYHA, New York Heart Association; PTCA, percutaneous transluminal coronary angioplasty; PVC, premature ventricular contraction; VF, ventricular fibrillation; VT, ventricular tachycardia

show efficacy of the ICD in patients with LQTS (57), Brugada syndrome (58), hypertrophic cardiomyopathy (59, 60), and arrhythmogenic RV dysplasia (61). Current guidelines support its use in selected patients with these disorders (54).

An evaluation of the cost-effectiveness of the ICD using a Markov model (62) revealed that prophylactic ICD implantation was both more effective and more expensive than control therapy. Consistent with the lower number needed to treat, the populations showing greatest cost-effectiveness of the ICD were those in MADIT I and MUSTT, with approximately $25,000 per life-year added. The ICD was less cost-effective in the MADIT II and SCD-HeFT populations, with an estimated cost of $40,000–$50,000 per life-year added, respectively. Direct data from SCD-HeFT showed a cost-effectiveness of just $30,000–$40,000, assuming that the mortality benefits extend to at least 8 years (63). Costs per quality-adjusted life-year ranged from $34,000 to $70,000 (62). Not surprisingly, lowering the cost of the device or increasing longevity would improve cost-effectiveness (62). These costs are well within the range considered acceptable to society (64).

3. ICD FUNCTION AND TECHNOLOGY

3.1. Treatment

The three main functions of the ICD are detection of arrhythmia (tachycardia or bradycardia), delivery of appropriate electrical therapy (high-voltage shock or low-energy pacing), and storage of diagnostic information, including electrograms and details of treated episodes. The device consists of two components: the pulse generator and the lead (electrode) system. Current ICDs are only slightly larger than a pacemaker (25–45 cm^3) and are similarly implanted in a subcutaneous pectoral pocket *(65)*. Leads are inserted transvenously through the subclavian, axillary, or cephalic vein into the right ventricular apex *(66)* (and the right atrial appendage for atrial sensing/pacing in dual-chamber systems). Lead characteristics are described in Table 6. Chest roentgenogram demonstrating positioning of the leads and generator is shown in Fig. 1.

Table 6
ICD electrode features

Type	*Comment*
Fixation mechanism	
Transvenous, passive fixation	Tines become lodged in trabeculations. Lower pacing threshold, higher dislodgement rate
Transvenous, active fixation	Helix or screw extends into the endocardial tissue to secure lead. Higher pacing thresholds, lower dislodgement rate
Epicardial	Surgically implanted on outer surface of heart. Typically higher pacing thresholds. May be used for patients with mechanical tricuspid valve, those with difficult coronary sinus access requiring LV pacing, or those with high defibrillation thresholds requiring epicardial patches
Insulation	
Polyurethane	Easier to pass, more rigid, less durable, thinner
Silicone	Higher coefficient of friction, therefore less "slippery," less rigid, more durable, thicker
Configuration	
Unipolar	Sensing and pacing between the lead tip (distal electrode) and the pacemaker pulse generator. Bigger "antenna," therefore more prone to oversensing
Bipolar	Sensing and pacing between two electrodes separated by several millimeters (proximal and distal) located on a single lead. Smaller "antenna," therefore less prone to oversensing
Connector type	
IS-1 bipolar, IS-1 unipolar, DF-1, IS-4	Lead connector and generator header must be compatible. IS-1 is the most common connector in use today for pace/sense connection; DF-1 is most commonly used for high-voltage connections

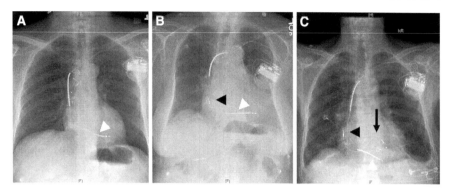

Fig. 1. Chest roentgenograms of standard ICD systems are shown. (**A**) Single-chamber ICD; (**B**) Dual-chamber ICD; (**C**) Biventricular ICD. Single-chamber systems consist of a right ventricular (RV) electrode (*white arrow head*). Dual-chamber systems have a right atrial (*black arrow head*) and RV electrode, while biventricular systems have a third lead positioned in the coronary sinus (*black arrow*).

The modern ICD combines high-energy defibrillation with two other electrical therapies, low-energy cardioversion and antitachycardia pacing (ATP), to terminate ventricular arrhythmias. Figure 2 shows a stored electrogram of a rapid ventricular tachycardia terminated with a high-energy shock. ATP terminates VT without delivering a painful shock by pacing at a rate faster than the intrinsic tachycardia, entering and interrupting the re-entrant circuit *(67, 68)*, as shown in Figs. 3 and 4. As shown in Fig. 5, demonstrating device programming options, tiered therapy allows programming these electrical modalities to treat tachycardias with rates within defined zones of detection *(69)*. For example, a slower arrhythmia might be treated by ATP followed by low-energy and then high-energy shock, if needed. VF falls in a faster zone,

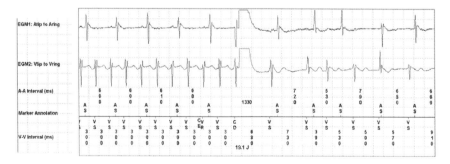

Fig. 2. Stored electrogram of a shock-terminated rapid ventricular tachycardia. *Top* tracing represents atrial electrogram, second tracing represents ventricular electrogram. Marker annotation describes device-defined event; "AS," atrial sensed event; "VS," ventricular sensed event; "CD," charge delivered.

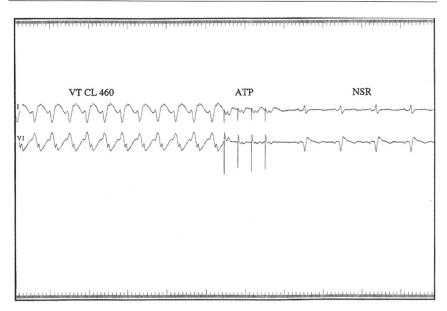

Fig. 3. Surface tracing recorded during standard ICD testing demonstrating anti-tachycardia pacing. Shown are surface leads I and V₁. One short burst (four beats) of antitachycardia pacing (ATP) is able to terminate a ventricular tachycardia (VT), restoring normal sinus rhythm (NSR).

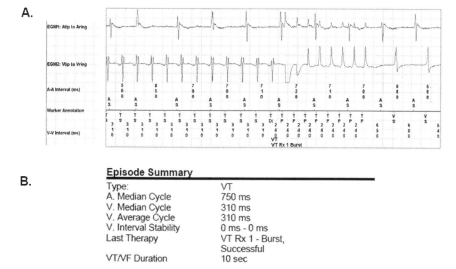

A.

B.

Episode Summary

Type:	VT
A. Median Cycle	750 ms
V. Median Cycle	310 ms
V. Average Cycle	310 ms
V. Interval Stability	0 ms - 0 ms
Last Therapy	VT Rx 1 - Burst, Successful
VT/VF Duration	10 sec

Fig. 4. (A) Stored electrogram of ATP-terminated ventricular tachycardia. "VT Rx 1 Burst" marks the beginning of delivered ATP. *Top* tracing represents atrial electrogram, second tracing represents ventricular electrogram. Marker annotation describes device-defined event; "AS," atrial sensed event; "TS," ventricular sensed event in "tachy" zone; "TD," arrhythmia has met tachycardia detection criteria; "TP," antitachycardia pacing, i.e., ATP; "VS," ventricular sensed event. **(B)** Text description of the same event with quantified cycle length and interval stability.

Device Parameter Summary						
VF	230 bpm 1.0 sec			31J⁄ # of Additional Max Shocks	31J⁄	31J 3
VT	170 bpm 2.5 sec		ATP1x 3 ATP2x Off	1.1J⁄	6J⁄	31J
VT-1	140 bpm 5.0 sec	Onset 16 % SRD 3:00 m:s	ATP1x 5 ATP2x Off	1.1J⁄	6J⁄	31J

Fig. 5. Printout of programming details for a device with three zones of therapy. Onset criteria are programmed for differentiation of VT from sinus tachycardia with sustained rate duration ("SRD") and the time-out variable set for 3 min.

prompting high-energy defibrillation. While ATP was initially used only to treat slower, stable VT, the recent Pacing Reduces Shocks for Fast VT II trial (PainFREE Rx II) *(70)* found that empirically programmed ATP delivered during device charging (a function available in some devices) could treat faster VTs, reducing shocks by 70% with no increase in adverse outcomes. Attempted ATP can accelerate VT into VF, leading to defibrillation.

3.2. Detection

As shown in Fig. 5, the primary criterion for arrhythmia detection is heart rate. However, other rhythms may result in heart rates above the defined rate cutoff, resulting in inappropriate shocks, occurring in up to 15% of patients with ICDs, and representing more than one-third of shocks received, regardless of ICD indication *(71)*. Figure 6 shows an example of atrial fibrillation with a rapid ventricular response triggering a high-energy shock. Programmable detection criteria, described in Table 7, can improve discrim-

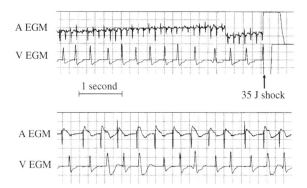

Fig. 6. Stored electrogram showing a shock received for atrial fibrillation with a rapid ventricular response. (*Top*) Atrial fibrillation with rapid ventricular response culminating in a 35 J shock. (*Bottom*) Postshock, sinus rhythm (sinus tachycardia) has been restored. A EGM, atrial electrogram; V EGM, ventricular electrogram.

Table 7
Arrhythmia discrimination

Discriminator	How it works	Clinical implications
Onset	Measures how sudden the arrhythmia onset was. Withholds therapy if onset is gradual	Effective at discriminating sinus tachycardia, which accelerates gradually, from VT, of usually sudden onset
Stability	Measures beat-to-beat variation in arrhythmia cycle length. Withholds therapy for irregular rhythms	Effective at discriminating between VT (regular) and rapid atrial fibrillation (irregular)
Morphology	Compares the QRS morphology during tachycardia to the baseline morphology. Withholds therapy if the tachycardia morphology is similar	Can discriminate supraventricular arrhythmias from VT
V>A	Compares the measured ventricular rate to the atrial rate. Treats as VT if ventricular rate greater than atrial	Can identify VT rapidly
AV interval (dual-chamber)	Evaluates the AV during tachycardia to differentiate sinus or atrial tachycardias (short P-R/long R-P interval) from VT (short R-P/long P-R)	Can differentiate supraventricular tachycardias from VT with retrograde conduction

VT – ventricular tachycardia.

ination between atrial and ventricular arrhythmias. For example, the device can be programmed to withhold therapy for a set amount of time if the onset of tachycardia is gradual, as is the case with sinus tachycardia (an example of this programming is shown in Fig. 5) In most, although not all studies, the dual-chamber ICD, incorporating a right atrial lead, can further decrease inappropriate shocks due to rapid supraventricular rhythms or physiologic sinus tachycardia using specific algorithms (72–74), such as those which analyze the relative timing of atrial and ventricular electrograms. Or, when the atrial sensed rate is faster than the ventricular rate, as in atrial fibrillation, ICD discharge may be inhibited (74).

Inappropriate detection, in which the device senses noncardiac electrical events, can occur due to either lead insulation disruption, as shown in Fig. 7, or electromagnetic interference (EMI) in the environment and can also result in inappropriate shock. Sources of environmental EMI that can be sensed by the ICD include medical procedures using cautery, radiofrequency abla-

A

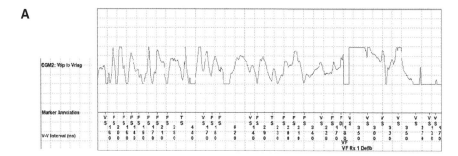

B

Observations
-V. pacing lead impedance is > 2000 ohms.
-726 V-V intervals have been sensed at 120 or 130ms since Dec 28, 2006 21:08:40. Check for sensing issues (e.g. double counting of R-waves, lead fracture, loose set screw).
-Patient Alert triggered -V. Pacing lead impedance >2000 ohms.
-2 VF episodes were longer than 30 seconds. Most recent was Episode #12, Dec 29, 2006 11:17:11.

Fig. 7. (A) Stored electrogram from shock delivered to otherwise asymptomatic patient. Electrogram clearly shows high-frequency variation in the signal consistent with electrical noise (noncardiac electrical activity) triggering the shock. **(B)** Observations recorded by the ICD at the time of interrogation demonstrating the electrogram above. High-pacing impedance implies lead fracture. Multiple, very short (120–130 ms) V–V intervals suggest inappropriate sensing of noise. VS, ventricular sensing; FS, sensing of ventricular signal in VF zone; TS, sensing of ventricular signal in VT zone; FD, detection criteria met to declare VF episode in progress.

tion, lithotripsy, or spinal stimulation; ICDs may need to be reprogrammed prior to these procedures. MRI is currently prohibited for patients with ICDs although precautions which may enhance the safety of MRI are under evaluation *(75)*. Other sources of EMI include antitheft devices *(76)* and machinery generating large magnetic fields *(77)*. Patients are advised to be cautious of potential EMI in the environment.

3.3. Management Issues in the Care of the CHF Patient with an ICD

3.3.1. PROGRAMMING OF THE ICD: BRADYCARDIA PACING

One concern following MADIT II was the higher rate of HF in the ICD group *(28, 78)*. The later Dual Chamber and VVI Implantable Defibrillator (DAVID) trial *(79)*, which randomized patients receiving ICDs to either dual- or single-chamber devices, showed higher incidence of HF with the dual-chamber device, and it was later determined that the percent of RV pacing was more important than pacing mode in determining adverse outcome (HF or death) *(80)*. The mechanism by which RV pacing effectively causes iatrogenic dyssynchrony likely explains the higher incidence of HF in ICD-treated patients in MADIT II, as this concern was not appreciated at that time. Based on these and other data showing deleterious effects of RV pacing *(81, 82)*, dual-chamber devices are now programmed to minimize RV pacing, using recently developed algorithms incorporating AV search hysteresis to provide atrial-based pacing *(83, 84)*.

3.4. Management of Frequent Shocks

While an ICD shock effectively terminates ventricular tachyarrhythmias and improves mortality, shocks are painful. One survey asking patients to describe the sensation of a shock yielded responses of "a blow to the body," "a punch in the chest," "being hit by a truck," "kicked by a mule," and "putting a finger in a light socket" *(85)*. In the Canadian Implantable Defibrillator Study (CIDS), patients who received 0–4 shocks had significant improvement in QOL over time, but those with 5 or more shocks did not improve *(86)*. Similarly, in the AVID trial, the occurrence of even one shock was associated with reduction in mental well-being and physical function, even after controlling for multiple clinical factors such as HF; the reduction in QOL grew greater as shocks were more frequent *(87)*. Thus, decreasing shock frequency is critical to maintaining quality of life in patients with ICDs.

In patients with ischemic cardiomyopathy, increases in BNP predict appropriate ICD shocks *(88)*, and therapies effective for HF decrease incidence of sudden cardiac death *(9, 10, 88)*. These findings suggest that the first step in the prevention of frequent shocks for patients with HF is maximization of heart failure therapy. For patients requiring specific antiarrhythmic therapy, amiodarone has been shown to decrease appropriate ICD shocks *(89)* and has neutral effects on survival in patients with heart failure *(29, 90)*. In patients suffering from shocks for atrial fibrillation, dofetilide also does not worsen survival or heart failure in patients with HF *(91)* and can be used safely as long as renal function and QT interval are normal. Class I antiarrhythmics, both Ia agents, such as quinidine and procainamide, and Ic agents, such as flecainide, increase mortality in patients with HF *(92)*.

3.5. Device Malfunction

With the expanse in device technology has come an increase in malfunctions resulting in advisories and recalls and with increasing indications for the ICD, the number of patients affected by advisories is expected to increase *(93)*. Actual device malfunction requiring device replacement, which can be due to either physical or mechanical factors or software failure, is estimated to be about 20 per 1000 implants *(94–96)*. Like ICD generators, leads may also experience performance concerns, most commonly due to insulation degradation or lead fractures *(97, 98)*. Fortunately, death due to device malfunction is rare *(59, 93, 99, 100)*. Each major ICD manufacturer has experienced product advisories and malfunctions *(101)*.

Patients and physicians faced with an advisory must weigh the risks of malfunction, the nature of the specific advisory, the patient's underlying arrhythmia and clinical condition, and the risks of replacement. The Heart Rhythm Society has published recommendations for management of device performance issues *(94)*, emphasizing greater transparency in postmarket surveillance, analysis, and reporting as well as cooperation among industry, regulators, and physicians. Further, ongoing efforts to improve detection, reporting, and management of device performance and malfunction information will improve patient safety *(102)*. Specific device algorithms to automatically measure performance-related variables such as lead and battery impedance on a regular basis, automated patient and physician alert systems, and the advent of remote ICD monitoring will further improve patient safety *(103)*.

3.6. *Management of the ICD in End-of-Life Care*

HF is a progressive disease with many interventions providing palliative, but not curative, benefit. The ACC/AHA heart failure guidelines stress that the possible reasons and process for potential deactivation of defibrillator features should be discussed long before functional capacity or outlook for survival is severely reduced *(54)*. The dying process of patients with ICDs can be accompanied by multiple shocks, to the distress of patient and family *(104, 105)*, and conversations between physicians and patients regarding the option of deactivation of the shocking functions have taken place only rarely, even among patients who have chosen a "do not resuscitate" order *(105)*. There is solid legal basis for deactivating an ICD should this be the patient's wishes *(106)*, and multidisciplinary strategies to identify patients with terminal illnesses and initiate withdrawal of ICD shock therapy as part of a comprehensive comfort care approach can decrease painful shocks as the patient ultimately succumbs to heart failure or another terminal illness *(107)*.

4. CONCLUSIONS

Preventing sudden SCD remains a major challenge for physicians treating patients with heart failure. ICDs are a remarkable technology, clinically and scientifically proven to improve survival in appropriately selected patients. Although the precise indications for ICD implantation continue to evolve, the therapy will undoubtedly remain an important complement to comprehensive medical treatment of patients with heart failure.

REFERENCES

1. Zipes DP, Wellens HJ. Sudden cardiac death. Circulation 1998; 98:2334–51.
2. Kannel WB, Schatzkin A. Sudden death: lessons from subsets in population studies. J Am Coll Cardiol 1985; 5:141B–9B.
3. Myerburg RJ, Kessler KM, Castellanos A. Sudden cardiac death: epidemiology, transient risk, and intervention assessment. Ann Intern Med 1993; 119:1187–97.
4. Luu M, Stevenson WG, Stevenson LW, Baron K, Walden J. Diverse mechanisms of unexpected cardiac arrest in advanced heart failure. Circulation 1989; 80:1675–80.
5. Huikuri HV, Castellanos A, Myerburg RJ. Sudden death due to cardiac arrhythmias. N Engl J Med 2001; 345:1473–82.
6. Bayes de Luna A, Coumel P, Leclercq JF. Ambulatory sudden cardiac death: mechanisms of production of fatal arrhythmia on the basis of data from 157 cases. Am Heart J 1989; 117:151–9.
7. Goldman S, Johnson G, Cohn JN, et al. Mechanism of death in heart failure: The vasodilator-heart failure trials. Circulation 1993; 87.suppl VI:VI24–31.
8. Uretsky BF, Sheahan RG. Primary prevention of sudden cardiac death in heart failure: will the solution be shocking? Journal of the American College of Cardiology 1997; 30:1589–97.
9. Anonymous. Effect of metoprolol CR/XL in chronic heart failure: Metoprolol CR/XL randomised intervention trial in congestive heart failure. Lancet 1999; 353:2001–7.
10. Anonymous. The cardiac insufficiency bisoprolol study II (Cibis II). Lancet 1999; 353:9–13.
11. Stevenson WG, Stevenson LW, Middlekauff HR, Saxon LA. Sudden death prevention in patients with advanced ventricular dysfunction. Circulation 1993; 88:2953–61.
12. Mirowski M, Reid PR, Mower MM, et al. Termination of malignant ventricular arrhythmias with an implanted automatic defibrillator in human beings. N Engl J Med 1980; 303:322–4.
13. The Antiarrhythmics versus Implantable Defibrillators (AVID) Investigators. A comparison of antiarrhythmic-drug therapy with implantable defibrillators in patients resuscitated from near-fatal ventricular arrhythmias. N Engl J Med 1997; 337:1576–83.
14. Kuck KH, Cappato R, Siebels J, Ruppel R. Randomized comparison of antiarrhythmic drug therapy with implantable defibrillators in patients resuscitated from cardiac arrest: the Cardiac Arrest Study Hamburg (CASH). Circulation 2000; 102:748–54.
15. Connolly SJ, Gent M, Roberts RS, et al. Canadian implantable defibrillator study (CIDS): a randomized trial of the implantable cardioverter defibrillator against amiodarone. Circulation 2000; 101:1297–302.
16. Nademanee K, Veerakul G, Mower M, et al. Defibrillator Versus beta-Blockers for Unexplained Death in Thailand (DEBUT): a randomized clinical trial. Circulation 2003; 107:2221–6.
17. Lau EW, Griffith MJ, Pathmanathan RK, et al. The Midlands Trial of Empirical Amiodarone versus Electrophysiology-guided Interventions and Implantable Cardioverter-defibrillators (MAVERIC): a multi-centre prospective randomised clinical trial on the secondary prevention of sudden cardiac death. Europace 2004; 6:257–66.
18. Connolly SJ, Hallstrom AP, Cappato R, et al. Meta-analysis of the implantable cardioverter defibrillator secondary prevention trials. AVID, CASH and CIDS studies. Antiarrhythmics vs Implantable Defibrillator study. Cardiac Arrest Study Hamburg. Canadian Implantable Defibrillator Study. Eur Heart J 2000; 21:2071–8.
19. Anderson JL, Hallstrom AP, Epstein AE, et al. Design and results of the antiarrhythmics vs implantable defibrillators (AVID) registry. The AVID Investigators. Circulation 1999; 99:1692–9.
20. Bigger JT. Expanding indications for implantable cardiac defibrillators. N Engl J Med 2002; 346:931–3.

21. de Vreede-Swagemakers JJ, Gorgels AP, Dubois-Arbouw WI, et al. Out-of-hospital cardiac arrest in the 1990s: a population-based study in the Maastricht area on incidence, characteristics and survival. J Am Coll Cardiol 1997; 30:1500–5.
22. Weaver WD, Hill D, Fahrenbruch CE, et al. Use of the automatic external defibrillator in the management of out-of-hospital cardiac arrest. N Engl J Med 1988; 319:661–6.
23. Bhandari AK, Widerhorn J, Sager PT, et al. Prognostic significance of programmed ventricular stimulation in patients surviving complicated acute myocardial infarction: a prospective study. Am Heart J 1992; 124:87–96.
24. Wilber DJ, Olshansky B, Moran JF, Scanlon PJ. Electrophysiological testing and nonsustained ventricular tachycardia. Use and limitations in patients with coronary artery disease and impaired ventricular function. Circulation 1990; 82:350–8.
25. Moss AJ, Hall WJ, Cannom DS, et al. Improved survival with an implanted defibrillator in patients with coronary disease at high risk for ventricular arrhythmia. Multicenter Automatic Defibrillator Implantation Trial Investigators. N Engl J Med 1996; 335:1933–40.
26. Buxton AE, Lee KL, Fisher JD, Josephson ME, Prystowsky EN, Hafley G. A randomized study of the prevention of sudden death in patients with coronary artery disease. Multicenter Unsustained Tachycardia Trial Investigators. N Engl J Med 1999; 341:1882–90.
27. Buxton AE, Lee KL, DiCarlo L, et al. Electrophysiologic testing to identify patients with coronary artery disease who are at risk for sudden death. Multicenter Unsustained Tachycardia Trial Investigators. N Engl J Med 2000; 342:1937–45.
28. Moss AJ, Zareba W, Hall WJ, et al. Prophylactic implantation of a defibrillator in patients with myocardial infarction and reduced ejection fraction. N Engl J Med 2002; 346:877–83.
29. Bardy GH, Lee KL, Mark DB, et al. Amiodarone or an implantable cardioverter-defibrillator for congestive heart failure. N Engl J Med 2005; 352:225–37.
30. Kadish A, Dyer A, Daubert JP, et al. Prophylactic defibrillator implantation in patients with nonischemic dilated cardiomyopathy. N Engl J Med 2004; 350:2151–8.
31. Bansch D, Antz M, Boczor S, et al. Primary prevention of sudden cardiac death in idiopathic dilated cardiomyopathy: the Cardiomyopathy Trial (CAT). Circulation 2002; 105:1453–8.
32. Strickberger SA, Hummel JD, Bartlett TG, et al. Amiodarone versus implantable cardioverter-defibrillator: randomized trial in patients with nonischemic dilated cardiomyopathy and asymptomatic nonsustained ventricular tachycardia–AMIOVIRT. J Am Coll Cardiol 2003; 41:1707–12.
33. Hohnloser SH, Kuck KH, Dorian P, et al. Prophylactic use of an implantable cardioverter-defibrillator after acute myocardial infarction. N Engl J Med 2004; 351:2481–8.
34. Coats AJ. MADIT II, the Multi-center Automatic Defibrillator Implantation Trial II stopped early for mortality reduction, has ICD therapy earned its evidence-based credentials. Int J Cardiology 2002; 82:1–5.
35. Buxton AE. Should everyone with an ejection fraction less than or equal to 30% receive an implantable cardioverter-defibrillator? Not everyone with an ejection fraction < or = 30% should receive an implantable cardioverter-defibrillator. Circulation 2005; 111:2537–49; discussion 2537–49.
36. Tung RT, Zimetbaum PJ, Josephson ME. A critical appraisal of implantable cardioverter-defibrillator therapy for the prevention of sudden cardiac death. J Am Coll Cardiol 2008 Sep 30;52(14):1111–21.
37. Epstein AE. Benefits of the implantable cardioverter-defibrillator. J Am Coll Cardiol 2008 Sep 30;52(14):1122–7.
38. Myerberg RJ. Implantable cardioverter-defibrillators after myocardial infarction. N Engl J Med 2008 359:2245–53.

39. Buxton AE, Lee KL, Hafley GE, et al. Relation of ejection fraction and inducible ventricular tachycardia to mode of death in patients with coronary artery disease: an analysis of patients enrolled in the multicenter unsustained tachycardia trial. Circulation 2002; 106:2466–72.
40. La Rovere MT, Pinna GD, Hohnloser SH, et al. Baroreflex sensitivity and heart rate variability in the identification of patients at risk for life-threatening arrhythmias: implications for clinical trials. Circulation 2001; 103:2072–7.
41. Bailey JJ, Berson AS, Handelsman H, Hodges M. Utility of current risk stratification tests for predicting major arrhythmic events after myocardial infarction. J Am Coll Cardiol 2001; 38:1902–11.
42. Kadish A. Prophylactic defibrillator implantation–Toward an evidence-based approach. N Engl J Med 2005; 352:285–6.
43. Buxton AE. The clinical use of implantable cardioverter defibrillators: where are we now? Where should we go? Ann Intern Med 2003; 138:512–4.
44. Reynolds MR, Josephson ME. MADIT II (second Multicenter Automated Defibrillator Implantation Trial) debate: risk stratification, costs, and public policy. Circulation 2003; 108:1779–83.
45. Bloomfield DM, Steinman RC, Namerow PB, et al. Microvolt T-wave alternans distinguishes between patients likely and patients not likely to benefit from implanted cardiac defibrillator therapy: a solution to the Multicenter Automatic Defibrillator Implantation Trial (MADIT) II conundrum. Circulation 2004; 110:1885–9.
46. Gold MR, Bloomfield DM, Anderson KP, et al. A comparison of T-wave alternans, signal averaged electrocardiography and programmed ventricular stimulation for arrhythmia risk stratification. J Am Coll Cardiol 2000; 36:2247–53.
47. Bigger JT, Jr. Prophylactic use of implanted cardiac defibrillators in patients at high risk for ventricular arrhythmias after coronary-artery bypass graft surgery. Coronary Artery Bypass Graft (CABG) Patch Trial Investigators. N Engl J Med 1997; 337:1569–75.
48. Solomon SD, Zelenkofske S, McMurray JJ, et al. Sudden death in patients with myocardial infarction and left ventricular dysfunction, heart failure, or both. N Engl J Med 2005; 352:2581–8.
49. Buxton AE. Sudden death after myocardial infarction – who needs prophylaxis, and when? N Engl J Med 2005; 352:2638–40.
50. Zareba W, Piotrowicz K, McNitt S, Moss AJ, MADIT II Investigators. Implantable cardioverter-defibrillator efficacy in patients with heart failure and left ventricular dysfunction (from the MADIT II population). Am J Cardiol 2005; 95:1487–91.
51. Bristow MR, Saxon LA, Boehmer J, et al. Cardiac-resynchronization therapy with or without an implantable defibrillator in advanced chronic heart failure. N Engl J Med 2004; 350:2140–50.
52. Gregoratos G, Abrams J, Epstein AE, et al. ACC/AHA/NASPE 2002 guideline update for implantation of cardiac pacemakers and antiarrhythmia devices: summary article. A report of the American College of Cardiology/American Heart Association Task Force on Practice Guidelines (ACC/AHA/NASPE Committee to Update the 1998 Pacemaker Guidelines). J Cardiovasc Electrophysiol 2002; 13:1183–99.
53. Zipes DP, Camm AJ, Borggrefe M, et al. ACC/AHA/ESC 2006 guidelines for management of patients with ventricular arrhythmias and the prevention of sudden cardiac death: A report of the American College of Cardiology/American Heart Association Task Force and the European Society of Cardiology Committee for Practice Guidelines. Circulation 2006; 114:e385–484.
54. Epstein AE, DiMarco JP, Ellenbogen KA, Estes NAM III, Freedman RA, Gettes LS, Gillinov AM, Gregoratos G, Hammill SC, Hayes DL, Hlatky MA, Newby LK, Page RL, Schoenfeld MH, Silka MJ, Stevenson LW, Sweeney MO. ACC/AHA/HRS 2008 guidelines for device-based therapy of cardiac rhythm abnormalities: a report of the American College of Cardiology/American Heart Association Task Force on Practice

Guidelines (Writing Committee to Revise the ACC/AHA/NASPE 2002 Guideline Update for Implantation of Cardiac Pacemakers and Antiarrhythmia Devices). J Am Coll Cardiol 2008;51:e1–62.

55. Heart Rhythm Society. National ICD Registry Becomes Official Database for Medicare. Accessed at: http://www.hrsonline.org/Policy/ICDRegistry/ICD_Registry_Official.cfm.

56. DiMarco JP. Implantable cardioverter-defibrillators. N Engl J Med 2003; 349:1836–47.

57. Zareba W, Moss AJ, Daubert JP, Hall WJ, Robinson JL, Andrews M. Implantable cardioverter defibrillator in high-risk long QT syndrome patients. J Cardiovasc Electrophysiol 2003; 14:337–41.

58. Watanabe H, Chinushi M, Sugiura H, et al. Unsuccessful internal defibrillation in Brugada syndrome: focus on refractoriness and ventricular fibrillation cycle length. J Cardiovasc Electrophysiol 2005; 16:262–6.

59. Maron BJ, Estes NA, 3rd, Maron MS, Almquist AK, Link MS, Udelson JE. Primary prevention of sudden death as a novel treatment strategy in hypertrophic cardiomyopathy. Circulation 2003; 107:2872–5.

60. Begley DA, Mohiddin SA, Tripodi D, Winkler JB, Fananapazir L. Efficacy of implantable cardioverter defibrillator therapy for primary and secondary prevention of sudden cardiac death in hypertrophic cardiomyopathy. Pacing Clin Electrophysiol 2003; 26:1887–96.

61. Corrado D, Leoni L, Link MS, et al. Implantable cardioverter-defibrillator therapy for prevention of sudden death in patients with arrhythmogenic right ventricular cardiomyopathy/dysplasia. Circulation 2003; 108:3084–91.

62. Sanders GD, Hlatky MA, Owens DK. Cost-effectiveness of implantable cardioverter-defibrillators. N Engl J Med 2005; 353:1471–80.

63. Mark DB, Nelson CL, Anstrom KJ, et al. Cost-effectiveness of defibrillator therapy or amiodarone in chronic stable heart failure: results from the Sudden Cardiac Death in Heart Failure Trial (SCD-HeFT). Circulation 2006; 114:135–42.

64. Goldman L. Cost-effectiveness in a flat world – can ICDs help the United States get rhythm? N Engl J Med 2005; 353:1513–5.

65. Kusumoto FM, Goldschlager N. Device therapy for cardiac arrhythmias. JAMA 2002; 287:1848–52.

66. Yee R, Klein GJ, Leitch JW, et al. A permanent transvenous lead system for an implantable pacemaker cardioverter-defibrillator. Nonthoracotomy approach to implantation. Circulation 1992; 85:196–204.

67. Saksena S, Krol RB, Kaushik RR. Innovations in pulse generators and lead systems: balancing complexity with clinical benefit and long-term results. Am Heart J 1994; 127:1010–21.

68. Estes NA, 3rd, Haugh CJ, Wang PJ, Manolis AS. Antitachycardia pacing and low-energy cardioversion for ventricular tachycardia termination: a clinical perspective. Am Heart J 1994; 127:1038–46.

69. Gollob MH, Seger JJ. Current status of the implantable cardioverter-defibrillator. Chest 2001; 119:1210–21.

70. Wathen MS, DeGroot PJ, Sweeney MO, et al. Prospective randomized multicenter trial of empirical antitachycardia pacing versus shocks for spontaneous rapid ventricular tachycardia in patients with implantable cardioverter-defibrillators: Pacing Fast Ventricular Tachycardia Reduces Shock Therapies (PainFREE Rx II) trial results. Circulation 2004; 110:2591–6.

71. Sweeney MO, Wathen MS, Volosin KJ, et al. Appropriate and inappropriate ventricular therapies, quality of life, and morality among primary and secondary prevention implantable cardioverter defibrillator patients. Circulation 2005; 111:2898–05.

72. Friedman PA, McClelland RL, Bamlet WR, et al. Dual-chamber versus single-chamber detection enhancements for implantable defibrillator rhythm diagnosis. Circulation 2006; 113:2871–79.

73. Stadler RW, Gunderson BD, Gillberg JM. An adaptive interval-based algorithm for withholding ICD therapy during sinus tachycardia. Pacing Clin Electrophysiol 2003; 26:1189–201.

74. Israel CW, Gronefeld G, Iscolo N, Stoppler C, Hohnloser SH. Discrimination between ventricular and supraventricular tachycardia by dual chamber cardioverter defibrillators: importance of the atrial sensing function. Pacing Clin Electrophysiol 2001; 24:183–90.

75. Gimbel JR, Bailey SM, Tchou PJ, Ruggier PM, Wilkoff BL. Strategies for the safe magnetic resonance imaging of pacemaker-dependent patients. PACE 2005; 28: 1041–6.

76. Santucci PA, Haw J, Trohman RG, Pinski SL. Interference with an implantable cardioverter defibrillator by an antitheft-surveillance device. N Engl J Med 1371; 339:1371–4.

77. Goldschlager N, Epstein AE, Friedman P, Gang E, Krol RB, Olshansky B. Environmental and drug effects on patients with pacemakers and implantable cardioverter defibrillators. Arch Intern Med 2001; 161:649–55.

78. Hurst TM, Hinrichs M, Breidenbach C, Katz N, Waldecker B. Detection of myocardial injury during transvenous implantation of automatic cardioverter-defibrillators. J Am Coll Cardiol 1999; 34:402–8.

79. Wilkoff BL, Cook JR, Epstein AE, et al. Dual-chamber pacing or ventricular backup pacing in patients with an implantable defibrillator: the Dual Chamber and VVI Implantable Defibrillator (DAVID) Trial. JAMA 2002; 288:3115–23.

80. Sharma AD, Rizo-Patron C, Hallstrom AP, et al. Percent right ventricular pacing predicts outcomes in the DAVID trial. Heart Rhythm 2005; 2:830–4.

81. Wonisch M, Lercher P, Scherr D, et al. Influence of permanent right ventricular pacing on cardiorespiratory exercise parameters in chronic heart failure patients with implanted cardioverter defibrillators. Chest 2005; 127:787–93.

82. Sweeney MO, Hellkamp AS, Ellenbogen KA, et al. Adverse effect of ventricular pacing on heart failure and atrial fibrillation among patients with normal baseline QRS duration in a clinical trial of pacemaker therapy for sinus node dysfunction. Circulation 2003; 107:2932–37.

83. Sweeney MO, Ellenbogen KA, Betzold R, et al. Multicenter, prospective, randomized trial of a new atrial-based managed ventricular pacing mode (MVP) in dual chamber ICDs. Circulation 2004; 110:III–444.

84. Sweeney MO, Shea JB, Fox V, et al. Randomized pilot study of a new atrial-based minimal ventricular pacing mode in dual chamber implantable cardioverter-defibrillators. Heart Rhythm 2004; 1:160–67.

85. Ahmad M, L B, Roelke M, Bernstein AD, Parsonnet V. Patients' attitudes toward implanted defibrillator shocks. PACE 2000; 23:934–38.

86. Irvine J, Dorian P, Baker B, et al. Quality of life in the Canadian implantable defibrillator study (CIDS). Am Heart J 2002; 144:282–9.

87. Schron E, Exner D, Yao Q, et al. Quality of life in the antiarrhythmics versus implantable defibrillators. Circulation 2002; 105:589–94.

88. Klingenberg R, Zugck C, Becker R, et al. Raised B-type natriuretic peptide predicts implantable cardioverter-defibrillator therapy in patients with ischaemic cardiomyopathy. Heart 2006; 92:1323–4.

89. Connolly SJ, Dorian P, Roberts R, et al. Comparison of beta-blockers, amiodarone plus beta-blockers, or sotalol for prevention of shocks from implantable cardioverter defibrillators: the OPTIC Study: a randomized trial. JAMA 2006; 295:165–71.

90. Doval HC, Nul DR, Grancelli HO, Perrone SV, Bortman GR, Curiel R. Randomised trial of low-dose amiodarone in severe congestive heart failure. Grupo de Estudio de la Sobrevida en la Insuficiencia Cardiaca en Argentina (GESICA). Lancet 1994; 344:493–8.

91. Torp-Pedersen C, Moller M, Bloch-Thomsen PE, et al. Dofetilide in patients with congestive heart failure and left ventricular dysfunction. Danish Investigations of Arrhythmia and Mortality on Dofetilide Study Group. N Engl J Med 1999; 341:857–65.
92. Pratt CM, Eaton T, Francis M, et al. The inverse relationship between baseline left ventricular ejection fraction and outcome of antiarrhythmic therapy: a dangerous imbalance in the risk–benefit ratio. Am Heart J 1989; 118:433–40.
93. Maisel WH, Sweeney MO, Stevenson WG, Ellison KE, Epstein LM. Recalls and safety alerts involving pacemakers and implantable cardioverter-defibrillator generators. JAMA 2001; 286:793–9.
94. Carlson MD, Wilkoff BL, Maisel WH, et al. Recommendations from the heart rhythm society task force on device performance policies and guidelines. Heart Rhythm 2006; 3:1250–73.
95. Maisel WH, Moynahan M, Zuckerman BD, Gross TP, Tovar OH, Tillman DB, Schultz DB. Pacemaker and ICD generator malfunctions: analysis of food and drug administration annual reports. JAMA 2006; 295: 1901–06.
96. Maisel WH. Pacemaker and ICD generator reliability: meta-analysis of device registries. JAMA 2006; 295: 1929–34.
97. Maisel WH, Kramer DB. Implantable cardioverter-defibrillator performance. Circulation 2008 May 27;117(21):2721–3.
98. Maisel WH. Semper fidelis – consumer protection for patients with implanted medical devices. N Engl J Med 2008; 358: 985–87.
99. Hauser RG, Kallinen L. Deaths associated with implantable cardioverter defibrillator failure and deactivation reported in the United States Food and Drug Administration Manufacturer and User Facility Device Experience Database. Heart Rhythm 2004; 1:399–405.
100. Hauser RG, Maron BJ. Lessons from the failure and recall of an implantable cardioverter-defibrillator. Circulation 2005; 112:2040–2.
101. Steinbrook R. The controversy over Guidant's implantable defibrillators. N Engl J Med 2005; 353:221–4.
102. Maisel WH, Hauser RG. Proceedings of the ICD performance conference. Heart Rhythm 2008 Sep;5(9):1331–8.
103. Vollmann D, Erdogan A, Himmrich E, et al. Patient Alert to detect ICD lead failure: efficacy, limitations, and implications for future algorithms. Europace 2006; 8:371–6.
104. Nambisan V, Chao D. Death and defibrillation: A shocking experience. Palliative Med 2004; 18:482–3.
105. Goldstein NE, Lampert R, Bradley E, Lynn J, Krumholz HM. Management of Implantable cardioverter defibrillators in end-of-life care. Ann Intern Med 2004; 141:835–38.
106. Gostin LO. Deciding life and death in the courtroom: From Quinlan to Cruzan, Glucksberg, and Vacco – A brief history and analysis of the constitutional protection of the "right to die". JAMA 1997; 278:1523–28.
107. Lewis WR, Luebke DL, Johnson NJ, Harrington MD, Costantini O, Aulisio MP. Withdrawing implantable defibrillator shock therapy in terminally ill patients. Am J Med 2006; 119:892–96.

7   Cardiac Resynchronization Therapy

Daniel Frisch, MD and Peter J. Zimetbaum, MD

CONTENTS

Abstract

A variety of medical therapies are clinically proven to improve symptoms and mortality in heart failure patients. However, some patients remain symptomatic despite optimal medical therapy. A subset of these patients may demonstrate electrical dyssynchrony which may contribute to hemodynamic and clinical deterioration. This chapter reviews the pathophysiology and clinical assessment of dyssynchrony, the clinical indications for cardiac resynchronization therapy, and a description of the devices and programming features currently available to heart failure patients.

Key Words: Heart failure; Dyssynchrony; Resynchronization; Implantable defibrillator.

From: *Contemporary Cardiology: Device Therapy in Heart Failure*
Edited by: W.H. Maisel, DOI 10.1007/978-1-59745-424-7_7
© Humana Press, a part of Springer Science+Business Media, LLC 2010

1. PATHOPHYSIOLOGY OF DYSSYNCHRONY AND DEFINITIONS

1.1. Context

Heart failure (HF) affects nearly 5 million patients in the United States and over 500,000 new diagnoses are made each year. Over the past decade, the rate of hospitalizations for heart failure has increased by over 150% and mortality can be as high as 40% at 1 year with severely symptomatic heart failure *(1, 2)*. Medicare spends more dollars for HF diagnosis and management than any other condition. Though multiple causes exist, the most common causes include coronary artery disease, hypertension, and idiopathic dilated cardiomyopathy *(2–4)*.

A variety of medical therapies have been introduced to optimize chamber loading, neurohormonal activation, and correct cellular abnormalities. These therapies, which include angiotensin-converting-enzyme (ACE) inhibitors *(5, 6)*, angiotensin-receptor antagonists *(7–9)*, beta-blockers *(10–15)*, spironolactone *(16)*, and coronary bypass surgery *(17, 18)* have been shown in multiple, large, randomized controlled clinical trials to improve functional class and survival (Fig. 1). In addition to myocardial abnormalities, electrical abnormalities occur in patients with cardiomyopathies and may contribute to hemodynamic and clinical deterioration.

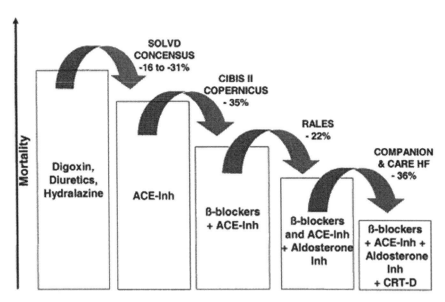

Fig. 1. A number of medications have been shown to reduce mortality in patients with heart failure as demonstrated by well-conducted scientific studies (above, *arrows*). In addition, cardiac resynchronization therapy with defibrillation (CRT-D) has been demonstrated to improve survival in patients already receiving optimal medical therapy for heart failure.

Approximately one third of patients with a low LV ejection fraction and New York Heart Association Class III to IV HF manifest a QRS duration greater than 120 ms *(2)*. Furthermore, the presence of a left bundle branch block (LBBB) has been associated with increased mortality in patients with HF *(19)*.

1.2. Electrical Timing

Under normal circumstances, the LV contracts synchronously with less than 40 ms difference between timing of contraction of the various walls *(20)*. This synchrony is important to maximize LV work performance. A segment of myocardium stimulated early is inefficient for chamber pumping function because little if any ejection of blood from the ventricle occurs with one segment contracting early. Late stimulation is wasted work as well because ejection will be compromised by the surrounding increased tension against which this contraction occurs and may affect other segments that are relaxing by exaggerating stretch *(20, 21)*. Such may be the case with bundle branch block or single-site pacing (e.g., RV apical pacing). Interventricular dyssynchrony may involve similar mechanisms by its effects on the interventricular septum *(22)*. Finally, atrioventricular coordination may contribute to sub-optimal ejection because of abnormal chamber filling and exacerbation of mitral regurgitation *(20)*. The role then of cardiac resynchronization therapy (CRT) may include optimization of these three areas of mechanical abnormalities: atrioventricular delay, interventricular dyssynchrony, and intra-left ventricular dyssynchrony (Table 1).

Small studies have evaluated different programmed AV delays on various hemodynamic parameters (Fig. 2). While positive effects have been shown in some *(23)*, including minimization of diastolic mitral regurgitation, other studies have failed to show any changes *(24)*. One explanation for the lack of benefit was the obligate right ventricular pacing during programmed AV delays shorter than the patients' baseline values.

Table 1
Mechanisms of dyssynchrony

Dyssynchrony location	Mechanism
Atrioventricular	Too short or too long an interval results in sub-optimal chamber filling and contributes to mitral regurgitation
Interventricular (RV/LV)	Part of the CRT response has been thought to be due to improvement in interventricular synchrony; QRS has been considered a marker
Intraventricular (LV septal/ posterior)	Not all patients with wide QRS respond to CRT; dyssynchronous stimulation (e.g., LBBB or RV pacing) creates regions of *early* and *late* contraction

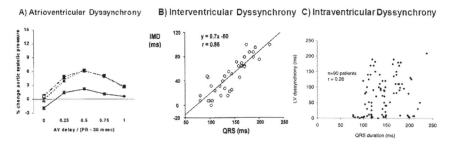

Fig. 2. (a) The effect of various programmed AV delay intervals on percentage change in systolic pressure is shown *(22)*; **(b)** interventricular mechanical delay (IMD) measured in milliseconds correlates with QRS duration *(23)*; **(c)** echocardiographic left ventricular dyssynchrony may not correlate with QRS duration in patients with congestive heart failure and a reduced LV ejection fraction *(25)*.

Correction of interventricular dyssynchrony has been considered to contribute to the response to CRT. The QRS duration has been identified as a marker of this abnormality and has been used to select patients for CRT *(22)*. However, when LV dyssynchrony is assessed by tissue Doppler echocardiography, QRS duration may correlate poorly. In one study, the relation between QRS duration and LV dyssynchrony (assessed by tissue Doppler imaging [TDI] in 90 patients with severe HF and LVEF <35%) revealed that LV dyssynchrony on TDI in patients with QRS durations of <120 ms, 120–150 ms, or >150 ms was present in 27%, 60%, and 70% of patients, respectively *(25)*. These results suggest that QRS duration as the sole measure of dyssynchrony would include patients who will not respond to therapy and exclude patient who might respond.

Nonetheless, the QRS duration is a marker of spatially dispersed mechanical activation and combining QRS information with imaging analysis of LV dyssynchrony (e.g., tissue Doppler echocardiography) may improve the ability to predict response to CRT *(26)*.

1.3. CRT Compared with Other Methods of Increasing Cardiac Output (Inotropes)

Patients who do respond to CRT have improved systolic performance. A concern that has been raised is the long-term effect of such a therapy compared with other therapies that alter hemodynamic parameters in a similar manner, notably pressors and inotropes. While agents such as milrinone *(27)* have been shown to acutely improve systolic performance, long-term efficacy and safety may be compromised by the increased metabolic demands of such therapies. In a hemodynamic study comparing the effects of dobutamine and LV pacing on ventricular and aortic pressure and myocardial oxygen consumption investigators found that systolic function rose substantially in both groups from LV pacing (43% and 37% increase in *dP/dt*(max) with LV pacing and dobutamine, respectively) *(28)*. However, myocardial oxygen consumption was significantly different among the groups with a decline of 8% in the pacing group and an increase of 22% in the dobutamine group ($P < 0.05$).

1.4. Mitral Regurgitation

Patients being considered for CRT have dilated ventricles and reduced systolic function. Mitral regurgitation (MR) is commonly associated. Often the MR is a functional problem related to one or more of at least three mechanisms: annular dilation, altered tethering and contractile forces, and atrioventricular delay *(20, 29–31)*. Though not considered a requirement for benefit from CRT, reduction of mitral regurgitation is an additional hemodynamic and clinical advantage.

Remodeling of the LV is a dynamic process which includes myocyte hypertrophy, fibrosis and deposition of extracellular matrix, and cellular necrosis and apoptosis. On the macroscopic level, LV dilation occurs and the chamber becomes more spherical. The remodeling process, which is an adaptation to preserve stroke volume, however, over time, causes loss of contractility and secondary MR *(32)*. Among the clinical and hemodynamic benefits of CRT, a reverse of this remodeling process has been observed with an 8–15% reduction in LV end-diastolic dimension and a 4–7% increase in LV ejection fraction *(1, 33)*.

Separate from improving chamber geometry, functional mitral regurgitation has been shown to be reduced by CRT in patients with HF and LBBB by altering contractile forces. By directly increasing the left ventricular *dP/dt*$_{max}$ and thus the transmitral pressure gradient, the mitral valve effective regurgitant orifice area is reduced *(31)*.

Too short or too long of an AV interval can contribute to MR. During long AV intervals, the mitral valve may attain an open configuration in late diastole, which may lead to regurgitation early in systole *(34)*. Optimizing the AV interval may mitigate this risk.

1.5. LV vs. BiV Pacing

Biventricular (BiV) and LV pacing result in different electrical activation and may provide different results in hemodynamic and clinical end points. Various investigators have tested the hypothesis that LV pacing alone confers the same benefit as BiV pacing despite the different electrical activation patterns. While larger clinical trials are ongoing, several of these studies have suggested that mechanical synchronization can be achieved equally with either approach *(35–37)*.

2. IMAGING MODALITIES TO IDENTIFY PATIENTS

2.1. Echocardiography

Echocardiography is the most often used tool to evaluate dyssynchrony, and various echocardiographic techniques can be used for this purpose *(38)*. Using M-mode echocardiography, time to peak contraction can be evaluated separately for the septal and posterior walls when the left ventricle is imaged in the parasternal short axis. The difference in timing has been used to identify intraventricular dyssynchrony. A septal to posterior difference of >130 ms has been proposed as a discriminator *(39)*. However, this value has not been validated in other studies *(40)*. Two-dimensional echocardiography has been evaluated to assess for dyssynchrony, but use of this technique has been largely supplanted by tissue Doppler imaging.

Tissue Doppler imaging (TDI) measures the velocity of contracting myocardial segments and allows relative timing of different left ventricular segments to be compared to the QRS and to each other. The necessary software is available in most echocardiographic packages. Specialized training is often required. Frequently, the time to peak systolic velocity is assessed. In one study, when the time to peak velocity was measured in the basal septal and lateral walls, a delay of ≥60 ms was considered predictive of a response to CRT *(41)*. In a four-segment model (septal, lateral, inferior, and anterior) ≥65 ms delay was shown to predict response to CRT *(42)*. Tissue synchronization imaging is a color-coded method to detect peak velocity and time to peak velocity based on tissue Doppler information. This technique tracks left ventricular segments from the time of aortic valve opening to the echocardiographic E wave.

The Predictors of Response to CRT (PROSPECT) trial evaluated 12 different echocardiographic parameters of dyssynchrony at 53 centers in 498 patients *(43)*. The ability of the 12 echocardiographic parameters to predict clinical response varied widely with sensitivity of the parameters ranging from 6% to 74% and the specificity ranging from 35% to 91%. There was large variability in the analysis of the dyssynchrony parameters and it was concluded that no single echocardiographic measure of dyssynchrony may be recommended to improve patient selection for CRT beyond current guidelines.

2.2. Other Imaging Techniques

Other imaging modalities have been used to support echocardiographic findings and add additional information. Nuclear and magnetic resonance imaging can be used for identification of non-viable myocardium (scar) that may be unsuitable for pacing. Computed tomographic and magnetic resonance angiography has been used to define coronary sinus anatomy prior to implantation procedures (Fig. 3). A summary of various imaging modalities is presented in Table 2.

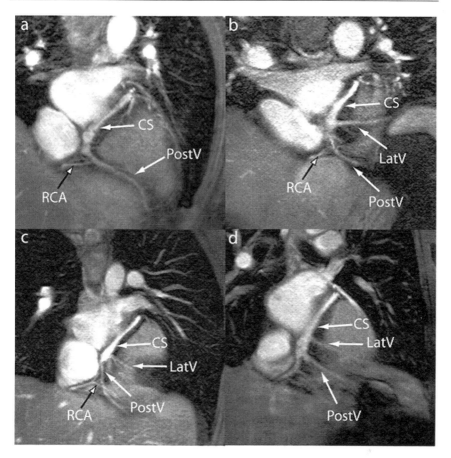

Fig. 3. Panels **a–d** demonstrate coronary sinus (CS) anatomy including posterior (PostV) and lateral (LatV) branches. The right coronary artery (RCA) is shown as well.

3. CLINICAL EVIDENCE

3.1. Trials

Based on the results of smaller CRT studies that evaluated hemodynamic and echocardiographic end points, a number of large randomized, clinical trials in CRT have been reported *(44–52)*. These trials have evaluated both functional and hard end points such as mortality and hospitalization for HF and form the basis for selecting candidates for CRT.

The Multisite Stimulation in Cardiomyopathy (MUSTIC) was a single-blinded randomized trial to examine CRT in HF *(47)*. In this study, 67 patients with sinus rhythm, a QRS duration greater than 150 ms, and New York Heart Association Class III HF due to left ventricular systolic dysfunction (LV ejection fraction < 0.35 and end-diastolic diameter > 6.0 cm) had BiV pacemakers implanted. The study was a single-blind, randomized,

Table 2
Various imaging modalities used to assess dyssnchrony

Imaging modality	Comment
M-mode echocardiography	Septal to posterior wall motion delay has been considered a marker of interventricular dyssynchrony in some studies but not others
Two-dimensional echocardiography	Has been largely replaced by tissue imaging
Tissue Doppler imaging (echocardiography)	Measures velocity of longitudinal cardiac motion in left ventricular walls
Tissue synchronization imaging (echocardiography)	Measures time to peak longitudinal velocity of left ventricular walls
Single-photon emission computed tomography (SPECT)	Can identify areas of scar
Computed tomography angiography (CTA)	Can identify coronary sinus anatomy
Magnetic resonance angiography (MRA)	Can identify areas of scar and coronary sinus anatomy

controlled crossover study and compared patient responses during 3 months of inactive pacing with 3 months biventricular pacing. The primary end point was the distance walked in 6 min and secondary end points included quality of life, peak oxygen consumption, hospitalizations for HF, and mortality rate. Of the 48 patients who completed both study phases, the mean distance walked in 6 min was 23% greater with active pacing, quality of life improved, peak oxygen uptake increased by 8%, and hospitalizations decreased by two thirds. Active pacing was preferred by 85% of the patients.

The Pacing Therapies in Congestive Heart Failure (PATH-CHF) study enrolled 41 patients with New York Heart Association Class III or IV symptoms for >6 months prior to enrollment, dilated cardiomyopathy of any etiology, sinus rhythm ≥ 55 beats/min, a QRS ≥ 120 ms, and a PR interval ≥ 150 ms. These patients received two pacemakers. The first was attached to a right atrial and right ventricular lead (both placed transvenously) and the second was attached to a right atrial lead (placed transvenously) and an LV epicardial lead (via thoracotomy). At implantation, hemodynamic testing was performed to select the optimal univentricular stimulation (LV or RV) and to determine the best AV delay as determined by the maximum rate of change in LV pressure and aortic pulse pressure. Patients were randomized to 4 weeks of univentricular or biventricular stimulation followed by 4 weeks of no treatment and then the opposite stimulation for another 4 weeks. The primary end points were measurements of exercise capacity. In 36 of 41, the LV was the optimal univentricular pacing site. The investigators found an improvement in 6 min walking distance and peak oxygen uptake over the course of the study and noted that clinical differences between hemodynamically optimized biventricular and univentricular (predominantly LV) resynchronization methods were not significant.

The Pacing Therapies in Congestive Heart Failure II (PATH-CHF II) study evaluated single-site LV pacing compared with no pacing and focused on the impact of baseline conduction delay. This trial enrolled 86 patients with New York Heart Association Class II CHF or worse, an LV ejection fraction of <0.3, sinus rhythm, and a QRS $\geq$120 ms. Investigators stratified patients by the baseline QRS interval into long (QRS >150 ms) and short (QRS 120–150 ms) groups. The groups were either paced or unpaced for 3 months and then crossed over to the other group for 3 months. The primary end point included peak oxygen consumption and distance walked in 6 min. The short QRS group did not improve in any end point with active pacing, while the long QRS group had an increase in peak oxygen consumption and distance walked in 6 min. This trial helped establish that patients with a longer QRS (i.e., >150 ms) derived the most benefit from LV pacing.

The Multicenter InSync Randomized Clinical Evaluation (MIRACLE) trial was a prospective, randomized, double-blind trial that evaluated 453 patients with moderate-to-severe symptoms of heart failure who had a LV ejection fraction <0.35 and a QRS interval of $\geq$ 130 ms *(44)*. All of the patients who had a successful biventricular pacemaker implantation (92%) were then randomized to CRT or to optimal medical therapy for 6 months. The primary end points were New York Heart Association functional class, quality of life, and the distance walked in 6 min. The patients in the CRT group had a significant improvement in the 6-min walk test (+39 m vs. +10 m), in functional class and quality of life, and in LV ejection fraction (+4.6% vs. –0.2%). A secondary end point was hospitalization for HF, and fewer patients in the CRT group required hospitalization (8% vs. 15%). Of note, 6 patients had major complications including death, refractory hypotension, bradycardia, and perforation of the coronary sinus requiring pericardiocentesis. Based on this study, the Medtronic InSync system was approved by the US Food and Drug Administration (FDA).

The Multicenter InSync ICD Randomized Clinical Evaluation (MIRACLE-ICD) trial was a prospective, randomized, double-blind trial designed similarly to the MIRACLE trial and included 369 patients with an indication for an ICD including cardiac arrest due to a ventricular tachyarrhythmia or to a spontaneous or induced sustained ventricular tachyarrhythmia. In both groups, the ICD was programmed on, but CRT was assigned randomly. Though functional class improved in the CRT group, there was no difference in the 6-min walk test between the groups nor was there a difference in LV ejection fraction, hospitalization for HF, survival, or proarrhythmia. Based on this study, the FDA approved the CRT–ICD device from this study.

The Cardiac Resynchronization Therapy for the Treatment of Heart Failure in Patients with Intraventricular Conduction Delay and Malignant Ventricular Tachyarrhythmias (CONTAK CD) trial randomized 490 patients with New York Heart Association Class II to IV HF, an LV ejection fraction ≤0.35, QRS interval ≥120 ms, and an indication for an ICD to CRT therapy programmed on or off for 6 months *(51)*. Patients were excluded if they had atrial tachyarrhythmias or had an indication for a permanent pacemaker. The primary end point was HF progression (defined as all-cause mortality, HF hospitalization, or ventricular tachyarrhythmias requiring device intervention). The study's secondary end points included peak oxygen consumption, distance walked in 6 min, New York Heart Association class, and quality of life. Though the primary end point was not statistically significantly different (approximately 15% lower in both groups), 6-min walk improved, LV ejection fraction improved, and LV dimension reduction occurred in the CRT-treated patients. The patients with Class III–IV HF had improvement in all of the functional end points.

The Cardiac Resynchronization Therapy with or without an Implantable Defibrillator in Advanced Chronic Heart Failure (COMPANION) trial tested the hypothesis that CRT with or without a defibrillator would reduce the risk of death and hospitalization among patients with advanced HF and intraventricular conduction delays *(49)*. Patients included had New York Heart Association Class III or IV heart failure resulting from either infarct-related or nonischemic causes, were hospitalized in the preceding 12 months, had an LV ejection fraction of ≤0.35, a QRS ≥120 ms, a PR interval ≥150 ms, sinus rhythm, and no clinical indication for a pacemaker or implantable defibrillator. In a 1:2:2 ratio, 1520 patients were assigned to medical therapy only, CRT with an ICD and CRT without an ICD. The primary end point was death or hospitalization for any cause. Implantation was successful in 87% of the patients in the pacemaker group and 91% of the patients in the ICD group. Both CRT groups had an approximately 20% reduction in annual risk of the primary end point. The 1-year mortality rate in the pharmacologic therapy group was 19%. In the CRT group without an ICD there was a 24% reduction ($P = 0.06$) and in the CRT group with an ICD there was a 36% reduction ($P = 0.003$). This large trial showed that CRT with or without an ICD reduced death or hospitalization.

The Effect of Cardiac Resynchronization on Morbidity and Mortality in Heart Failure (CARE-HF) study was designed to evaluate the effect of CRT without an ICD on morbidity and mortality in patients with New York Heart Association Class III or IV HF despite optimal medical therapy, with an LV ejection fraction ≤0.35, with an LV end-diastolic dimension ≥3.0 cm (indexed to height), and with a QRS ≥120 ms *(46)*. A unique feature of this trial was that patients with a QRS 120–149 ms were required to meet two of three additional echocardiographic criteria for dyssynchrony. These criteria were an aortic preejection delay of >140 ms, an interventricular mechanical delay of >40 ms, and delayed activation of the posterolateral

LV wall. The primary end point was death from any cause or hospitalization for a cardiovascular event. Death from any cause was a secondary end point. Patients were followed for an average of 29.4 months. Among the 813 patients enrolled, 55% in the medical therapy arm reached the primary end point while 36% reached it in the CRT arm ($P < 0.001$). There was a 30% mortality rate in the medial therapy arm and a 20% mortality rate in the CRT arm ($P < 0.002$). Of note, CRT reduced the end-systolic volume index and mitral regurgitant volume and increased the LV ejection fraction. A summary of the patient characteristics, QRS findings, and principle results are noted in Tables 3, 4, and 5.

Table 3
Patient characteristics in selected cardiac resynchronization trials

Study (year)	Number of patients	NYHA class	LVEF	LVEDD (cm)	Cardiomyopathy
MUSTIC (2001)	67	III	0.23	7.3	n/a
MIRACLE (2002)	453	III, IV	0.22	6.9	IRC: 50–58%
PATH-CHF (2002)	42	III, IV	0.21	7.3	IRC: 29% DCM:71%
CONTAK-CD (2003)	490	II, III, IV	0.21	7.1	IRC: 67–71%
MIRACLE-ICD (2003)	369	III, IV	0.24	7.6	IRC: 64–74% DCM:26–36%
PATH-CHF II (2003)	101	II, III, IV	0.23	n/a	CAD: 24–44%
COMPANION (2004)	1520	III, IV	0.22	6.7	IRC: 55–59%
CARE-HF (2005)	813	III, IV	0.25	n/a	IRC: 43–48% DCM:36–40%

IRC, infarct-related cardiomyopathy; DCM, dilated cardiomyopathy; CAD, coronary artery disease

3.2. Patient Characteristics/Subsets

Notable characteristics of patients enrolled in CRT trials include LV ejection fractions substantially lower than 0.35, enlarged LV end-diastolic dimensions (frequently > 6.0 cm), similar benefits in patients with infarct-related and dilated cardiomyopathies, and QRS durations considerably longer than 120 ms (frequently > 160 ms and predominantly LBBB).

Within the CARE-HF population, age, sex, cause of cardiomyopathy, and LV ejection fraction did not discriminate responders from non-responders. However, patients with New York Heart Association Class III HF, a QRS $\geq$ 160 ms, an echocardiographic interventricular mechanical delay

Table 4
QRS morphology in selected cardiac resynchronization
trials

Study	Mean QRS (ms)	Morphology
MUSTIC	175	87% LBBB
MIRACLE	165	Not stated
PATH-CHF	175	93% LBBB 7% RBBB
CONTAK-CD	160	54% LBBB 32% IVCD 14% RBBB
MIRACLE-ICD	165	13% RBBB
PATH-CHF II	155	88% LBBB
COMPANION	160	70% LBBB 10% RBBB
CARE-HF	160	Not stated

LBBB = left bundle branch block; RBBB = right bundle
branch block; IVCD = intraventricular conduction delay

≥ 49.2 ms, and/or a mitral regurgitation area ≥0.22 had statistically significant benefit from CRT when these cutoffs were used *(46)*. In the COMPANION study, patients with NYHA Class IV HF had a significant reduction in death rate compared with NYHA Class III patients. The same was true for those with LV ejection fractions ≤ 0.2 (compared with > 0.2), QRS ≥148 ms (compared with < 147 ms), and LBBB (compared with other conduction delays) *(49)*.

3.3. QRS Morphology

The majority, but not the entirety, of patients included in the major clinical CRT trials had LBBB. While no trials have prospectively compared non-LBBB QRS morphology with LBBB morphology, retrospective analysis has been performed on patients with RBBB. In an analysis of the patients with RBBB in the MIRACLE and CONTAK CD trials, there were trends toward improvement in 6-min walk distance, quality-of-life scores, and norepinephrine levels, but they were not statistically significant *(53)*. These investigators did note an improvement in NYHA HF, however, control patients also showed significant improvement in NYHA class. These researchers concluded that CRT therapy in patients with RBBB was not

Table 5
Results of selected cardiac resynchronization clinical trials

Study	Findings	All-cause mortality or HF hospitalization
MUSTIC	Improved 6-min walk with CRT	N/A
MIRACLE	Improved quality of life, NYHA class, and 6-min walk	20% Med Rx 12% CRT-P
PATH-CHF	No significant differences between hemodynamically optimized biventricular and univentricular (predominantly LV) resynchronization	N/A
CONTAK-CD	Improved 6-min walk with CRT but no difference in NYHA class or peak oxygen consumption	38% Med Rx 32% CRT-D
MIRACLE-ICD	Improved quality of life, NYHA class, and peak oxygen consumption with CRT-D	26% Med Rx 26% CRT-D
PATH-CHF II	QRS >150 ms group (but not QRS 120–150 ms group) had an increase in peak oxygen consumption and 6-min walk compared to no pacing	N/A
COMPANION	Both CRT-P and CRT-D had significant reduction in all-cause mortality and hospitalization compared to Med Rx (improved survival only seen in CRT-D)	45% Med Rx 31% CRT-P 29% CRT-D
CARE-HF	Improved survival in CRT group and improved LVEF, chamber dimensions, and quality of life compared to Med Rx	33% Med Rx 18% CRT-P

HF = heart failure; CRT = cardiac resynchronization therapy; N/A = not available; NYHA = New York Heart Association Classification; Med Rx = medical treatment; CRT-P = cardiac resynchronization therapy with pacing only; CRT-D = cardiac resynchronization therapy with defibrillation

supported by available data. Others have postulated that echocardiographic evaluation is superior to QRS duration in selecting patients for CRT *(54–56)*. In small studies, patients with narrow QRS duration (<120 ms) with echocardiographic dyssynchrony were found to derive equal benefit from CRT as their counterparts with similar echocardiographic dyssynchrony but prolonged QRS duration. The Cardiac Resynchronization Therapy in Patients with Heart Failure and Narrow QRS (RethinQ) study was a double-blind clinical trial evaluating the efficacy of CRT in patients with a standard indication for an ICD (ischemic or nonischemic cardiomyopathy and an ejection fraction of 35% or less), NHYA Class III heart failure, a QRS interval of less than 130 ms, and evidence of mechanical dyssynchrony as measured on echocardiography *(57)*. In a prespecified subgroup with a QRS interval of 120 ms or more, the peak oxygen consumption increased in the CRT group ($P = 0.02$), but it was unchanged in a subgroup with a QRS interval of less than 120 ms ($P = 0.45$). There were 24 heart failure events requiring intravenous therapy in 14 patients in the CRT group (16.1%) and 41 events in 19 patients in the control group (22.3%), but the difference was not significant. The study authors concluded that CRT did not improve peak oxygen consumption in patients with moderate-to-severe heart failure, providing evidence that patients with heart failure and narrow QRS intervals may not benefit from CRT.

3.4. Atrial Fibrillation

Although most clinical trials have excluded patients with atrial fibrillation, atrial fibrillation is a common arrhythmia in patients with heart failure occurring in up to 50% of patients with advanced HF *(58)*. Small studies have examined the use of CRT in this patient population and have reported functional benefit *(59–61)*. Concomitant performance of an atrioventricular junctional ablation to ensure >85% biventricular pacing may improve results compared to use of CRT in patients with native conduction *(59)*.

3.5. Cost-Effectiveness

While device implantation is expensive, improved survival and functional improvement may offset these costs. A cost-effective analysis was performed on the COMPANION patient population. Investigators noted that the incremental cost of CRT therapy with or without an ICD was within accepted benchmarks cost-effectiveness *(62)*. However, when comparing CRT without a defibrillator to CRT with an ICD, the additional cost may be substantial *(63)*. In the absence of a head-to-head trial, the true cost-effectiveness cannot be determined.

The American Heart Association issued a science advisory based on the published clinical trials incorporating the results into a statement about patient selection for CRT (Table 6) *(64)*.

4. HARDWARE

4.1. Leads and Delivery Systems

Essential to transvenous placement of a lead for left ventricular pacing is cannulation of the coronary sinus. A variety of techniques and aids have been developed to facilitate gaining access to the coronary sinus including the use of guidewires, guiding sheaths, sub-selective sheaths (used within the guiding sheath to direct the guidewire into the coronary sinus), and steerable catheters/sheaths.

Table 6
Patient selection for cardiac resynchronization therapy

Sinus rhythm
LV ejection fraction ≤ 0.35
Infarct-related or idiopathic dilated cardiomyopathy
QRS duration ≥ 120 ms
NYHA functional Class III or IV
Maximal pharmacologic therapy for CHF

Each major CRT device manufacturer has accessories designed to facilitate LV lead placement (Fig. 4). Medtronic Attain™ system includes preformed shaped catheters that can be integrated with soft-tipped subselective telescoping catheters to engage the coronary sinus and its branches. The Boston Scientific system (Guidant RAPIDO™) contains an outer guide catheter that is used to cannulate the coronary sinus, while inner catheters may be used to facilitate branch vessel selection. The St. Jude Medical lead delivery system offers various different preformed shaped catheters to account for variable cardiac and coronary sinus anatomy.

4.2. Technical Considerations

Once in place, occlusive coronary sinus venography is frequently performed to identify potential target branches. A variety of leads are available to match branch anatomy and increase the chance of acute successful placement and secure longevity. Specific considerations include size, lead delivery, lead shape, fixation, and pacing electrode polarity (Table 7).

Choosing the appropriate lead requires knowledge of the target vessel size and matching the vessel size with the pacing electrode. Unipolar leads tend to be narrower in diameter. A number of over-the-wire leads are available for CS pacing (Table 8).

Initially, LV leads were placed via stylet-driven systems. The development of LV pacing leads that could be placed via an over-the-wire technique facilitated lead placement and improved rates of successful LV lead placement. The technique uses a guiding wire (ranging from softer to stiffer compositions depending on the clinical need) to cannulate a target vein and serve as the guide for advancement of the pacing electrode.

Lead shape is often an additional consideration to ensure stability and appropriate lead orientation (Fig. 5). Leads with varying tip angulation and preformed curves (S curve and corkscrew configurations) are available. Generally, large veins require larger curved leads and smaller, tortuous veins may require smaller caliber leads for stability. Because LV pacing electrodes sit within vein branches and not directly on atrial or ventricular endocardium, fixation is passive. Some leads, however, do contain tines to increase stability by wedging within the target vessel.

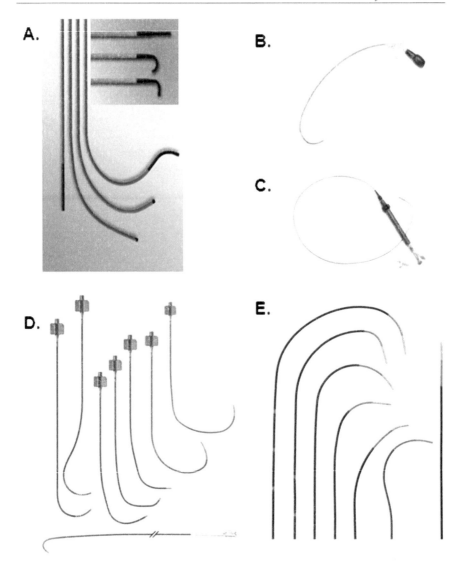

Fig. 4. A variety of sheaths and LV lead delivery systems are displayed. (**A**) Medtronic Attain Select Guide Catheters; (**B**) Medtronic Attain Deflectable Catheter Delivery System; (**C**) Medtronic Prevail Steerable Catheter; (**D**) Boston Scientific (Guidant) Rapido Dual-Catheter System; (**E**) St. Jude Medical Cardiac Positioning System.

Inability to successfully place a lead in the desired coronary sinus branch occurs occasionally and lead dislodgement may occur in up to 12% of patients despite initial successful placement *(38, 44, 46, 47)*. When biventricular pacing is desired but transvenous lead placement is unattainable, surgical LV lead placement remains an option. Epicardial leads are

Table 7
LV Lead selection factors

Size
Lead delivery
Lead shape
Fixation
Pacing electrode polarity
Coronary sinus anatomy

available in unipolar or bipolar configurations and attach by active fixation. These leads are typically implanted in pairs to ensure pacing if one fails.

4.3. Devices

4.3.1. PACING CONFIGURATIONS

Pacemakers and ICDs designed to deliver biventricular pacing offer a multitude of programming options to support optimal delivery of therapy. Programmable parameters include pacing polarity, algorithms to maximize biventricular pacing, and functions to assure pacing with an adequate pacing threshold.

Not all devices offer all possible pacing configurations. In addition, choices may be limited by the LV lead implanted (unipolar vs. bipolar, for example) or by the patient's anatomy (for example, if the tip electrode paces adequately but the proximal ring electrode of a bipolar lead has a high threshold or does not capture due to cardiac scar). In general, most modern CRT devices offer a variety of pacing configurations. The advantage of this is the potential to minimize pacing threshold to conserve battery life and avoid diaphragmatic capture. For example, some CRT-D devices offer three LV pacing polarities when a bipolar lead is implanted: LV tip to RV coil, LV tip to LV ring, and LV ring to RV coil. In many cases, the RV–LV timing is adjustable such that pacing one chamber can be programmed to precede the other by up to 80 ms (see below). Many devices also include algorithms to automatically optimize A-V and V-V intervals, based on data extracted from clinical trials and echo-guided substudies.

4.3.2. MAXIMIZING LV PACING

At its most basic, CRT devices sense the intrinsic atrial depolarization and then deliver timed signals to the right and left ventricles resulting in coordinated, atrial synchronous biventricular pacing. A variety of arrhythmias can undermine the devices ability to perform in this manner, including atrial fibrillation and ventricular ectopic beats. Because these arrhythmias often

Table 8

Selected over-the-wire leads available for coronary sinus pacing

Lead	Connector/polarity	Maximum body and tip diameter (French)	Length (cm)	Insulation	Fixation/shape
4193 Attain (Medtronic)	IS-1 Unipolar	(tip 5.4)	78, 88, 103	Polyurethane (55D)	Canted tip
4194 Attain (Medtronic)	IS-1 Bipolar	6.0 (tip 5.4)	78, 88	Polyurethane (55D)	Canted tip
1056 K Quicksite (St. Jude Medical)	IS-1 Unipolar	6.0 (tip 5.0)	75, 86	Polyurethane, Silicone	Blunt tip 8 mm S-curve
1056T Quicksite (St. Jude Medical)	IS-1 Bipolar	6.0 (tip 5.0)	75, 86	Polyurethane, Silicone	Blunt tip 8 mm S-curve
1058T Quicksite (St. Jude Medical)	IS-1 Bipolar	6.0 (tip 5.0)	75, 86	Polyurethane, Silicone	Blunt tip 16 mm S-curve
4510, 4511, 4512, 4513 Easytrak	LV-1 Unipolar	6.0 (tip 4.8)	65, 72, 80, 90	Polyurethane	Tined
4537, 4538 Easytrak (Boston Scientific)	IS-1 Unipolar	6.0 (tip 4.8)	80, 90	Polyurethane, Silicone	
4515, 4517, 4518, 4520 Easytrak2	LV-1 Bipolar	6.0 (tip 5.7)	65, 80, 90, 100	Polyurethane, Silicone	Tined
4542, 4543, 4544 Easytrak2 (Boston Scientific)	IS-1 Bipolar	6.0 (tip 5.7)	80, 90, 100		
4522, 4524, 4525, 4527 Easytrak3	LV-1 Bipolar	6.0 (tip 5.8)	65, 80, 90, 100	Polyurethane, Silicone	Pigtail
4548, 4549, 4550 Easytrak3 (Boston Scientific)	IS-1 Bipolar		80, 90, 100		

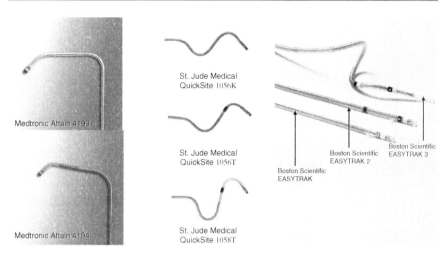

Fig. 5. Selected leads used for left ventricular pacing via the coronary sinus are shown. A variety of sizes and shapes are available to accommodate variable patient anatomy.

occur in patients with heart failure, algorithms have been designed to maximize the frequency of biventricular pacing in order to deliver the greatest therapeutic benefit to patients.

For example, patient who develop atrial fibrillation may stop LV pacing due to an intrinsic conducted ventricular rate greater than the lower programmed pacing rate of the device. This would result in the absence of LV pacing and loss of therapeutic benefit. Many devices now may be programmed to trigger LV pacing upon sensing of an intrinsic RV signal. This can restore (at least partially) resynchronization of the RV and LV pacing and may be utilized during atrial fibrillation or periods of ventricular ectopy. It should be noted, however, that in some patients LV pacing may be proarrhythmia and increase the frequency of ventricular events.

4.3.3. OTHER DIAGNOSTICS

Several additional diagnostic options have been incorporated into many modern CRT devices in an effort to better monitor heart failure status. While the precise methodology and function of these additional features varies from manufacturer to manufacturer and device to device, each attempts to provide some physiologic measurement of the patient's clinical status. For example, Medtronic's OptiVol system measures intrathoracic impedance using an electrical impulse vector between the RV lead and the CRT generator, which has been shown to correlate with the patient's overall volume status. Some Boston Scientific devices offer an autonomic balance monitor, heart rate variability counter, and an activity log to assist in patient clinical evaluation. Heart rate histograms, like those present in some St. Jude Medical CRT devices permit a physiologic assessment of patient status.

4.4. CRT Defibrillators vs. CRT Pacemakers

Because most patients who meet guideline criteria for CRT devices also meet criteria for implanted defibrillators, CRT devices without defibrillation capability (CRT-P) are implanted much less often. The most common reasons for selection of a CRT-P rather than a CRT-D device are (1) patient and physician preference to avoid defibrillator shocks and (2) the desire to improve quality but not necessarily quantity of life. That being said, well-conducted clinical trials suggest that resynchronization therapy, even in the absence of defibrillation improves survival in appropriately selected patients. Each of the major device manufacturers that offers CRT-D also offer devices that deliver CRT-P with defibrillation.

5. TROUBLESHOOTING/OPTIMIZATION

Hemodynamic and clinical changes can be anticipated in patients implanted with CRT devices. Hemodynamic changes include increased cardiac output, increased systolic blood pressure, decreased pulmonary capillary wedge pressure, and decreased chamber size (65, 66). Clinical changes include improvement in New York Heart Association Heart Failure class, improved 6-min walk tests, fewer hospitalizations, and improved survival (44, 46). Some patients notice improvement within a few days, others feel improvement after several months, and still others notice no change or progression of symptoms. When HF symptoms persist, however, a series of troubleshooting steps should be employed to optimize the device function (Fig. 6).

Routine follow-up is required for every patient with an implantable device, and a number of specific issues should be addressed in patients with CRT devices. The patient's symptoms, volume status, heart rhythm, comorbidities, and medications should be evaluated (66). When ischemia, a volume abnormality (i.e., fluid overload or hypovolemia), supraventricular tachycardia, or other important clinical developments are noted, these conditions merit specific and often immediate attention.

5.1. ECG Patterns

A 12-lead electrocardiogram (ECG) is a simple, inexpensive test that can assess the presence or absence of appropriate biventricular pacing. In patients with an R/S ratio $\geq$ 1 in lead VI and an R/S ratio $\leq$ 1 in lead I, biventricular pacing can be confirmed with a sensitivity of 94% and a specificity of 93% (Fig. 7) (67). Confirming ECG findings with device interroga-

Clinical Evaluation After CRT Device Implantation

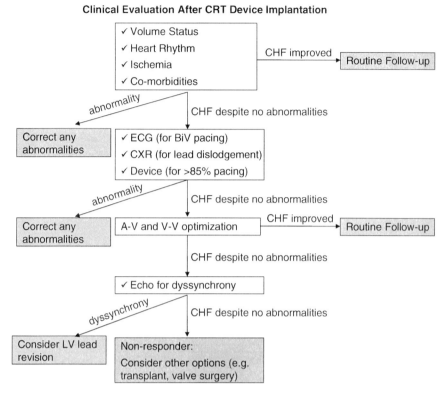

Fig. 6. An algorithm for the approach to clinical management of patients with cardiac resynchronization devices (CRT) is shown. For patients that respond well to therapy, routine follow-up are advised. Further clinical assessment and additional testing or device optimization may be warranted for non-responders *(44)*.

tion will identify sensing, pacing, and programming abnormalities. Patients with CRT devices should undergo biventricular pacing close to 100% of the time. Less than 85% pacing should prompt programming changes or other actions (e.g., AVJ ablation in patients with atrial fibrillation) *(57)*. When lead parameters are abnormal, a chest x-ray to identify lead position is indicated.

5.2. AV Optimization

When patients continue to have clinical HF symptoms despite adequate device function, pacing parameters should be reviewed for optimal programming *(66)*. In particular, atrioventricular (AV) and interventricular (VV) timing should be carefully reviewed. Lack of atrioventricular coordination may contribute to sub-optimal ejection due to abnormal chamber filling and exacerbation of mitral regurgitation *(21)*. Several techniques to adjust AV delay to maximize left ventricular performance have been described (Table 9)

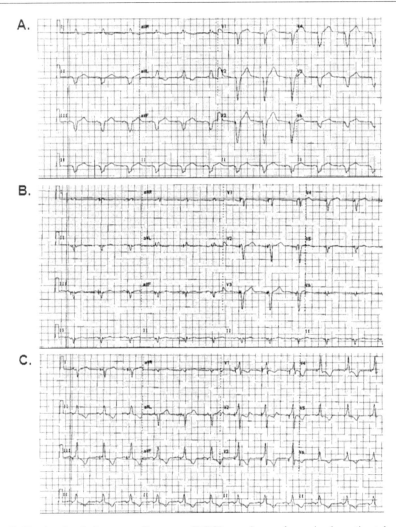

Fig. 7. Twelve-lead electrocardiograms (ECG) are shown for a single patient during
(**a**) RV only pacing, (**b**) RV and LV simultaneous pacing, and (**C**) LV only pacing. If
an R/S ratio ≥ 1 is present in lead VI and an R/S ratio ≤ 1 is present in lead I, then
biventricular pacing can be confirmed with a sensitivity of 94% and a specificity of
93%.

(68–70) A common and practical method uses echocardiography to measure
continuous wave Doppler flow across the mitral valve to examine the E and
A waves. The AV delay is set as short as possible without truncating the
A wave. This method minimizes isovolumic contraction time during which
diastolic mitral regurgitation can occur. By allowing full inscription of the A
wave, full contribution of atrial contraction to ventricular filling can occur.
With any of the described techniques to optimize AV timing, echocardiog-

Table 9
Selected methods of AV optimization

Method	Comment
Aortic velocity time integral (VTI) method : Maximum increase aortic VTI using continuous wave Doppler	Optimized AV delay may increase in aortic VTI more than mitral inflow method
Mitral inflow method : Shortest AV delay that does not compromise the transmitral A wave using continuous wave Doppler	Requires visualization of A wave
Left Ventricular dP/dt method : Initial downslope of mitral regurgitation jet using continuous wave Doppler	Requires mitral regurgitation

raphy (or another mode of hemodynamic monitoring) is requisite. Reports have suggested improvement in the aortic velocity time integral of up to 19% and an increase in LV ejection fraction by up to 5% *(69, 70)*.

5.3. VV Optimization

Because most modern CRT devices permit programming of variable V-V (right ventricular stimulation to left ventricular stimulation) timing, the opportunity exists to optimize an individual patient's programming. One method measures continuous Doppler flow across the aortic valve at different programmed V-V settings to determine the maximum velocity time integral as a correlate of stroke volume. Some investigators have noted improvement in LV ejection fraction of up to 8% while others have noted no change from empiric simultaneous RV and LV pacing *(71, 72)*. Of note, in one study, 50% of patients benefited from RV pacing prior to LV pacing while the other 50% benefited from the reverse timing *(73)*.

5.4. Additional Evaluation

When HF persists despite optimized volume status, exclusion of arrhythmias and ischemia, adequate device function, and optimized timing settings, repeat evaluation for dyssynchrony can be considered *(66)*. If dyssynchrony is present then LV lead revision may be necessary either via the transvenous or transthoracic approach. When dyssynchrony is not present, other management options for severe HF may be required including transplant evaluation or, in the case of valvular heart disease, valve repair or replacement.

6. GUIDELINES

Published Clinical Guidelines from professional organization including the American Heart Association, the American College of Cardiology, and the Heart Rhythm Society have categorized recommendations into three classes. Class I includes conditions for which there is evidence and/or general agreement that a given procedure or treatment is beneficial, useful, and effective. Class II includes conditions for which there is conflicting evidence and/or a divergence of opinion about the usefulness/efficacy of a procedure or treatment. The Class II recommendations are further divided into Class IIa and Class IIb. The Class IIa label is applied when the weight of evidence/opinion is in favor of usefulness/efficacy, and the Class IIb distinction is used when usefulness/efficacy is less well established by evidence/opinion. Class III conditions are those for which there is evidence and/or general agreement that a procedure/treatment is not useful/effective and in some cases may be harmful. Furthermore, the degree of evidence is

Table 10
AHA/ACC/HRS Guidelines for cardiac resynchronization therapy

Recommendation class	Level of evidence	Recommendation
I	A	For patients with LVEF ≤35%, QRS duration ≥ 0.12 s, and *sinus rhythm*, CRT and/or an ICD is indicated for the treatment of NYHA functional Class III or ambulatory Class IV HF symptoms on OMT.
IIa	B	For patients who have LVEF ≤ 35%, QRS duration ≥ 0.12 s, and *AF*, CRT and/or an ICD is reasonable for the treatment of NYHA functional Class III or ambulatory Class IV heart failure symptoms on OMT.
	C	For patients with LVEF ≤ 35% with NYHA functional Class III or ambulatory Class IV symptoms on OMT and *who have frequent dependence on ventricular pacing*, CRT is reasonable
IIb	C	For patients with LVEF ≤ 35% with NYHA functional Class I or II symptoms on OMT and who are undergoing implantation of a permanent pacemaker and/or ICD with anticipated frequent ventricular pacing, CRT may be considered
III	B	CRT is not indicated for asymptomatic patients with reduced LVEF in the absence of other indications for pacing
	C	CRT is not indicated for patients whose functional status and life expectancy are limited predominantly by chronic noncardiac conditions

AF = atrial fibrillation or atrial flutter; CRT = cardiac resynchronization therapy; HF = heart failure; LVEF = left ventricular ejection fraction; NYHA = New York Heart Association; OMT = optimal medical therapy divided into three levels. Level of Evidence A is data derived from multiple randomized clinical trials or meta-analyses. Level B is data derived from a single randomized trial or nonrandomized studies, and Level C is consensus opinion of experts, case studies, or standard of care in the absence of the above.

In guidelines published that address CRT, prolonged QRS duration, an electrocardiographic representation of abnormal cardiac conduction, has been used to identify patients with left ventricular dyssynchrony *(74, 75)*. To date, no well-established consensus definition of cardiac dyssynchrony (e.g., an echocardiographic description) has been formed.

Generally, guidelines suggest that the use of an ICD in combination with CRT should be based on the indications for ICD therapy while noting that the majority of CRT trials have primarily enrolled patients in normal sinus rhythm, and acknowledging that further investigation of patients with atrial fibrillation, right-bundle branch block, and obligate right ventricular pacing are ongoing.

The ACC/AHA/HRS 2008 Guidelines for Device-Based Therapy of Cardiac Rhythm Abnormalities categorizes CRT with or without an ICD for patients with a left ventricular ejection fraction $\leq$ 35%, QRS duration $\geq$ 120 ms, and NYHA Class III or ambulatory Class IV on optimal medical therapy as Class I for patients in normal sinus rhythm, and Class IIa for patients with atrial fibrillation or for patients who ventricularly pace frequently. Comprehensive recommendations are displayed in Table 10[74].

7. CONCLUSIONS

Cardiac resynchronization therapy (CRT) has been well studied and is proven to improve clinical outcomes and quality of life, and reduce mortality, in selected patients with heart failure and reduced ejection fraction. A variety of devices are available to deliver this important therapy to patients. Ongoing investigations will continue to refine the subset of patients most likely to benefit from this important therapy.

REFERENCES

1. Jessup M, Brozena S, Heart failure. N Engl J Med, 2003;348(20): 2007–18.
2. Hunt SA, et al. ACC/AHA 2005 Guideline update for the diagnosis and management of chronic heart failure in the adult: a report of the American College of Cardiology/American Heart Association Task Force on practice guidelines (writing committee to update the 2001 guidelines for the evaluation and management of heart failure): Developed in Collaboration With the American College of Chest Physicians and the International Society for Heart and Lung Transplantation: Endorsed by the Heart Rhythm Society. Circulation, 2005;112(12): e154–235.
3. Ho KK, et al. The epidemiology of heart failure: the Framingham study. J Am Coll Cardiol, 1993;22(4 Suppl A): 6A–13A.
4. Schocken DD, et al. Prevalence and mortality rate of congestive heart failure in the United States. J Am Coll Cardiol, 1992;20(2): 301–6.

5. Ball SG, Cardioprotection and ACE inhibitors. Clin Physiol Biochem, 1992;9(3): 98–104.

6. The SOLVD Investigators. Effect of enalapril on survival in patients with reduced left ventricular ejection fractions and congestive heart failure. N Engl J Med, 1991;325(5): 293–302.

7. Boucher M, Ma J, Heart failure: is there a role for angiotensin II receptor blockers? Issues Emerg Health Technol, 2002;38: 1–4.

8. Maggioni AP, et al., Effects of valsartan on morbidity and mortality in patients with heart failure not receiving angiotensin-converting enzyme inhibitors. J Am Coll Cardiol, 2002;40(8): 1414–21.

9. Pfeffer MA, et al., Valsartan, captopril, or both in myocardial infarction complicated by heart failure, left ventricular dysfunction, or both. N Engl J Med, 2003;349(20): 1893–906.

10. Fowler MB, Carvedilol prospective randomized cumulative survival (COPERNICUS) trial: carvedilol in severe heart failure. Am J Cardiol, 2004;93(9A): 35B–9B.

11. Keating GM, Jarvis B, Carvedilol: a review of its use in chronic heart failure. Drugs, 2003;63(16): 1697–741.

12. Fowler M, Beta-adrenergic blocking drugs in severe heart failure. Rev Cardiovasc Med, 2002;3(Suppl 3): S20–6.

13. Wollert KC, Drexler H, Carvedilol prospective randomized cumulative survival (COPERNICUS) trial: carvedilol as the sun and center of the beta-blocker world? Circulation, 2002;106(17): 2164–6.

14. Singh BN, CIBIS, MERIT-HF, and COPERNICUS trial outcomes: do they complete the chapter on beta-adrenergic blockers as antiarrhythmic and antifibrillatory drugs? J Cardiovasc Pharmacol Ther, 2001;6(2): 107–10.

15. Louis A, et al., Clinical Trials Update: CAPRICORN, COPERNICUS, MIRACLE, STAF, RITZ-2, RECOVER and RENAISSANCE and cachexia and cholesterol in heart failure. Highlights of the Scientific Sessions of the American College of Cardiology. Eur J Heart Fail, 2001;3(3): 381–7.

16. Dieterich HA, Wendt C, Saborowski F, Cardioprotection by aldosterone receptor antagonism in heart failure. Part I. The role of aldosterone in heart failure. Fiziol Cheloveka, 2005;31(6): 97–105.

17. Killip T, Passamani E, Davis K, Coronary artery surgery study (CASS): a randomized trial of coronary bypass surgery. Eight years follow-up and survival in patients with reduced ejection fraction. Circulation, 1985;72(6 Pt 2): V102–9.

18. Myers WO, et al., CASS Registry long term surgical survival. Coronary Artery Surgery Study. J Am Coll Cardiol, 1999;33(2): 488–98.

19. Baldasseroni S, et al., Left bundle-branch block is associated with increased 1-year sudden and total mortality rate in 5517 outpatients with congestive heart failure: a report from the Italian network on congestive heart failure. Am Heart J, 2002;143(3): 398–405.

20. Leclercq C, Kass DA, Retiming the failing heart: principles and current clinical status of cardiac resynchronization. J Am Coll Cardiol, 2002;39(2): 194–201.

21. Prinzen FW, et al., Mapping of regional myocardial strain and work during ventricular pacing: experimental study using magnetic resonance imaging tagging. J Am Coll Cardiol, 1999;33(6): 1735–42.

22. Rouleau F, et al., Echocardiographic assessment of the interventricular delay of activation and correlation to the QRS width in dilated cardiomyopathy. Pacing Clin Electrophysiol, 2001;24(10): 1500–6.

23. Auricchio A, et al., Effect of pacing chamber and atrioventricular delay on acute systolic function of paced patients with congestive heart failure. The Pacing Therapies for Congestive Heart Failure Study Group. The Guidant Congestive Heart Failure Research Group. Circulation, 1999;99(23): 2993–3001.

24. Gold MR, et al., Dual-chamber pacing with a short atrioventricular delay in congestive heart failure: a randomized study. J Am Coll Cardiol, 1995;26(4): 967–73.

25. Bleeker GB, et al., Relationship between QRS duration and left ventricular dyssynchrony in patients with end-stage heart failure. J Cardiovasc Electrophysiol, 2004;15(5): 544–9.

26. Nelson GS, et al., Predictors of systolic augmentation from left ventricular preexcitation in patients with dilated cardiomyopathy and intraventricular conduction delay. Circulation, 2000;101(23): 2703–9.

27. Packer M, et al., Effect of oral milrinone on mortality in severe chronic heart failure. The PROMISE Study Research Group. N Engl J Med, 1991;325(21):1468–75.

28. Nelson GS, et al., Left ventricular or biventricular pacing improves cardiac function at diminished energy cost in patients with dilated cardiomyopathy and left bundle-branch block. Circulation, 2000;102(25): 3053–9.

29. Kaji S, et al., Annular geometry in patients with chronic ischemic mitral regurgitation: three-dimensional magnetic resonance imaging study. Circulation, 2005;112(9 Suppl): I409–14.

30. Breithardt OA, Kuhl HP, Stellbrink C, Acute effects of resynchronisation treatment on functional mitral regurgitation in dilated cardiomyopathy. Heart, 2002;88(4): 440.

31. Breithardt OA, et al., Acute effects of cardiac resynchronization therapy on functional mitral regurgitation in advanced systolic heart failure. J Am Coll Cardiol, 2003;41(5): 765–70.

32. Vogt J, et al., Electrocardiographic remodeling in patients paced for heart failure. Am J Cardiol, 2000;86(9, Supplement 1): K152–6.

33. Donal E, et al., Effects of cardiac resynchronization therapy on disease progression in chronic heart failure. Eur Heart J, 2006;27(9): 1018–25.

34. David D, et al., Diastolic "locking" of the mitral valve: the importance of atrial systole and intraventricular volume. Circulation, 1983;67(3): 640–5.

35. Gasparini M, et al., Comparison of 1-year effects of left ventricular and biventricular pacing in patients with heart failure who have ventricular arrhythmias and left bundle-branch block: The Bi vs Left Ventricular Pacing: An International Pilot Evaluation on Heart Failure Patients with Ventricular Arrhythmias (BELIEVE) multicenter prospective randomized pilot study. Am Heart J, 2006;152(1): 155.e1–155.e7.

36. Leclercq C, et al., Biventricular vs. left univentricular pacing in heart failure: rationale, design, and endpoints of the B-LEFT HF study. Europace, 2006;8(1): 76–80.

37. Leclercq C, et al., Systolic improvement and mechanical resynchronization does not require electrical synchrony in the dilated failing heart with left bundle-branch block. Circulation, 2002;106(14): 1760–63.

38. Bax JJ, et al., Cardiac resynchronization therapy: Part 1–issues before device implantation. J Am Coll Cardiol, 2005;46(12): 2153–67.

39. Pitzalis MV, et al., Ventricular asynchrony predicts a better outcome in patients with chronic heart failure receiving cardiac resynchronization therapy. J Am Coll Cardiol, 2005;45(1): 65–9.

40. Marcus GM, et al., Septal to posterior wall motion delay fails to predict reverse remodeling or clinical improvement in patients undergoing cardiac resynchronization therapy. J Am Coll Cardiol, 2005;46(12): 2208–14.

41. Bax JJ, et al., Left ventricular dyssynchrony predicts benefit of cardiac resynchronization therapy in patients with end-stage heart failure before pacemaker implantation. Am J Cardiol, 2003;92(10): 1238–40.

42. Bax JJ, et al., Left ventricular dyssynchrony predicts response and prognosis after cardiac resynchronization therapy. J Am Coll Cardiol, 2004;44(9): 1834–40.

43. Chung ES, Leon AR, Tavazzi L, Sun J-P, Nihoyannopoulos P, Merlino J, et al. Results of the predictors of response to CRT (PROSPECT) trial. Circulation, 2008;117: 2608–16.

44. Abraham WT, Fisher WG, Smith AL, et al. Cardiac resynchronization in chronic heart failure. N Engl J Med, Jun 13 2002;346(24):1845–53.
45. Auricchio A, Stellbrink C, Sack S, et al. Long-term clinical effect of hemodynamically optimized cardiac resynchronization therapy in patients with heart failure and ventricular conduction delay. J Am Coll Cardiol, Jun 19 2002;39(12):2026–33.
46. Cleland JG, Daubert JC, Erdmann E, et al. The effect of cardiac resynchronization on morbidity and mortality in heart failure. N Engl J Med, Apr 14 2005;352(15):1539–49.
47. Cazeau S, Leclercq C, Lavergne T, et al. Effects of multisite biventricular pacing in patients with heart failure and intraventricular conduction delay. N Engl J Med, Mar 22 2001;344(12):873–80.
48. Young JB, Abraham WT, Smith AL, et al. Combined cardiac resynchronization and implantable cardioversion defibrillation in advanced chronic heart failure: the MIRA-CLE ICD Trial. JAMA, May 28 2003;289(20):2685–94.
49. Bristow MR, Saxon LA, Boehmer J, et al. Cardiac-resynchronization therapy with or without an implantable defibrillator in advanced chronic heart failure. N Engl J Med, May 20 2004;350(21):2140–50.
50. Auricchio A, Stellbrink C, Butter C, et al. Clinical efficacy of cardiac resynchronization therapy using left ventricular pacing in heart failure patients stratified by severity of ventricular conduction delay. J Am Coll Cardiol, Dec 17 2003;42(12):2109–16.
51. Higgins SL, Hummel JD, Niazi IK, et al. Cardiac resynchronization therapy for the treatment of heart failure in patients with intraventricular conduction delay and malignant ventricular tachyarrhythmias. J Am Coll Cardiol, Oct 15 2003;42(8): 1454–59.
52. McAlister, FA, Ezekowitz J, Hooton N, Vandermeer B, Spooner C, Dryden DM, et al. Cardiac resynchronization therapy for patients with left ventricular systolic dysfunc-tion – a systematic review. JAMA, 2007;297:2502–14
53. Egoavil CA, Ho RT, Greenspon AJ, et al. Cardiac resynchronization therapy in patients with right bundle branch block: Analysis of pooled data from the MIRACLE and Contak CD trials. Heart Rhythm, 2005;2(6):611–5.
54. Bleeker GB, Holman ER, Steendijk P, et al. Cardiac resynchronization therapy in patients with a narrow QRS complex. J Am Coll Cardiol, 2006;48(11):2243–50.
55. Yu C-M, Chan Y-S, Zhang Q, et al. Benefits of cardiac resynchronization therapy for heart failure patients with narrow QRS complexes and coexisting systolic asynchrony by echocardiography. J Am Coll Cardiol, 2006;48(11):2251–57.
56. Kashani A, Barold SS. Significance of QRS complex duration in patients with heart failure. J Am Coll Cardiol, Dec 20 2005;46(12):2183–92.
57. Beshai JF, Grimm RA, Nagueh SF, Baker II JH, Beau SL, Greenberg SM, Pires LA, Tchou PJ, for the RethinQ Study Investigators. Cardiac-resynchronization therapy in heart failure with narrow QRS complexes. N Engl J Med, 2007;357:2461–71.
58. Maisel WH, Stevenson LW. Atrial fibrillation in heart failure: epidemiology, pathophys-iology, and rationale for therapy. Am J Cardiol, 2003;91(6, Supplement 1):2–8.
59. Gasparini M, Auricchio A, Regoli F, et al. Four-year efficacy of cardiac resynchroniza-tion therapy on exercise tolerance and disease progression: the importance of performing atrioventricular junction ablation in patients with atrial fibrillation. J Am Coll Cardiol, Aug 15 2006;48(4):734–43.
60. Doshi RN, Daoud EG, Fellows C, et al. Left ventricular-based cardiac stimulation post AV nodal ablation evaluation (the PAVE study). J Cardiovasc Electrophysiol, Nov 2005;16(11):1160–65.
61. Molhoek SG, Bax JJ, Bleeker GB, et al. Comparison of response to cardiac resynchro-nization therapy in patients with sinus rhythm versus chronic atrial fibrillation. Am J Cardiol, Dec 15 2004;94(12):1506–09.
62. Feldman AM, de Lissovoy G, Bristow MR, et al. Cost effectiveness of cardiac resyn-chronization therapy in the Comparison of Medical Therapy, Pacing, and Defibrilla-

tion in Heart Failure (COMPANION) trial. J Am Coll Cardiol, Dec 20 2005;46(12): 2311–21.

63. Hlatky MA. Cost effectiveness of cardiac resynchronization therapy. J Am Coll Cardiol, Dec 20 2005;46(12):2322–24.

64. Strickberger SA, Conti J, Daoud EG, et al. Patient selection for cardiac resynchronization therapy: from the Council on Clinical Cardiology Subcommittee on Electrocardiography and Arrhythmias and the Quality of Care and Outcomes Research Interdisciplinary Working Group, in collaboration with the Heart Rhythm Society. Circulation, Apr 26 2005;111(16):2146–50.

65. Leclercq C, et al., Acute hemodynamic effects of biventricular DDD pacing in patients with end-stage heart failure. J Am Coll Cardiol, 1998;32(7): 1825–31.

66. Aranda JM, Jr., et al., Management of heart failure after cardiac resynchronization therapy: integrating advanced heart failure treatment with optimal device function. J Am Coll Cardiol, 2005;46(12): 2193–8.

67. Ammann P, et al., An electrocardiogram-based algorithm to detect loss of left ventricular capture during cardiac resynchronization therapy. Ann Intern Med, 2005;142(12 Pt 1): 968–73.

68. Meluzin J, et al., A fast and simple echocardiographic method of determination of the optimal atrioventricular delay in patients after biventricular stimulation. Pacing Clin Electrophysiol, 2004;27(1): 58–64.

69. Kerlan JE, et al., Prospective comparison of echocardiographic atrioventricular delay optimization methods for cardiac resynchronization therapy. Heart Rhythm, 2006;3(2): 148–54.

70. Morales MA, et al., Atrioventricular delay optimization by Doppler-derived left ventricular dP/dt improves 6-month outcome of resynchronized patients. Pacing Clin Electrophysiol, 2006;29(6): 564–8.

71. Boriani G, et al., Randomized comparison of simultaneous biventricular stimulation versus optimized interventricular delay in cardiac resynchronization therapy: The Resynchronization for the HemodYnamic Treatment for Heart Failure Management II implantable cardioverter defibrillator (RHYTHM II ICD) study. Am Heart J, 2006;151(5): 1050–58.

72. Sogaard P, et al., Sequential versus simultaneous biventricular resynchronization for severe heart failure: evaluation by tissue Doppler imaging. Circulation, 2002;106(16): 2078–84.

73. Porciani MC, et al., Echocardiographic examination of atrioventricular and interventricular delay optimization in cardiac resynchronization therapy. Am J Cardiol, 2005;95(9): 1108–10.

74. Epstein AE, DiMarco JP, Ellenbogen KA, Estes NAM III, Freedman RA, Gettes LS, et al. ACC/AHA/HRS 2008 guidelines for device-based therapy of cardiac rhythm abnormalities: a report of the American College of Cardiology/American Heart Association Task Force on Practice Guidelines (Writing Committee to Revise the ACC/AHA/NASPE 2002 Guideline Update for Implantation of Cardiac Pacemakers and Antiarrhythmia Devices). Circulation, 2008;117:e350–e408.

75. Zipes DP, et al., ACC/AHA/ESC 2006 guidelines for management of patients with ventricular arrhythmias and the prevention of sudden cardiac death: a report of the American College of Cardiology/American Heart Association Task Force and the European Society of Cardiology Committee for Practice Guidelines (writing committee to develop Guidelines for Management of Patients With Ventricular Arrhythmias and the Prevention of Sudden Cardiac Death): developed in collaboration with the European Heart Rhythm Association and the Heart Rhythm Society. Circulation, 2006;114(10): e385–484.

8

Pacing and Defibrillation for Atrial Arrhythmias

Joshua M. Cooper, MD

CONTENTS

Abstract

Atrial arrhythmias and heart failure frequently coexist. A number of device-based therapies are available for the diagnosis, prevention, and treatment of these arrhythmias. This chapter reviews the clinical impact of atrial and ventricular pacing on atrial arrhythmias, the diagnosis of atrial arrhythmias via device-based data retrieval, the value of alternate site atrial pacing algorithms for prevention of atrial fibrillation, and the treatment of atrial arrhythmias with device-based pacing and defibrillation.

Key Words: Atrial fibrillation; Heart failure; Pacemaker; Defibrillation.

From: *Contemporary Cardiology: Device Therapy in Heart Failure*
Edited by: W.H. Maisel, DOI 10.1007/978-1-59745-424-7_8
© Humana Press, a part of Springer Science+Business Media, LLC 2010

1. MECHANISMS OF ATRIAL ARRHYTHMIAS AND INTERACTION WITH ELECTRICAL PACING

Normal atrial electrical activity initiates in the sinus node, which is located along the epicardial surface of the mid-to-high lateral right atrium. With each generated impulse from the sinus node, an electrical wavefront sequentially sweeps across the right and left atrium, with the most prominent interatrial electrical connections being located in the high posterior interatrial septum, the region of the fossa ovalis, and around the coronary sinus ostium. Atrial arrhythmias result from either impulse generation at alternative sites, or abnormalities in wavefront propagation across the atria, or an interplay between these two mechanisms.

Ectopic atrial foci may be located anywhere in the atria but tend to predominate in specific anatomic locations, such as the crista terminalis, the tricuspid and mitral annuli, the eustachian ridge, the fossa ovalis, and in the pulmonary veins. An ectopic focus may fire sporadically, resulting in atrial premature depolarizations (APDs), or continuously, resulting in an atrial tachycardia. Depending on the responsiveness of an ectopic focus to catecholamines and autonomic tone, as well as competition with sinus node activity, atrial ectopy may be more prominent at rest, when the sinus node is at its slowest, or with exertion, when circulating catecholamines may stimulate ectopic atrial firing to a greater degree than sinus node acceleration.

As the atrial myocardium ages, collagen deposition between myocytes progressively disrupts organized wavefront propagation, with countless microscopic electrical barriers increasing the complexity of atrial activation. In addition, the variation in myofibril orientation, conduction velocities, cellular coupling, and refractory periods each impact local electrical propagation direction and velocity. Any hemodynamic derangement that increases atrial filling pressure, such as valvular stenosis or regurgitation, systolic or diastolic ventricular dysfunction, and restrictive or constrictive cardiac physiology, will result in myocardial stretching and atrial dilation. The combination of atrial enlargement and local disorganization of wavefront propagation creates an ideal substrate for electrical reentry. All the aforementioned mechanisms are active in patients with congestive heart failure, which explains why atrial arrhythmias are so commonly seen in the heart failure population.

Interactions between implanted devices and atrial arrhythmias fall into three main categories: (1) impact of atrial pacing on the electrical environment of the atria, (2) impact of atrial and ventricular pacing on atrial hemodynamics and remodeling, and (3) ability of an implanted device to detect and terminate atrial arrhythmias. While these interactions are relevant to all atrial arrhythmias, including atrial tachycardia, atrial flutter, and atrial fibrillation, it is the latter arrhythmia to which most attention has been given. The mechanisms of atrial tachycardia and atrial flutter are well understood, and, consequently, the pharmacologic and catheter ablation treatment options are highly effective in achieving arrhythmia control or cure. The complexity of atrial fibrillation, including its heterogeneous mechanisms, its disorganized and constantly changing electrical pattern, and its evolution over time, has led to the investigation of implanted devices for the prevention and treatment of this arrhythmia.

2. ATRIAL FIBRILLATION IN PATIENTS WITH PACEMAKERS

Several retrospective, non-randomized studies made the initial observation that patients with dual-chamber pacemakers developed atrial fibrillation at a significantly lower rate (0–3% per year) than those with single-chamber ventricular pacemakers (6–15% per year) (1–3). The theoretical mechanisms by which the addition of atrial pacing might reduce the incidence of atrial fibrillation are both electrical and hemodynamic. Atrial pacing prevents episodes of bradycardia that might facilitate atrial fibrillation by prolonging the atrial refractory period and affecting the regional variation in refractoriness (known as "dispersion of refractoriness") and atrial pacing might also serve to suppress ectopic atrial foci that serve as triggers of atrial fibrillation. Regardless of whether atrial sensing or atrial pacing predominates, the addition of an atrial lead also allows for mechanical atrioventricular synchrony and eliminates the episodic increases in atrial pressure that result from atrioventricular dissociation. It should be noted that these initial observational studies exclusively examined a population of patients with sinus node dysfunction; when a mixed population was used, there was a far greater antiarrhythmic benefit of dual-chamber pacing seen in the sinus node dysfunction patients than in those with AV block. The strong correlation between the development of atrial fibrillation and sinus node dysfunction suggests a possible mechanistic link between the two conditions.

Prompted by the findings of retrospective studies, several large randomized prospective trials were conducted to better investigate the benefits of dual-chamber pacing on the risk of developing atrial fibrillation (4–14). These studies varied in the patient populations studied (sinus node dysfunction vs. AV block), the mode of atrial-based pacing (AAI vs. DDD), the cohort size (67–2568 patients), and the follow-up time frame (2–6 years). There were, however, some consistent findings with regard to pacing mode and development of atrial fibrillation. In patients with sinus node dysfunction, an atrial-based pacing mode was almost always found to be associated with a lower rate of atrial fibrillation in follow-up than a ventricular-only-based pacing mode. Statistical differences were generally not seen in patients with AV block without sinus node dysfunction. A meta-analysis of these prospective trials, which incorporated nearly 35,000 patient-years of follow-up, showed that an atrial-based pacing mode was associated with a hazard ratio (HR) of 0.76 [95% confidence interval (CI) 0.67–0.86] for development of atrial fibrillation in patients with sinus node dysfunction and 0.90 (95% CI 0.74–1.09) in those without sinus node dysfunction (15). There was no statistical benefit on mortality or heart failure hospitalization in this population, but there was a borderline significant reduction in risk for stroke with dual-chamber pacing in the full cohort (Fig. 1).

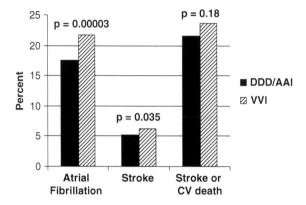

Fig. 1. Summary of findings from a meta-analysis of studies comparing "physiologic" dual-chamber pacing (AAI or DDD) with ventricular-only pacing (VVI) *(15)*. Over a mean follow-up of 2 years, physiologic pacing was associated with less atrial fibrillation and stroke than ventricular-only pacing, and there was a trend toward improvement in the combined endpoint of stroke and cardiovascular death.

An important caveat with regard to the population of patients with dual-chamber pacemakers, with or without AV block, is the potentially harmful effect of ventricular pacing that might counteract the benefit of AV synchrony. A greater appreciation of the detrimental impact of ventricular pacing on mechanical synchrony and intracardiac hemodynamics has developed in the years following these pacemaker trials. A retrospective analysis of the Mode Selection Trial (MOST), which prospectively randomized 2010 patients with sinus node dysfunction to single-chamber or dual-chamber pacing, revealed that the cumulative percentage of ventricular pacing correlated with the development of atrial fibrillation *(16)*. This relationship held true in both arms of the study, with the risk of atrial fibrillation increasing by 0.7–1% for each 1% increase in the cumulative percentage of ventricular pacing in the VVIR and DDDR groups, respectively, up to approximately 85% ventricular pacing, where the rates tapered off. The correlation between ventricular pacing and atrial fibrillation was not affected when other predictors of atrial fibrillation were taken into account. It may therefore be fortuitous that the benefit of maintaining atrioventricular synchrony in such studies outweighed the detriment from desynchronizing ventricular contraction with ventricular pacing, to the point where the benefit of dual-chamber pacing was able to be recognized.

The discovery that right ventricular pacing has detrimental effects on the incidence of not only atrial fibrillation but also heart failure hospitalization and mortality *(17)* has prompted further investigation of novel dual-chamber pacing modalities *(18)* and algorithms to lengthen the paced atrioventricular delay *(19)* in an effort to reduce the amount of ventricular pacing in dual-chamber devices. Most recently, the SAVE-PACe Trial *(20)* randomized 1065 patients with sinus node dysfunction but intact AV conduction to conventional dual-chamber pacing vs. dual-chamber pacing with programming features designed to minimize ventricular pacing. This study demonstrated a dramatic decrease in the median percentage of heart beats that were ventricularly paced (9.1% vs. 99.0%, $P < 0.001$) and a 40% relative risk reduction for developing persistent atrial fibrillation at 1.7 years (7.9% vs. 12.7%, HR 0.60, 95% CI 0.41–0.88, $P = 0.009$). It is therefore proving possible to capitalize on the advantages of dual-chamber devices without paying the price that comes with ventricular pacing. Implantation of an atrial lead is recommended in patients with sinus node dysfunction who require pacing in order to reduce the risk of future atrial fibrillation, but careful attention must be paid to device programming in order to minimize the amount of ventricular pacing delivered *(21)*.

3. DIAGNOSIS OF ATRIAL ARRHYTHMIAS IN PATIENTS WITH PACEMAKERS

Implanted devices with atrial leads can serve as long-term monitors for the development of atrial arrhythmias. In contrast to Holter monitors, event monitors, and home telemetry monitors, which provide either continuous or short segments of surface recordings for hours or days, pacemakers are able to automatically detect and report atrial arrhythmias over the time frame of years. This information could be used to track the success of antiarrhythmic therapy in a patient with known atrial fibrillation or to assess the potential contribution of atrial arrhythmias to a patient's heart failure status. In addition, pacemakers can be used to make a new diagnosis of atrial fibrillation, which might warrant the initiation of anticoagulation to reduce the risk of stroke.

Pacemakers can be programmed to respond in various ways to an atrial tachyarrhythmia. With regard to pacing mode, the pacemaker can be programmed to switch from a dual-chamber pacing mode (DDD or DDDR) to a ventricular-only pacing mode (VVI or VVIR) when an atrial high rate episode is detected. This automatic mode switch avoids the potential problem of the pacemaker attempting to "track" atrial fibrillation, which would result in ventricular pacing at the upper programmed pacing limit. When the atrial rate falls back below the programmed atrial high rate cutoff, thereby signifying a return to sinus rhythm, the pacemaker will switch back to a dual-chamber pacing mode. In addition, most pacemakers can keep track of the number, frequency, and duration of atrial high rate episodes, typically in the form of a graph and/or an event log (Fig. 2). Some pacemakers have the additional option of storing atrial electrograms from detected events, which

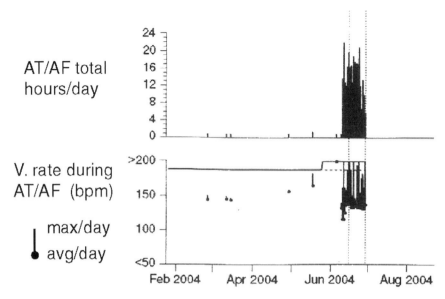

Fig. 2. Sample printout from a patient who presented with worsening heart failure at the end of June. The device reports a dramatic increase in the burden of atrial fibrillation (AF) starting approximately 2 weeks prior to presentation, with very little AF prior to mid-June, and many hours of AF daily since then (*top plot*). Mean ventricular response rates were approximately 130–140 beats per minute (bpm), with peak heart rates during AF up to 200 bpm (*bottom plot*).

comes at the expense of a minor reduction in battery longevity. This feature may initially prove useful for the physician to differentiate between true atrial arrhythmias and false atrial high rate events that are triggered by far-field oversensing of the ventricular electrogram (Figs. 3 and 4). Careful device programming is essential to minimize the possibilities of undersensing atrial activity during atrial fibrillation or far-field R-wave oversensing, which would result in false-negative and false-positive data. With sound device programming, pacemakers have been demonstrated to be reliable diagnostic devices for detection of atrial tachyarrhythmias *(22, 23)*.

Published studies have reported a high prevalence of atrial high rate episodes in patients with pacemakers, which includes short events lasting seconds to hours *(24–26)*. The rates of newly diagnosed atrial fibrillation range from 35 to 70% over the first 2 years of pacemaker implantation, with higher rates seen in patients with sinus node dysfunction. In a substudy of the MOST trial, the clinical significance of atrial high rate episodes longer than 5 min was evaluated. Over a median follow-up of 27 months, 51% of the 312 patients in the substudy were found to have atrial high rate events. The presence of atrial high rate episodes was an independent predictor of total mortality (HR 2.48, 95% CI 1.25–4.91), death or nonfatal stroke (HR 2.79, 95% CI 1.51–5.15), and atrial fibrillation (HR 5.93, 95% CI 2.88–12.2) *(27)*.

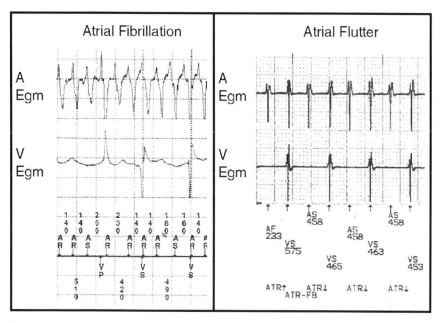

Fig. 3. Sample stored electrograms (Egm) from the atrium (A) and ventricle (V) retrieved from implanted devices in patients who had prior episodes of atrial fibrillation (*left panel*) and atrial flutter (*right panel*). The device interpretation of the intracardiac signals is noted at the bottom of each tracing, with company-specific nomenclature used.

The question, however, of thromboembolic risk in patients with atrial high rate episodes exclusively shorter than 24 h remains unanswered, especially when the potential risks of initiating anticoagulation are taken into account. To address this question, a large prospective clinical trial is being conducted in older patients with hypertension and a standard pacemaker indication to evaluate the clinical significance of asymptomatic atrial high rate episodes without overt atrial fibrillation, with a particular focus on the risk of stroke and other vascular events *(28)*.

4. ALTERNATE SITE ATRIAL PACING

Multiple models and explanations for the mechanism of atrial fibrillation exist, and wavelet reentry is a common theme among them. In order for reentry to occur in atrial tissue, different regions of the atrium must have different recovery times. The greater the local variation in refractory period (dispersion of refractoriness), the greater the susceptibility to reentry and atrial fibrillation *(29)*. In patients with atrial fibrillation, abnormalities in the atrial myocardium result in slower electrical conduction, local barriers to wavefront propagation, and more varied repolarization times, all of which increase the dispersion of refractoriness. The decreased electrical

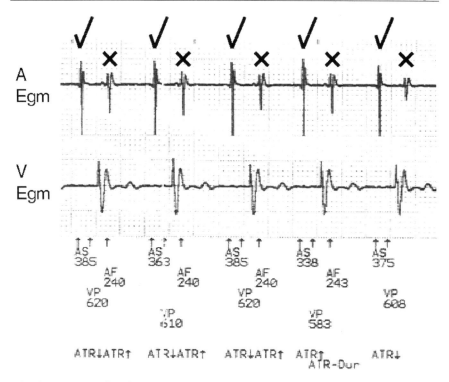

Fig. 4. Example of an incorrect device diagnosis of atrial arrhythmia due to double counting of true atrial events (*check marks*) and oversensed "far-field" ventricular events (denoted with an "x"). The atrial lead had been implanted close to the tricuspid annulus where it was able to sense electrical events from the nearby ventricular myocardium. The device interpretation of the intracardiac signals is noted at the bottom of each tracing, with company-specific nomenclature used. ATR indicates atrial tachy response, a manufacturer-specific term that indicates that the device believes that a true atrial arrhythmia is occurring.

coordination of diseased atrial myocardium can be seen on the surface ECG as a broader P wave, reflecting the longer time required to complete the electrical depolarization of both atria.

The traditional location for placement of an atrial pacing lead is in the right atrial appendage or on the lateral wall of the right atrium. Impulse generation at these sites results in sequential activation first across the right atrium and then the left atrium. Theoretically, if the atria were activated more simultaneously rather than sequentially, the global dispersion of refractoriness could be reduced, with potential implications on the ability of atrial fibrillation to initiate. Placement of the atrial lead on the interatrial septum, particularly at sites of preferential electrical communication between the right and the left atrium, results in more simultaneous atrial depolarization during atrial pacing, reflected by a narrower P wave (Fig. 5) *(30–32)*.

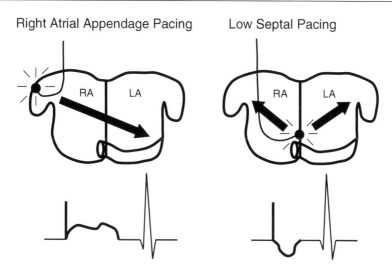

Fig. 5. Comparison of wavefront propagation (*arrows*) across the right and the left atrium (RA, LA) and P-wave morphology (shown *below*) when pacing from the right atrial appendage (*left*) vs. pacing from the interatrial septum near the coronary sinus ostium (*right*). Pacing from the right atrial appendage is associated with sequential activation of the RA and then the LA, and is associated with a broad P wave. Pacing from the low interatrial septum is associated with more simultaneous activation of the RA and the LA, and is associated with a narrower P wave. In this case, the P wave is superiorly directed due to the atrial lead location being low on the septum, near the coronary sinus ostium.

Several small studies have been conducted to evaluate the antifibrillatory effect of atrial pacing near the coronary sinus ostium or at Bachmann's bundle, which are two sites on the interatrial septum where electrical communication between the right and left atria is more prominent *(33–36)*. These clinical studies showed a decreased propensity to progression of atrial fibrillation, including a reduction in the daily burden of atrial fibrillation episodes.

An alternative strategy for electrically "synchronizing" the atria is to pace from two different atrial sites simultaneously (Fig. 6). Several studies have investigated the electrical effects of simultaneous pacing from the high right atrium and either the proximal or the distal coronary sinus *(37, 38)*, as well as the feasibility of placing a left atrial pacing lead in the coronary sinus *(39–41)*. Dual-site atrial pacing is feasible and results in a decrease in total atrial activation time with a shorter P-wave duration, particularly when the distal coronary sinus is used to pace from the lateral portion of the left atrium. With regard to the effect on atrial fibrillation, dual-site atrial pacing has been demonstrated in small studies to result in improvement of atrial fibrillation burden in select patients, particularly when used in combination with antiarrhythmic drug therapy *(42, 43)*, but large, long-term multicenter trials have not been conducted to answer this question *(44)*.

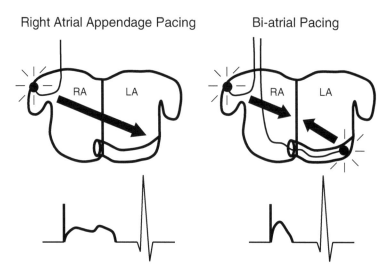

Fig. 6. Comparison of wavefront propagation (*arrows*) across the right and the left atrium (RA, LA) and P-wave morphology (shown *below*) when pacing from a single site in the right atrial appendage (*left*) vs. pacing from both the right atrial appendage and the distal coronary sinus simultaneously (*right*). Pacing from the right atrial appendage is associated with sequential activation of the RA and then the LA, and is associated with a broad P wave. Pacing from the RA and the LA simultaneously results in the generation of two simultaneous wavefronts, more simultaneous activation of the atria, and a narrower P wave.

From a practical standpoint, placement of a single atrial lead on the interatrial septum is more technically challenging, might be associated with a higher risk for lead dislodgement, and is associated with a greater risk of far-field oversensing of ventricular signals as the lead is placed closer to the tricuspid annulus. Multisite pacing results in the placement of additional intracardiac hardware, and there is the additional problem of "double counting" intrinsic atrial events with the risk of provoking inappropriate pacemaker behavior. With the current status of device and lead technology, coupled with the lack of large multicenter trials to demonstrate clear benefit of alternate site or dual-site atrial pacing, these treatment options remain unproven and the current standard of care for patients with paroxysmal atrial fibrillation and sinus node dysfunction is the implantation of a standard dual-chamber pacemaker (*21, 45*).

5. PACING ALGORITHMS TO PREVENT ATRIAL FIBRILLATION

With basic pacemaker programming, atrial pacing will occur only if the native atrial rate falls below the programmed lower pacemaker rate. If the rate–response feature is activated, then the pacemaker will pace faster in response to movement (accelerometer or piezoelectric crystal sensor) and/or more rapid breathing (minute ventilation sensor), in an attempt to reproduce the physiologic increase in heart rate with exertion. The ability of atrial pacing to affect dispersion of refractoriness or suppress atrial ectopy is dependent on atrial pacing being delivered. A higher percentage of atrial pacing has been shown to correlate with fewer atrial arrhythmias in prospective studies that evaluated atrial arrhythmia burden in patients with pacemakers *(46)*. With standard pacemaker programming, the amount of atrial pacing depends on the interplay between the intrinsic atrial rate and the lower pacing rate (and/or sensor rate). A greater percentage of atrial pacing could be delivered by increasing the lower pacing rate, but this strategy would commit the patient to continuous faster pacing that might result in symptoms from a persistently elevated heart rate, more rapid pacemaker battery depletion, and possibly even cause harm by worsening left ventricular ejection fraction and exacerbating heart failure symptoms if the patient is paced continuously at rates significantly over 100 pulses per minute.

In order to increase the percentage of atrial pacing while maintaining a more physiologic heart rate profile, different pacing algorithms have been developed that drive atrial pacing slightly faster than the intrinsic sinus rate. The algorithms developed by different pacemaker manufacturers vary, but they all result in faster atrial pacing after detection of intrinsic sinus beats, premature atrial beats, or after sporadic assessment of the underlying heart rate. To avoid excessive pacing rates, pacing is gradually slowed back down until native atrial activity is again seen, which triggers another increase in the pacing rate (Fig. 7). The goals of these algorithms are to prevent brady-

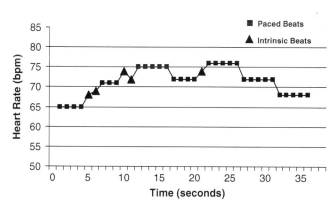

Fig. 7. Schematic of a hypothetical overdrive atrial pacing algorithm. The pacemaker increases its pacing rate (shown as *squares*) after intrinsic atrial beats (shown as *triangles*) are detected. After five beats at the faster pacing rate in this hypothetical algorithm, the pacemaker slows down the pacing rate toward the lower pacing limit until more intrinsic beats are seen. In this manner, atrial pacing predominates without necessitating sustained rapid atrial pacing rates.

cardia, promote a high percentage of atrial pacing, as well as eliminate the short–long intervals that would ordinarily result from premature atrial depolarizations. In addition, these algorithms usually include a postmode switch overdrive pacing component, where faster atrial pacing is delivered for a fixed period of time following reversion from atrial fibrillation back to sinus rhythm. It is during this postconversion time period that the atria might be most susceptible to recurrent fibrillation, and atrial ectopy is also more frequent immediately after reversion to sinus rhythm.

Studies of overdrive atrial pacing have clearly shown that predominant atrial pacing can be achieved, but the impact on atrial fibrillation has yielded variable results (47–53). With atrial overdrive algorithms turned on, over 80–90% atrial pacing is easily achieved, but suppression of atrial arrhythmias seems to be patient-specific, with some patients experiencing a significant reduction in atrial fibrillation and others experiencing no decrease or even an increased number of episodes. In the larger trials, there appears to be an average 25–35% reduction in the burden of atrial tachyarrhythmias with atrial overdrive pacing, typically defined as a decrease in the number of episodes on a daily basis. In the studies that showed this effect, the clinical impact was not clear, as there was no reported change in pharmacologic management and frequently no significant reduction in symptom burden. Trials of atrial preventative pacing algorithms have generally suffered from the use of small patient cohorts, different definitions of atrial tachyarrhythmias and of arrhythmia burden, and variable use of antiarrhythmic medications (54–56). Similarly, studies that have combined atrial overdrive pacing with alternative or dual-site atrial pacing have not convincingly demonstrated a dramatic benefit of preferential atrial pacing (57–59). A major possible confounder for all these studies is the percentage of ventricular pacing, which was generally not reported and yet likely has a deleterious effect on the development and progression of atrial arrhythmias. Future studies of atrial overdrive pacing will make use of newer device software algorithms that minimize ventricular pacing in order to investigate the beneficial effects of atrial pacing without paying the price that comes with increased ventricular pacing.

6. TERMINATION OF ATRIAL ARRHYTHMIAS: ANTITACHYCARDIA PACING AND CARDIOVERSION

Pace termination of a tachyarrhythmia occurs when a paced beat penetrates the excitable gap within a reentry circuit, resulting in a collision of wavefronts and termination of the tachycardia. The location and specific electrical properties of the circuit, such as conduction velocity and recovery time of the tissue, determine the likelihood of success of antitachycardia pacing. Electrical rhythms that involve multiple circuits or changing patterns of activation are far less likely to respond to antitachycardia pacing and are more likely to require a shock for cardioversion back to sinus rhythm.

Implanted devices have been designed to deliver both types of therapy to terminate atrial arrhythmias. The rationale for automatic device treatment of atrial arrhythmias is based both on prompt alleviation of symptoms, such as palpitations, dyspnea, and congestive heart failure, and on the principle that the persistence of atrial arrhythmias can provoke changes in the atrial myocardium that facilitate arrhythmia recurrence *(60)*.

While atrial fibrillation, per se, is not a rhythm that responds to antitachycardia pacing, patients with atrial fibrillation frequently also have episodes of more organized atrial tachyarrhythmias, such as atrial flutter and atrial tachycardia. These latter arrhythmias may either directly initiate or degenerate into atrial fibrillation, or they may appear after spontaneous or antiarrhythmic, drug-induced organization of atrial fibrillation. Pacemakers with antitachycardia pacing capabilities can terminate some atrial arrhythmias in patients with atrial fibrillation, presumably with the highest likelihood of success occurring during periods of greatest arrhythmia organization (Fig. 8). Randomized trials have demonstrated an approximate 35–50% success rate for antitachycardia pacing termination of atrial arrhythmias, but the overall favorable impact on arrhythmia burden has been disappointing *(61–66)*.

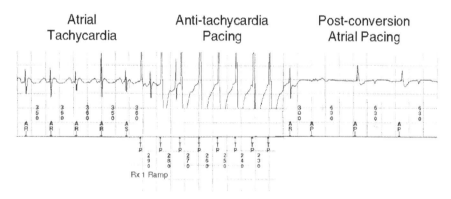

Fig. 8. Example of pace termination of an atrial tachycardia. An atrial electrogram, as recorded by an implanted pacemaker, is shown. On the left-hand side of the panel, the atrial arrhythmia (atrial tachycardia) is detected. Each intracardiac signal is recognized by the device (denoted "AR") and the time (in milliseconds) between beats is noted by the device (350–360 ms). A train of eight pacing stimuli (denoted "TP") is delivered at a rate faster than the atrial tachycardia. The atrial arrhythmia terminates and the pacemaker paces (denoted "AP") at 95 pulses per minute (630 ms) after tachycardia termination in an attempt to suppress atrial ectopy that might result in early recurrence of the arrhythmia.

Cardioversion from an implanted device is associated with a much higher success rate of restoration of sinus rhythm, usually over 90% (Fig. 9), but the main limitations of this therapy are arrhythmia recurrence and the pain

Atrial   Shock

Tachycardia   Delivery   Atrial Pacing

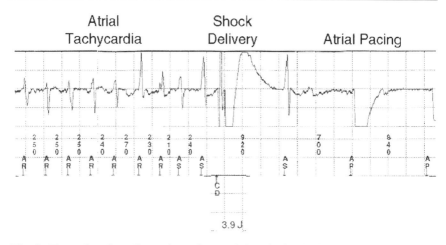

Fig. 9. Example of cardioversion of an atrial arrhythmia from an implanted cardioverter/defibrillator. Atrial tachycardia is detected (denoted "AR" and "AS") with cycle length of 210–270 ms. A 4 J shock is delivered (denoted "CD"), which successfully restores sinus rhythm.

associated with shock delivery. Both dedicated atrial defibrillators, with a shocking coil placed in the coronary sinus, and traditional defibrillators, with the distal coil in the right ventricle, have been studied for the treatment of patients with recurrent symptomatic atrial fibrillation *(67–69)*. These devices can be programmed either to deliver patient-triggered shocks after a short delay, allowing the patient to premedicate with an analgesic or sedating medication, or to deliver a nocturnal shock while the patient is asleep. Nighttime shock delivery in the absence of sedation tends to be associated with sleep disturbances and concerns about future pain from shocks; however, daytime patient-triggered cardioversion after premedication is well tolerated in a motivated subpopulation of symptomatic atrial fibrillation patients, and an improved quality of life has been demonstrated in this cohort *(70–72)*. The main impact of device-based cardioversion of atrial fibrillation is on duration of episodes and reduction in symptoms, but atrial arrhythmia recurrence is common and there is little evidence for reduction in the number of episodes *(73–75)*.

7. CONCLUSIONS

Implanted pacemakers and defibrillators can help in the management of atrial arrhythmias from both diagnostic and treatment perspectives (Table 1). Device detection of atrial fibrillation, with detailed reports of frequency, duration, and burden of atrial arrhythmias, can be of diagnostic help in the management of patients with congestive heart failure exacerbation. Dual-chamber pacing is clearly superior to ventricular pacing in patients with sinus node dysfunction with regard to progression of atrial fibrillation, but

Table 1

Device-based features in the management of atrial fibrillation

Device feature	Function in atrial fibrillation management
Log of atrial high rate episodes	Detection/diagnosis of AF
Atrial electrogram storage	Detection/diagnosis of AF
Dual-chamber pacing (i.e., DDD vs. VVI)	Prevention of AF
Alternate site atrial pacing (i.e., Bachmann's bundle, coronary sinus ostium, distal coronary sinus)	Prevention of AF
Dual-site atrial pacing	Prevention of AF
Algorithms to increase percentage of atrial pacing	Prevention of AF
Algorithms to promote intrinsic AV conduction (i.e., automatic AV delay extension or alternating AAI/DDD pacing mode)	Prevention of AF
Overdrive pacing algorithm after reversion to sinus rhythm	Prevention of AF
Antitachycardia pacing therapy	Treatment of AF
Patient-controlled cardioversion (i.e., shock delivery)	Treatment of AF

alternate site atrial pacing and preventative pacing algorithms do not currently play a major role in atrial arrhythmia management *(21)*. Right ventricular pacing has proven to worsen both heart failure and atrial arrhythmias, and pacing algorithms to minimize ventricular pacing are now being incorporated into most implanted devices. Antitachycardia pacing and cardioversion therapies have not been demonstrated to impact overall atrial fibrillation burden or stroke, but they can improve the quality of life in a select subset of highly symptomatic patients whose atrial arrhythmias are not well controlled with other pharmacologic and ablative therapies. Current ongoing and future trials are needed to further clarify the role of device therapies in the various subgroups of paroxysmal and persistent atrial fibrillation patients with and without congestive heart failure *(76)*.

REFERENCES

1. Stangl K, Seitz K, Wirtzfeld A, Alt E, Blomer H. Differences between atrial single chamber pacing (AAI) and ventricular single chamber pacing (VVI) with respect to prognosis and antiarrhythmic effect in patients with sick sinus syndrome. Pacing Clin Electrophysiol 1990;13:2080–5.
2. Hesselson AB, Parsonnet V, Bernstein AD, Bonavita GJ. Deleterious effects of long-term single-chamber ventricular pacing in patients with sick sinus syndrome: the hidden benefits of dual-chamber pacing. J Am Coll Cardiol 1992;19:1542–9.
3. Sgarbossa EB, Pinski SL, Maloney JD, et al. Chronic atrial fibrillation and stroke in paced patients with sick sinus syndrome: relevance of clinical characteristics and pacing modalities. Circulation 1993;88:1045–53.

4. Andersen HR, Thuesen L, Bagger JP, Vesterlund T, Thomsen PEB. Prospective randomised trial of atrial versus ventricular pacing in sick-sinus syndrome. Lancet 1994;344:1523–8.

5. Andersen HR, Nielsen JC, Thomsen PEB, et al. Long-term follow-up of patients from a randomised trial of atrial versus ventricular pacing for sick-sinus syndrome. Lancet 1997;350:1210–6.

6. Gillis AM, Wyse DG, Connolly SJ, et al. Atrial pacing periablation for prevention of paroxysmal atrial fibrillation. Circulation 1999;99:2553–8.

7. Gillis AM, Connolly SJ, Lacombe P, et al. Randomized crossover comparison of DDDR versus VDD pacing after atrioventricular junction ablation for prevention of atrial fibrillation. Circulation 2000;102:736–41.

8. Connolly SJ, Kerr CR, Gent M, et al. Effects of physiologic pacing versus ventricular pacing on the risk of stroke and death due to cardiovascular causes. N Engl J Med 2000;342:1385–91.

9. Skanes AC, Krahn AD, Yee R, et al. Progression to chronic atrial fibrillation after pacing: the Canadian Trial of Physiologic Pacing. J Am Coll Cardiol 2001;38:167–72.

10. Lamas GA, Orav J, Stambler BS, et al. Quality of life and clinical outcomes in elderly patients treated with ventricular pacing as compared with dual-chamber pacing. N Engl J Med 1998;338:1097–104.

11. Wharton JM, Sorrentino RA, Campbell P, et al. Effect of pacing modality on atrial tachyarrhythmia recurrence in the tachycardia–bradycardia syndrome: preliminary results of the Pacemaker Atrial Tachycardia Trial. Circulation 1998;98:I-494. Abstract.

12. Lamas GA, Lee KL, Sweeney MO, et al. Ventricular pacing or dual-chamber pacing for sinus-node dysfunction. N Engl J Med 2002;346:1854–62.

13. Toff WD, Camm AJ, Skehan JD. Single-chamber versus dual-chamber pacing for high-grade atrioventricular block. N Engl J Med 2005;353:145–55.

14. Charles RG, McComb JM. Systematic trial of pacing to prevent atrial fibrillation (STOP-AF). Heart 1997;78:224–5.

15. Healey JS, Toff WD, Lamas GA, et al. Cardiovascular outcomes with atrial-based pacing compared with ventricular-based pacing: Meta-analysis of randomized trials, using individual patient data. Circulation 2006;114:11–7.

16. Sweeney MO, Hellkamp AS, Ellenbogen KA, et al. Adverse effect of ventricular pacing on heart failure and atrial fibrillation among patients with normal baseline QRS duration in a clinical trial of pacemaker therapy for sinus node dysfunction. Circulation 2003;107:2932–7.

17. Wilkoff BL, Cook JR, Epstein AE, et al. Dual-chamber pacing or ventricular backup pacing in patients with an implantable defibrillator: the Dual Chamber and VVI Implantable Defibrillator (DAVID) Trial. J Am Med Assoc 2002;288:3115–23.

18. Sweeney MO, Ellenbogen KA, Miller EH, et al. The managed ventricular pacing versus VVI 40 pacing (MVP) trial: clinical background, rationale, design, and implementation. J Cardiovasc Electrophysiol 2006;17:1295–8.

19. Olshansky B, Day JD, Moore S, et al. Is dual-chamber programming inferior to single-chamber programming in an implantable cardioverter-defibrillator? Results of the INTRINSIC RV (Inhibition of Unnecessary RV Pacing with AVSH in ICDs) study. Circulation 2007;115:9–16.

20. Sweeney MO, Bank AJ, Nsah E, Koullick M, Zeng QC, Hettrick D, Sheldon T, Lamas GA. Search AV Extension and Managed Ventricular Pacing for Promoting Atrioventricular Conduction (SAVE PACe) Trial. N Engl J Med 2007 Sep 6;357(1):1000–8.

21. Epstein AE, DiMarco JP, Ellenbogen KA, Estes NAM III, Freedman RA, Gettes LS, Gillinov AM, Gregoratos G, Hammill SC, Hayes DL, Hlatky MA, Newby LK, Page RL, Schoenfeld MH, Silka MJ, Stevenson LW, Sweeney MO. ACC/AHA/HRS 2008 guidelines for device-based therapy of cardiac rhythm abnormalities: a report of the American College of Cardiology/American Heart Association Task Force on Practice

Guidelines (Writing Committee to Revise the ACC/AHA/NASPE 2002 Guideline Update for Implantation of Cardiac Pacemakers and Antiarrhythmia Devices). J Am Coll Cardiol 2008;51:e1–62

22. Seidl K, Meisel E, VanAgt E, et al. Is the atrial high rate episode diagnostic feature reliable in detecting paroxysmal episodes of atrial tachyarrhythmias? Pacing Clin Electrophysiol 1998;21:694–700.

23. Pollak WM, Simmons JD, Interian A Jr, et al. Clinical utility of intraatrial pacemaker stored electrograms to diagnose atrial fibrillation and flutter. Pacing Clin Electrophysiol 2001;24:424–9.

24. Defaye P, Dournaux F, Mouton E. Prevalence of supraventricular arrhythmias from the automated analysis of data stored in the DDD pacemakers of 617 patients: the AIDA study. Pacing Clin Electrophysiol 1998;21:250–5.

25. Gillis AM, Morck M. Atrial fibrillation after DDDR pacemaker implantation. J Cardiovasc Electrophysiol 2002;13:542–7.

26. Orlov MV, Ghali JK, Araghi-Niknam M, et al., for the Atrial High Rate Trial Investigators. Asymptomatic atrial fibrillation in pacemaker recipients: incidence, progression, and determinants based on the Atrial High Rate Trial. Pacing Clin Electrophysiol 2007;30:404–11.

27. Glotzer TV, Hellkamp AS, Zimmerman J, et al., for the MOST Investigators. Atrial high rate episodes detected by pacemaker diagnostics predict death and stroke: report of the atrial diagnostics ancillary study of the Mode Selection Trial (MOST). Circulation 2003;107:1614–9.

28. Hohnloser SH, Capucci A, Fain E, et al. Asymptomatic atrial fibrillation and stroke evaluation in pacemaker patients and the atrial fibrillation reduction atrial pacing trial (ASSERT). Am Heart J 2006;152:442–7.

29. Ramdat Misier AR, Opthof T, van Hemel NM, et al. Increased dispersion of "refractoriness" in patients with idiopathic paroxysmal atrial fibrillation. J Am Coll Cardiol 1992;19:1531–5.

30. Spencer WH 3rd, Zhu DW, Markowitz T, Badruddin SM, Zoghbi WA. Atrial septal pacing: a method for pacing both atria simultaneously. Pacing Clin Electrophysiol 1997;20:2739–45.

31. Katsivas A, Manolis AG, Lazaris E, Vassilopoulos C, Louvros N. Atrial septal pacing to synchronize atrial depolarization in patients with delayed interatrial conduction. Pacing Clin Electrophysiol 1998;21:2220–5.

32. Rothinger FX, Abou-Harb M, Pachinger O, Hintringer F. The effect of the atrial pacing site on the total atrial activation time. Pacing Clin Electrophysiol 2001;24:316–22.

33. Papageorgiou P, Anselme F, Kirchhof CJ, et al. Coronary sinus pacing prevents induction of atrial fibrillation. Circulation 1997;96:1893–8.

34. Duytschaever M, Danse P, Eysbouts S, Allessie M. Is there an optimal pacing site to prevent atrial fibrillation?: an experimental study in the chronically instrumented goat. J Cardiovasc Electrophysiol 2002;13:1264–71.

35. Bailin SJ, Adler S, Giudici M. Prevention of chronic atrial fibrillation by pacing in the region of Bachmann's bundle: results of a multicenter randomized trial. J Cardiovasc Electrophysiol 2001;12:912–7.

36. Padeletti L, Pieragnoli P, Ciapetti C, et al. Randomized crossover comparison of right atrial appendage pacing versus interatrial septum pacing for prevention of paroxysmal atrial fibrillation in patients with sinus bradycardia. Am Heart J 2001;142:1047–55.

37. Prakash A, Delfaut P, Krol RB, Saksena S. Regional right and left atrial activation patterns during single- and dual-site atrial pacing in patients with atrial fibrillation. Am J Cardiol 1998;82:1197–1204.

38. Gilligan DM, Fuller IA, Clemo HF, et al. The acute effects of biatrial pacing on atrial depolarization and repolarization. Pacing Clin Electrophysiol 2000;23:1113–20.

39. Mirza I, Holt P, James S. Permanent left atrial pacing: a 2-year follow-up of coronary sinus leads. Pacing Clin Electrophysiol 2004;27:314–7.

40. Ouali S, Anselme F, Hidden F, et al. Effective long-term left atrial pacing using regular screw-in lead implanted within the coronary sinus. Pacing Clin Electrophysiol 2003;26:1873–7.

41. Levy T, Walker S, Rex S, Paul V. A comparison between passive and active fixation leads in the coronary sinus for biatrial pacing: initial experience. Europace 2000;2:228–32.

42. Mirza I, James S, Holt P. Biatrial pacing for paroxysmal atrial fibrillation: a randomized prospective study into the suppression of paroxysmal atrial fibrillation using biatrial pacing. J Am Coll Cardiol 2002;40:457–63.

43. Saksena S, Prakash A, Ziegler P, et al., for the DAPPAF Investigators. Improved suppression of recurrent atrial fibrillation with dual-site right atrial pacing and antiarrhythmic drug therapy. J Am Coll Cardiol 2002;40:1140–50.

44. Ellenbogen K. Pacing therapy for prevention of atrial fibrillation. Heart Rhythm 2007;4(Suppl 1):S84–7.

45. Knight BP, Gersh BJ, Carlson MD, et al., for the AHA Writing Group. Role of permanent pacing to prevent atrial fibrillation. Circulation 2005;111:240–3.

46. Defaye P, Dournaux F, Mouton E, et al., for the AIDA Multicenter Study Group. Prevalence of supraventricular arrhythmias from the automated analysis of data stored in the DDD pacemakers of 617 patients: the AIDA study. Pacing Clin Electrophysiol 1998;21:250–5.

47. Israel CW, Lawo T, Lemke B, Gronefeld G, Hohnloser SH. Atrial pacing in the prevention of paroxysmal atrial fibrillation: first results of a new combined algorithm. Pacing Clin Electrophysiol 2000;23:1888–90.

48. Funck RC, Adamec R, Lurje L, et al., on behalf of the PROVE Study Group. Atrial overdriving is beneficial in patients with atrial arrhythmias: first results of the PROVE study. Pacing Clin Electrophysiol 2000;23:1891–3.

49. Carlson MD, Ip J, Messenger J, et al. A new pacemaker algorithm for the treatment of atrial fibrillation: results of the Atrial Dynamic Overdrive Pacing Trial (ADOPT). J Am Coll Cardiol 2003;42:627–33.

50. Hemels ME, Wiesfeld AC, Inberg B, et al. Right atrial overdrive pacing for prevention of symptomatic refractory atrial fibrillation. Europace 2006;8:107–12.

51. Lewalter T, Yang A, Pfeiffer D, et al. Individualized selection of pacing algorithms for the prevention of recurrent atrial fibrillation: results from the VIP registry. Pacing Clin Electrophysiol 2006;29:124–34.

52. Blanc JJ, De Roy L, Mansourati J, et al., for the PIPAF Investigators. Atrial pacing for prevention of atrial fibrillation: assessment of simultaneously implemented algorithms. Europace 2004;6:371–9.

53. Schuchert A, Rebeski HP, Peiffer T, Bub E, Dietz A, Mortensen K, Aydin MA, Camm J, Gazarek S, Meinertz T; 3:4 Study Group. Effects of continuous and triggered atrial overdrive pacing on paroxysmal atrial fibrillation in pacemaker patients. Pacing Clin Electrophysiol 2008 Aug;31(8):929–34.

54. Konz KH, Danilovic D, Brachmann J, et al. The influence of concomitant drug therapy on the efficacy of atrial overdrive stimulation for prevention of atrial tachyarrhythmias. Pacing Clin Electrophysiol 2003;26:272–7.

55. Israel CW, Gronefeld G, Ehrlich JR, Hohnloser SH. Suppression of atrial tachyarrhythmias by pacing. J Cardiovasc Electrophysiol 2002;13:S31–9.

56. Ricci RP, Boriani G, Grammatico A, Santini M. Optimization of pacing algorithms to prevent and treat supraventricular tachyarrhythmias. Pacing Clin Electrophysiol 2006;29:S61–72.

57. Lau CP, Tse HF, Yu CM, et al., for the NIPP-AF Investigators. Dual-site atrial pacing for atrial fibrillation in patients without bradycardia. Am J Cardiol 2001;88:371–5.

58. De Simone A, Senatore G, Donnici G, et al. Dynamic and dual-site atrial pacing in the prevention of atrial fibrillation: the Stimolazione Atrial Dinamica Multisito (STADIM) Study. Pacing Clin Electrophysiol 2007;30:S71–4.

59. Padeletti L, Purerfellner H, Adler SW, et al., for the Worldwide ASPECT Investigators. Combined efficacy of atrial septal lead placement and atrial pacing algorithms for prevention of paroxysmal atrial tachyarrhythmia. J Cardiovasc Electrophysiol 2003;14:1189–95.

60. Wijffels MCEF, Kirchhof CJHJ, Dorland R, Allessie MA. Atrial fibrillation begets atrial fibrillation: a study in awake chronically instrumented goats. Circulation 1995;92: 1954–68.

61. Israel CW, Hugl B, Unterberg C, et al., for the AT500 Verification Study Investigators. Pace-termination and pacing for prevention of atrial tachyarrhythmias: results from a multicenter study with an implantable device for atrial therapy. J Cardiovasc Electrophysiol 2001;12:1121–8.

62. Lee MA, Weachter R, Pollack S, et al., for the ATTEST Investigators. The effect of atrial pacing therapies on atrial tachyarrhythmia burden and frequency: results of a randomized trial in patients with bradycardia and atrial tachyarrhythmias. J Am Coll Cardiol 2003;41:1926–32.

63. Gulizia M, Mangiameli S, Orazi S, et al., for the PITAGORA investigators. Randomized comparison between Ramp and Burst+ atrial antitachycardia pacing therapies in patients suffering from sinus node disease and atrial fibrillation and implanted with a DDDRP device. Europace 2006;8:465–73.

64. Hugl B, Israel CW, Unterberg C, et al., for the AT500 Verification Study Investigators. Incremental programming of atrial anti-tachycardia pacing therapies in bradycardia-indicated patients: effects on therapy efficacy and atrial tachyarrhythmia burden. Europace 2003;5:403–9.

65. Gillis AM, Unterberg-Buchwald C, Schmidinger H, et al., for the GEM III AT Worldwide Investigators. Safety and efficacy of advanced atrial pacing therapies for atrial tachyarrhythmias in patients with a new implantable dual chamber cardioverter-defibrillator. J Am Coll Cardiol 2002;40:1653–9.

66. Hemels ME, Ruiter JH, Molhoek GP, Veeger NJ, Wiesfeld AC, Ranchor AV, van Trigt M, Pilmeyer A, Van Gelder IC; Features in AT500TM Study. Chances for patients with episodes of atrial tachyarrhythmia without bradycardia indication for pacing (FACET) investigators right atrial preventive and antitachycardia pacing for prevention of paroxysmal atrial fibrillation in patients without bradycardia: a randomized study. Europace 2008 Mar;10(3):306–13.

67. Jung W, Wolpert C, Esmailzadeh B, et al. Clinical experience with implantable atrial and combined atrioventricular defibrillators. J Interv Card Electrophysiol 2000;4:S185–95.

68. Geller JC, Reek S, Timmermans C, et al. Treatment of atrial fibrillation with an implantable atrial defibrillator – long term results. Eur Heart J 2003;24:2083–9.

69. Daoud EG, Timmermans C, Fellows C, et al., for the METRIX Investigators. Initial clinical experience with ambulatory use of an implantable atrial defibrillator for conversion of atrial fibrillation. Circulation 2000;102:1407–13.

70. Boodhoo L, Mitchell A, Ujhelyi M, Sulke N. Improving the acceptability of the atrial defibrillator: patient-activated cardioversion versus automatic night cardioversion with and without sedation (ADSAS 2). Pacing Clin Electrophysiol 2004;27:910–7.

71. Burns JL, Serber ER, Keim S, Sears SF. Measuring patient acceptance of implantable cardiac device therapy: initial psychometric investigation of the Florida Patient Acceptance Survey. J Cardiovasc Electrophysiol 2005;16:384–90.

72. Newman DM, Dorian P, Paquette M, et al., for the Worldwide Jewel AF-Only Investigators. Effect of an implantable cardioverter defibrillator with atrial detection and shock therapies on patient-perceived, health-related quality of life. Am Heart J 2003;145; 841–6.

73. Schwartzman D, Musley SK, Swerdlow C, et al. Early recurrence of atrial fibrillation after ambulatory shock conversion. J Am Coll Cardiol 2002;40:93–9.
74. Spurrell P, Mitchell A, Kamalvand K, et al. Does sinus rhythm beget sinus rhythm? Long-term follow-up of the patient activated atrial defibrillator. Pacing Clin Electrophysiol 2004;27:175–81.
75. Schwartzman D, Gold M, Quesada A, et al., for the Worldwide Jewel AF-Only Investigators. Serial evaluation of atrial tachyarrhythmia burden and frequency after implantation of a dual-chamber cardioverter-defibrillator. J Cardiovasc Electrophysiol 2005;16: 708–13.
76. Funck RC, Boriani G, Manolis AS, Püererfellner H, Mont L, Tukkie R, Pisapia A, Israel CW, Grovale N, Grammatico A, Padeletti L; MINERVA Study Group. The MINERVA study design and rationale: a controlled randomized trial to assess the clinical benefit of minimizing ventricular pacing in pacemaker patients with atrial tachyarrhythmias. Am Heart J 2008 Sep 1;156(3):445–51.

9 Atrial Fibrillation Ablation

John V. Wylie, MD and Mark E. Josephson, MD

CONTENTS

Abstract

Due to the toxicities and limited efficacy of medical therapy, nonpharmaco-logic strategies for the management of atrial fibrillation in patients with heart failure are often employed. This chapter describes the techniques, clinical indications, and the devices utilized to perform catheter-based ablation of atrial fibrillation, including pulmonary vein isolation and left atrial substrate ablation.

Key Words: Atrial fibrillation; Heart failure; Ablation; Pulmonary veins.

1. ATRIAL FIBRILLATION – PREVALENCE AND MORBIDITY

Atrial fibrillation (AF) is the most common cardiac rhythm disorder, affecting nearly 1% of the general population *(1)*. The prevalence of AF in patients with heart failure (HF) is much higher, with reported rates of 4–50% in clinical heart failure trials *(2–7)*. Worsening heart failure promotes AF, and AF often exacerbates HF, leading to significant morbidity and mortality.

The prevalence of AF increases in proportion to the severity of HF *(8)*. An analysis of 4228 patients with New York Heart Association (NYHA) functional class I and II and left ventricular ejection fraction (LVEF) $\leq 35\%$ enrolled in the Studies of Left Ventricular Dysfunction (SOLVD) Prevention

From: *Contemporary Cardiology: Device Therapy in Heart Failure*
Edited by: W.H. Maisel, DOI 10.1007/978-1-59745-424-7_9
© Humana Press, a part of Springer Science+Business Media, LLC 2010

trial demonstrated a 4% prevalence of atrial fibrillation *(3)*. In the treatment arm of the trial, which enrolled patients with more symptomatic heart failure, the prevalence of atrial fibrillation was 10%. The MERIT-HF trial enrolled patients with primarily NYHA class II and III heart failure, representing an intermediate disease severity, and reported a prevalence of atrial fibrillation of 17% *(2, 9)*. Two studies of patients with more severe heart failure, the ADHERE database and the CONSENSUS trial, which enrolled patients with decompensated and advanced heart failure, reported a prevalence of atrial fibrillation of 31 and 49.8%, respectively *(6, 7)*.

In patients with HF, atrial fibrillation appears to be an independent risk factor for morbidity and mortality *(10)*. In the Candesartan in Heart Failure–Assessment of Reduction in Mortality and Morbidity (CHARM) study, which enrolled 7599 patients with heart failure and a range of ejection fractions, atrial fibrillation was an independent predictor of mortality in patients with a reduced ejection fraction and in patients with heart failure and preserved systolic function *(4)*. A subgroup analysis of the SOLVD study also demonstrated an independent association of atrial fibrillation with mortality *(5)*. Analysis of the original Framingham Study cohort of 5209 subjects revealed that the lifetime incidence of AF was over 10% and was independently associated with mortality *(11)*.

2. TREATMENT OPTIONS

2.1. Pharmacologic Therapy

Given the high prevalence of AF and its significant contribution to morbidity and mortality in patients with heart failure, investigators have recently focused on comparison of treatment strategies. Two large trials, the Atrial Fibrillation Follow-up Investigation of Rhythm Management (AFFIRM) and the Rate Control versus Electrical Cardioversion (RACE) trials, compared a "rate control" strategy for management of AF with a "rhythm control" strategy, in which patients were prescribed antiarrhythmic medications and elective cardioversion as needed *(12, 13)*. Neither trial showed any significant benefit from rhythm control in the management of AF. However, both trials enrolled older patients with asymptomatic or minimally symptomatic AF, limiting their generalizability to symptomatic patients *(14)*.

The Atrial Fibrillation in Congestive Heart Failure (AF-CHF) trial compared rate control versus rhythm control strategies in patients with AF, symptomatic HF, and an LVEF of 35% or less. It also showed no significant clinical benefit to the maintenance of sinus rhythm over rate control *(15)*.

For patients with symptomatic atrial fibrillation, a rate control strategy often does not relieve symptoms, and therapies to restore sinus rhythm are indicated. Antiarrhythmic medications and direct current cardioversion are generally considered first-line therapy for restoration and maintenance of sinus rhythm in patients with symptomatic atrial fibrillation *(16)*.

Antiarrhythmic medications for maintenance of sinus rhythm must be used with caution in patients with heart failure, and the choice of medications with an adequate safety profile is limited. Current guidelines recommend using only dofetilide or amiodarone for maintenance of sinus rhythm in patients with heart failure, based on their established safety in clinical trials (17–19). Unfortunately, these medications are limited by significant potential toxicities and a relatively low efficacy for maintaining sinus rhythm, with success rates of approximately 50–60% (18, 20).

2.2. Nonpharmacologic Therapy

Due to the toxicities and limited efficacy of medical therapy, nonpharmacologic strategies for the management of AF in patients with heart failure are often employed. For patients with highly symptomatic AF with a poorly controlled rapid ventricular rate, atrioventricular nodal ablation may be an option. This procedure involves catheter ablation of the atrioventricular conduction system and obligate implantation of a pacemaker. In selected patients, this therapy is highly effective and may improve quality of life (21). Patients with atrial fibrillation and heart failure undergoing atrioventricular junction ablation and pacemaker implantation may benefit more from biventricular or left ventricular pacing than right ventricular pacing alone (22).

3. CATHETER ABLATION OF ATRIAL FIBRILLATION

The observation by Haissaguerre et al. that focal triggers originating in the pulmonary veins may initiate atrial fibrillation led to a new catheter-based approach to the treatment of AF (23). Early procedures employing focused catheter ablation of ectopic foci found in pulmonary veins had limited success. More extensive ablation in the pulmonary veins was complicated by pulmonary vein stenosis due to scarring of the proximal veins (24). This led to the development of techniques employing wider ablations at the ostia of the pulmonary veins and in the left atrial wall. Recently, the technique of catheter ablation of AF has become more standardized, and two general strategies have become widely accepted.

The first strategy, segmental pulmonary vein isolation (PVI), is based on the principle that pulmonary vein triggers initiate AF in the left atrium. Ablation is performed around the ostium of each pulmonary vein with the goal of achieving conduction block at the left atrium–pulmonary vein border, thus electrically isolating each vein and preventing pulmonary vein triggers from reaching the left atrium to initiate and perpetuate AF (25, 26). This procedure requires that at least two catheters be placed in the left atrium via transseptal access to allow for electrical mapping and ablation around the pulmonary vein ostia.

The second strategy, circumferential left atrial catheter ablation (LACA) or substrate-based ablation, involves the creation of empiric anatomic ablation lines around the pulmonary veins (27). Conduction block is not usually assessed, and longer ablation times and larger lesions are often employed in this technique *(28)*. This procedure generally employs only a single transseptal catheter in the left atrium used for electroanatomic mapping and ablation.

No clear consensus exists as to which of these approaches are superior, and each has certain advantages. Reported success rates in the literature for each approach are similar, and the two published studies directly comparing them produced conflicting results *(26, 28)*. The larger of these two studies reported a significantly higher success rate with PVI compared with LACA (66% vs. 42%) during 6-month follow-up with 7-day Holter monitoring *(28)*.

Several variations on these two strategies have been developed and are gaining wider acceptance. It has been postulated that nonpulmonary venous structures entering the atria are alternative triggers of atrial fibrillation, and ablation of regions around the SVC, the ligament of Marshall, and the coronary sinus is performed by many operators as adjunctive therapy to PVI *(29)*. Enhancement of the LACA procedure has involved both targeting of fractionated electrograms in the posterior left atrium and ablation of vagal ganglia adjacent to the pulmonary veins, which are also hypothesized to facilitate initiation and maintenance of AF *(30, 31)*.

Due to the invasive nature of catheter ablation of AF, in most cases it is considered a second-line therapy for patients who do not respond to medical therapy with antiarrhythmic drugs *(16, 32, 33)*. Given the low efficacy of medications and the high success rates of catheter ablation published by many centers, this procedure is occasionally considered first-line therapy for patients who do not wish to take antiarrhythmic medications. However, randomized trials comparing antiarrhythmic medications with catheter ablation have shown catheter ablation to be significantly superior despite significant crossover in the studies *(34–36)*.

AF ablation has been rapidly growing in popularity, with the number of procedures increasing more than 100-fold since the mid-1990s *(36)*. Published success rates vary widely, ranging from 42 to 88% for patients with paroxysmal AF in studies with adequate follow-up available *(28, 35–37)*. Success rates for patients with persistent AF are much lower, reported at approximately 50% in most studies. Variation in success rates is partially due to procedural differences at different centers but seems primarily to relate to the intensity of follow-up and electrocardiographic monitoring. In addition, limited long-term follow-up is available at this time. Reported complication rates for catheter ablation of AF are 6% in the worldwide survey, with tamponade, pulmonary vein stenosis, stroke, and access site complications being the most common adverse outcomes *(36)*.

The efficacy of AF ablation in HF patients with depressed ejection fraction has been evaluated *(38)*. Patients with an ejection fraction less than 45% and NYHA class II or higher HF undergoing AF ablation were compared with a matched control group of patients with normal left ventricular function undergoing AF ablation. The reported success rate for patients with HF after 1 year was 69%, which was not significantly different than the success rate of 71% in the control group. In addition, left ventricular function, exercise capacity, and functional class all improved significantly after AF ablation in the patients with HF compared with baseline.

A randomized trial comparing pulmonary vein isolation (PVI) with atrioventricular node ablation and biventricular pacing in patients with symptomatic, drug-resistant AF, an LVEF ≤40%, and NYHA class II or III HF demonstrated improved quality of life, 6-min walk distance, and ejection fraction in the PVI group. In all, 88% of PVI patients receiving antiarrhythmic drugs and 71% of those not receiving drugs were free of AF at 6 months *(39)*.

These dramatic results have led to the use of AF ablation in selected patients with HF and structural heart disease.

3.1. Clinical Guidelines for Atrial Fibrillation Ablation

The Heart Rhythm Society (HRS), European Heart Rhythm Association (EHRA), and the European Cardiac Arrhythmia Society (ECAS) published a consensus statement pertaining to catheter and surgical ablation of atrial fibrillation *(32, 33)*. The consensus recommendations are presented in Table 1.

Table 1
HRS/EHRA/ECAS consensus recommendations for catheter ablation of atrial fibrillation (AF)

Recommendations
Catheter ablation of AF, in general, should not be considered first-line therapy
The primary indication for catheter AF ablation is the presence of symptomatic AF refractory intolerant to at least one Class I or III antiarrhythmic medication
In rare clinical situations, it may be appropriate to perform catheter ablation of AF as first-line therapy
Catheter ablation of AF is appropriate in selected symptomatic patients with HF and/or reduced ejection fraction
The presence of LA thrombus is a contraindication to catheter ablation

AF, atrial fibrillation; HF, heart failure; LA, left atrial.

3.2. Devices Used for Catheter Ablation of AF

As described above, there are several strategies for catheter ablation of AF, but all have several common elements and use similar cardiovascular devices. Transseptal puncture is required for left atrial access in all techniques, and intracardiac ultrasound is often used to guide the puncture procedure as well as to visualize the pulmonary veins. Both the PVI and the LACA method generally use fluoroscopic and three-dimensional electroanatomic mapping techniques. Radiofrequency ablation via a steerable catheter is used to create left atrial lesions, though several other new technologies using alternative energy sources are under investigation. A review of selected devices used for this procedure is provided below.

3.2.1. INTRACARDIAC ECHOCARDIOGRAPHY

Intracardiac echocardiography (ICE) is used in the AF ablation procedure to visualize the interatrial septum and fossa ovalis to guide transseptal puncture as well as to visualize the left atrium and pulmonary veins during ablation. Transseptal puncture is traditionally guided by fluoroscopy, but anatomic variations, particularly atrial enlargement, which is common in patients with atrial fibrillation, can make the fluoroscopic landmarks less reliable. Potential complications of transseptal puncture include atrial perforation with subsequent pericardial effusion and aortic root puncture. Imaging the fossa ovalis during transseptal puncture provides real-time, precise anatomical guidance, thus improving the safety of this procedure *(40)* (Fig. 1).

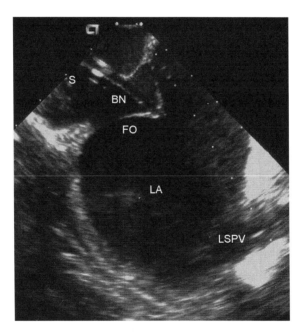

Fig. 1. Phased-array intracardiac echo image of Brockenbrough transseptal needle "tenting" the fossa ovalis during transseptal puncture procedure. BN, Brockenbrough needle; FO, fossa ovalis; LA, left atrium; LSPV, left superior pulmonary vein; S, sheath.

Two types of ICEs are available for use with invasive electrophysiologic procedures (Table 2). The first, mechanical ICE, uses a rapidly rotating transducer (up to 1800 rpm) which provides a 360° image perpendicular to the

Table 2
Selected intracardiac echocardiography catheters

Type	Transducer	Frequency (MHz)	Tissue penetration	Doppler	Uses
Mechanical	Ultra-ICE (Boston Scientific, Natick, MA, USA)	9–12	5–8 cm radius	No	Transseptal puncture Pulmonary vein isolation (when placed in LA) Sinus node modification
Phased-array	Acunav (Acuson Corp., Mountain View, CA, USA)	5–10	12–15 cm	Pulsed wave Continuous wave Color flow Tissue Doppler	Transseptal puncture Pulmonary vein isolation (placed in RA) Sinus node modification

axis of the catheter. Imaging frequencies used in these catheters vary from 9 to 12 MHz, which provide good resolution of objects close to the transducer but have limited tissue penetration (41). These catheters are generally non-steerable.

The second type of transducer available is phased-array ICE. This catheter employs a 64-element ultrasound transducer mounted at the end of an 8F or 10F catheter using imaging frequencies of 5–10 MHz. This catheter is steerable in two planes, which allows for more focused imaging of intracardiac structures. The tissue penetration is significantly deeper than that with mechanical ICE, with good visualization of structures 12–15 cm from the transducer (42, 43). In addition, this transducer has the capacity for full Doppler imaging, including pulsed-wave, continuous-wave, color Doppler flow, and tissue Doppler imaging. The greater versatility of this catheter has made it more popular for use during AF ablations, and it is compatible with many standard echocardiography workstations. Both types of transducers are advanced to the heart via venous sheaths.

Mechanical ICE is primarily used to guide transseptal puncture, as its limited tissue penetration does not allow adequate visualization of the left atrium from the right atrium. However, some operators advance the mechanical ICE catheter into the left atrium via a transseptal sheath and directly visualize the pulmonary veins from the left atrium (44). This technique allows for close monitoring of ablation catheter position and stability during radiofrequency ablation.

Phased-array transducers are more widely used in AF ablation procedures due to their greater tissue penetration, steerability, and ability to perform Doppler imaging *(45)*. Visualization of the pulmonary vein ostia and measurement of pulmonary vein inflow velocity before and after ablation are possible using pulsed-wave Doppler with this catheter. Though pulmonary vein stenosis can be identified by ICE, one study has suggested that increased velocity after ablation represents acute inflammation and may not be correlated with chronic stenosis *(46)*.

Phased-array transducers are able to image accurately complex pulmonary vein anatomy, which has significant variability in the population *(47)*. The ICE is also able to monitor lasso catheter position at each pulmonary vein ostium during the procedure, which is required for effective pulmonary vein isolation. In addition, ablation catheter position and stability can be monitored in real time during ablation. Catheter tissue heating can also be monitored through observation of bubble formation from the site of ablation. Formation of dense bubbles, or "Type II" bubbles, heralds high tissue temperatures and impedance rise and necessitates termination of ablation to avoid myocardial damage *(48)*.

3.2.2. BROCKENBROUGH TRANSSEPTAL PUNCTURE NEEDLE

After the introduction of standard pacing and recording catheters into the right atrium, the next step in an atrial fibrillation ablation procedure is transseptal puncture. Due to the difficulty and risks of left atrial mapping via the retrograde arterial approach, transseptal access from the right atrium is the standard method for mapping and ablation in the left atrium. Long guiding sheaths with a distal curve (or steerable tip) are advanced to the right atrium, and a Brockenbrough needle (multiple manufacturers) is used to puncture the interatrial septum *(49)*. The standard needle is 71 cm, but two different curvatures (BRK and BRK-1) and several lengths are available to accommodate different right atrial anatomies and different transseptal sheath lengths.

As noted above, intracardiac echocardiography (ICE) is often used to guide this procedure. ICE effectively visualizes the fossa ovalis and allows the operator to see the needle "tenting" this structure before puncture (Fig. 1). Other methods of guidance used are fluoroscopic imaging and contrast dye injection to confirm that the catheter is appropriately positioned. The transseptal sheath is then passed over the needle into the left atrium and the needle is withdrawn from the body.

3.2.3. TRANSSEPTAL SHEATHS

As described above, a guiding sheath introduced into the femoral vein is advanced over the Brockenbrough needle across the interatrial septum in order to gain left atrial access. The sheath is used to guide catheter placement in the left atrium and to provide stable access to the left atrium. A variety of transseptal sheaths are available on the market (see Table 3). Standard Mullins sheaths were initially developed for this purpose *(50)*. Newer sheaths have deflectable tips that are primarily intended for facilitating

Table 3
Selected transseptal sheaths

Sheath	Manufacturer	Curves available	Comments
Mullins	Bard EP, Lowell, MA, USA and Medtronic, Inc., Minneapolis, MN, USA	Standard Mullins curve	8 French, 60 cm sheath with 67 cm dilator is the standard transseptal sheath.
Fast-Cath/Swartz	St. Jude Medical, Minnetonka, MN, USA	SR0, SR1, SR2, SR3, SL0, SL1, SL2, SL3, and 6-cm diameter curve	8 French and 8.5 French sheaths available, SR sheaths have posterior curve which may facilitate access to pulmonary veins
Preface	Biosense Webster, Diamond Bar, CA, USA	Multipurpose, anterior, posterior	8 French. Posterior multipurpose curve may facilitate access to pulmonary veins
Convoy	Boston Scientific, San Jose, CA, USA	15–120° curves	8.5 French diameter with five different curves
TeleSheath	St. Jude Medical, Minnetonka, MN, USA	Compound curve, braided inner sheath	Telescoping sheath design – sheath within sheath allows increased range of motion. External diameter is 11 French
Agilis NXT	St. Jude Medical, Minnetonka, MN, USA	Deflectable	Deflectable sheath facilitates access to right pulmonary veins. Outer diameter is 11.5 French. Requires a 98-cm Brockenbrough needle
Channel	Bard EP, Lowell, MA, USA	Deflectable	Deflectable sheath facilitates access to right pulmonary veins. Outer diameter is 11.4 French, inner diameter 8.3 French. Requires an 89 cm Brockenbrough needle

manipulation of the ablation catheter in the left atrium during pulmonary vein isolation. The angle from the point of transseptal puncture to the right pulmonary veins can be quite acute, and deflectable sheaths are used in order to direct the ablation catheter these locations. Disadvantages of these newer sheaths include a larger outer diameter, which increases bleeding risk, and increased cost. Other fixed curve sheaths have a secondary posterior curve, which may also facilitate access to the pulmonary veins.

3.2.4. NONFLUOROSCOPIC THREE-DIMENSIONAL MAPPING TECHNIQUES

Atrial fibrillation ablation procedures require extensive catheter manipulation in the left atrium to precise locations around the pulmonary veins. Atrial anatomy is often distorted by left atrial enlargement in patients with atrial fibrillation, and pulmonary venous anatomy can be quite variable among patients. These issues make precise catheter navigation to specific anatomical sites within the left atrium quite challenging. Standard biplane fluoroscopic views enable the operator to track catheter movement accurately but do not allow visualization of left atrial structures. Pulmonary venography may be performed with injection of radio-opaque contrast dye into each pulmonary vein via a luminal catheter. Biplane images of each venogram can then be stored as digital images for reference later in the procedure to assist in localizing each pulmonary vein for catheter ablation. Use of this method alone does not allow full visualization of left atrial anatomy, however, and is limited by the potential for contrast nephropathy and the requirement for prolonged fluoroscopy times with this technique. As noted above, intracardiac echocardiography can be a useful adjunctive imaging modality which can visualize left atrial structures and be used to assist in catheter manipulation. While this is used by some operators as the only additional imaging tool beyond fluoroscopy, most employ one of several available nonfluoroscopic mapping systems (Table 4).

Three-dimensional mapping of the left atrium is a nonfluoroscopic technique used to define left atrial anatomy and guide catheter manipulation. There are several different technologies which allow a three-dimensional "shell" of the left atrium to be created from points acquired by intracardiac catheters. As catheters are moved into the left atrium, a virtual image of the structure is created. As the pulmonary veins, the left atrial appendage, and the mitral annulus are mapped, a functional three-dimensional model of the left atrium is created, which can then be used to guide catheter manipulation in real time.

3.2.5. CARTO

The CARTO system (Biosense Webster, Diamond Bar, CA, USA) is a widely used electroanatomic mapping system based on the principles of interaction of a metal coil within an electromagnetic field. Three low-power magnetic fields are generated beneath the patient and are used to track the

Table 4
Electroanatomic mapping systems

System	Three-dimensional technique	Catheter	Comments
CARTO (Biosense Webster, Diamond Bar, CA, USA)	Electroanatomic mapping within a magnetic field	Proprietary catheter only	Creates a 3D model of the cardiac chamber Provides voltage and activation mapping Displays only the proprietary mapping/ablation catheter CARTOMERGE allows integration of MRI or CT data with 3D chamber model
EnSite NavX (St. Jude Medical, Minnetonka, MN, USA)	Electrical field impedance	Standard catheters (up to 64 electrodes)	Creates 3D model of the cardiac chamber Provides voltage and activation mapping Displays multiple standard catheters at once EnSite Verismo system able to display 3D model segmented from MRI or CT data side by side with electroanatomic map
LocaLisa (Medtronic, Inc., Minneapolis, MN, USA)	Electrical field voltage	Standard catheters (up to 10 electrodes)	Creates 3D model of the cardiac chamber Catheter navigation without the use of fluoroscopy Displays multiple standard catheters at once Does not provide voltage or activation mapping

movement of the tip of a proprietary catheter (Navistar) in three dimensions relative to a fixed reference sensor attached to the patient's back. The deflectable catheter is placed at known anatomic sites under fluoroscopic guidance, and using these reference points, additional endocardial surface points are collected. The system records the position, the electrogram voltage, and the timing of each acquired endocardial "point." As multiple points are acquired, a three-dimensional shell is constructed (Fig. 2). Catheter movement is tracked in real time in the computer model

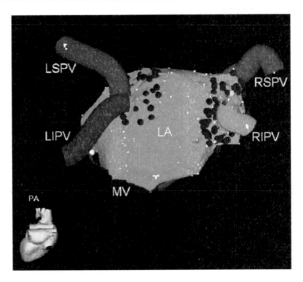

Fig. 2. Three-dimensional electroanatomic CARTO (Biosense Webster, Diamond Bar, CA, USA) image of the left atrium during pulmonary vein isolation. The shell is created by point-by-point mapping of endocardial sites in the left atrium. The colored tubes represent the pulmonary veins and the *red dots* mark points of radiofrequency ablation. LA, left atrium; LIPV, left inferior pulmonary vein; LSPV, left superior pulmonary vein; MV, mitral valve; RIPV, right inferior pulmonary vein; RSPV, right superior pulmonary vein.

generated, and this model can be used to guide catheter positioning for ablation, thus dramatically reducing the need for fluoroscopy in ablation procedures *(51)*.

Advantages of the CARTO system include its reported high spatial resolution of 0.7 mm *(52)*, its ability to display true measured electrograms from the endocardium, and the capacity to provide voltage and activation mapping in addition to anatomy. Due to the high spatial resolution and the ability to display voltage and activation timing simultaneously, this system is widely used for AF ablation procedures *(53)*. Recently, software has been developed which allows integration of the electroanatomic model with three-dimensional imaging data from computed tomography (CT) scans or cardiac magnetic resonance (CMR) imaging (CARTOMERGE, Biosense Webster, Diamond Bar, CA, USA and Siemens AG, Munich, Germany) *(54)*. Once fixed anatomic reference points (such as the aorta) are identified on electroanatomic mapping, these points can be registered with the three-dimensional CT or CMR images. Further electroanatomic mapping of the left atrium is then performed to calibrate the images further with the computer model, and a virtual "merged" image is created which may more accurately reflect an individual patient's anatomy to guide catheter manipulation more accurately (Fig. 3).

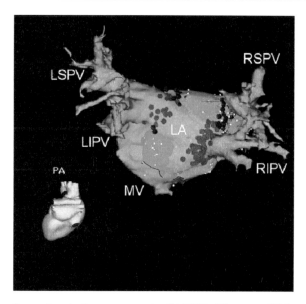

Fig. 3. Three-dimensional electroanatomic CARTO (Biosense Webster, Diamond Bar, CA, USA) image of the left atrium during pulmonary vein isolation with integration of a CT scan image of the left atrium using proprietary CARTOMERGE (Biosense Webster) software. This is the same patient as shown in Fig. 2. The *light green* surfaces are segmented images from a prior CT scan and the *darker green* surfaces are the endocardial shell created by 3D mapping. LA, left atrium; LIPV, left inferior pulmonary vein; LSPV, left superior pulmonary vein; MV, mitral valve; RIPV, right inferior pulmonary vein; RSPV, right superior pulmonary vein.

A disadvantage of the CARTO system is that it requires a proprietary catheter for use with the system. Other catheters are not compatible and the system records only data gathered from the mapping catheter. Because data are typically collected from only a single bipolar catheter, mapping of a structure such as the left atrium requires sequential point-to-point mapping, which often requires over 100 points to create an accurate electroanatomic map. This can add significant time to a procedure and makes accurate mapping dependent upon operator experience *(55)*.

3.2.6. ENSITE NAVX

Another three-dimensional mapping system is the EnSite NavX system (St. Jude Medical, Minnetonka, MN, USA). This system uses measured impedance from a 5.7-kHz electrical signal emitted from three surface electrodes to map intracardiac catheters in three dimensions. This system is able to map up to 64 electrodes at once and does not require the use of proprietary catheters. Data from each electrode in relation to a fixed reference electrode are measured and recorded on a computer model of the left

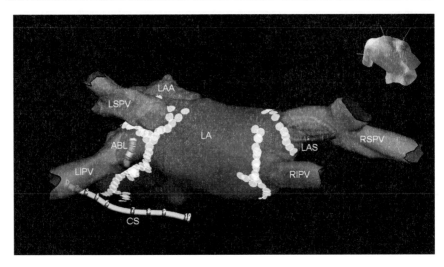

Fig. 4. Three-dimensional electroanatomic EnSite NavX (St. Jude Medical, Minnetonka, MN, USA) image of the left atrium during pulmonary vein isolation. In addition to the left atrial structures, the catheters used during the procedure can be seen in real time. The circumferential lasso catheter (LAS) is seen in the right superior pulmonary vein (RSPV), the coronary sinus (CS) catheter is shown in position along the mitral valve, and the ablation catheter (ABL) is shown below the left inferior pulmonary vein (LIPV). The *white dots* mark points of radiofrequency ablation. LA, left atrium; LAA, left atrial appendage; LSPV, left superior pulmonary vein; RIPV, right inferior pulmonary vein.

atrium. Catheter movement is visualized in real time and can be used to guide ablations around the pulmonary veins (Fig. 4).

One of the chief advantages of the NavX system is the ability to visualize multiple catheters in real time. For the pulmonary vein isolation technique, a multielectrode catheter placed in the os of a pulmonary vein can be visualized and used to guide the placement of the ablation catheter around the multielectrode catheter in the computer model. In addition, the system is able to monitor the movement of the multielectrode catheter and confirm stable position in the os of the pulmonary vein. Use of this system in AF ablation procedures has been studied and may reduce fluoroscopy exposure *(56)*. Three-dimensional data from CT and CMR imaging can also be used with this system. Though it does not register the images directly with electroanatomic mapping data, the three-dimensional image can be reconstructed and viewed side by side with the electroanatomic model to facilitate understanding of the anatomy.

The EnSite system can also be used with a multielectrode array probe for noncontact mapping. This is a "balloon" catheter with 64 electrodes that can be advanced through a guiding sheath and deployed in a cardiac chamber. After endocardial anatomy is defined by a conventional mapping catheter, the multielectrode array can be used to create an activation map of the entire chamber from a single cardiac cycle. Using the Laplace equation and a proprietary algorithm, endocardial activation is extrapolated and the electrical timing of any point in the atrium can be identified. While use of this multielectrode catheter can allow identification of left atrial triggers and left atrial tachycardia foci *(57)*, its large size and cost limits its use in atrial fibrillation ablation procedures, and it is not commonly used for this procedure.

A disadvantage of the NavX system is its lack of precision in localizing catheters in three dimensions. The reported accuracy is 4 ± 3.2 mm, which can be quite significant when attempting to create precise lesions around the pulmonary veins *(58)*. In addition, effective use of this system can be quite complex and often requires dedicated technical support.

3.2.7. LocaLisa

Another nonfluoroscopic three-dimensional mapping system is the LocaLisa system (Medtronic, Inc., Minneapolis, MN, USA). Like the EnSite NavX system, this system uses skin electrodes to apply a low-power current across the body in three orthogonal planes. Endocardial catheters receive this 30-kHz signal and by integrating the signal strength from each plane, relative endocardial catheter position in three dimensions is able to be determined. This system is able to localize catheters with an accuracy of less than 2 mm and provide real-time assessment of catheter position, which is stable over the course of a procedure *(59)*. This system can be used for AF ablation and has been shown to be able to provide accurate localization of circumferential mapping and ablation catheters in the left atrium, allowing shorter fluoroscopy exposure and shorter time to completion of ablation lesions *(60, 61)*.

Like the EnSite NavX system, a chief advantage of this system is the ability to use standard catheters and visualize multiple catheters in real time. The reported accuracy of catheter location is higher than that of the NavX system and nearly comparable to CARTO. The disadvantage of this system is that only navigational anatomic information is recorded. Electrogram voltage and activation is not recorded on the three-dimensional maps created in the LocaLisa system. In addition, this system is currently able to track only 10 electrodes simultaneously, somewhat lessening the advantages of tracking multiple electrodes in real time.

3.2.8. Remote Magnetic Catheter Navigation

A catheter navigation system (Niobe, Stereotaxis, St. Louis, MO, USA) which uses permanent magnets to guide a catheter remotely within the heart is approved. Two large magnets controlled by a computer system are adjusted to vary the orientation of a 0.08-T magnetic field centered on the patient's chest. A soft flexible catheter with a magnetic tip can then be steered remotely by adjusting the orientation of the magnetic field. The catheter is advanced and retracted by means of a small motor drive unit (Cardiodrive, Sterotaxis, St. Louis, MO, USA) attached just proximal to the point of entry into the introducer sheath. Using a single-plane fluoroscopic unit, the entire system can be remotely controlled by the operator. The system allows storage of navigation points, allowing the operator to return to previously marked endocardial positions with a reported accuracy of less than 1 mm *(62–64)*. It has been shown to be an effective device for guiding ablation of supraventricular tachycardias and in AF ablations *(65–67)*.

There are several advantages to this system. The ability to navigate remotely and return to stored positions reduces fluoroscopic exposure for both the operator and the patient. Magnetic navigation with a flexible catheter provides more accurate and stable catheter positioning and may allow more effective ablation lesions due to the improved contact *(65)*. Experimental studies in animals suggest that magnetic navigation is safe, as attempts to navigate the catheter outside the right atrium were unable to cause cardiac damage or perforation in one report *(64)*. After an early learning curve, the system has been shown to decrease ablation times for AF ablation procedures *(67)*. The complex anatomy of the left atrium and prolonged fluoroscopy times usually required for this procedure make this tool quite promising for use in AF ablations. Disadvantages of the system are primarily cost and the large space required for the unit. A proprietary catheter is required and is available only in limited sizes. In addition, the current design allows for only single-plane fluoroscopy with limitations on camera movement of less than 30° in the left and right anterior oblique angulations.

The remote Robotic Navigation System (Hansen Medical, Inc., Mountain View, CA) offers similar potential benefits and risks. A mapping/ablation catheter is placed within a two-sheath robotic system, and a software interface allows the operator to remotely navigate the catheter with precision. The internal sheath contains four pull wires located at each quadrant; the range of motion includes deflection in 360° and provides the ability to insert/withdraw the sheath. The external sheath contains a single pull wire to permit deflection and to provide the ability to rotate and insert/withdraw. These movements allow a broad range of motion in virtually any direction. This steerable sheath system can be used in the same way as conventional sheaths with different mapping/ablation catheters inserted through the guide lumen. The sheath system is attached to the remote robotic arm unit that can be fixed to the foot of a standard X-ray procedure table. A joystick allows the operator to remotely drive the catheter tip using a software interface. This interface translates movements of the joystick into the complex series of manipulation by the pull wires governing sheath motion. The operator can decide whether to individually manipulate the internal or the external sheath *(68)*. Clinical feasibility studies have demonstrated the potential for this system to serve as an adjunct to pulmonary vein isolation procedures *(69)*.

3.2.9. Multielectrode Catheters for Electrical Mapping of the Pulmonary Veins

The pulmonary vein isolation technique for ablation of atrial fibrillation requires the recording of electrical signals within the pulmonary veins simultaneously with recording of left atrial signals. A variety of catheters have been designed to map the electrical signals at the pulmonary vein ostium in order to guide this process (Table 5). A standard circular "lasso" catheter has 10–20 electrodes with a fixed or variable diameter. This catheter is placed

Table 5
Selected multielectrode mapping catheters

Catheter	Shape	Electrodes	Comments
Lasso (Biosense Webster, Diamond Bar, CA, USA)	Circular "lasso" with fixed and adjustable loops	10 or 20	Fixed diameters of 12–30 mm as well as variable loop which adjusts from 15 to 25 mm are available. When placed at the pulmonary vein ostium, it can be used to determine pulmonary vein–atrium conduction
Orbiter PV (Bard EP, Lowell, MA, USA)	Circular "lasso" with adjustable loop	14	Loop diameter adjusts from 14.5 to 25 mm. When placed at the pulmonary vein ostium, it can be used to determine pulmonary vein–atrium conduction
Spiral HP (St. Jude Medical, Minnetonka, MN, USA)	Circular "lasso" with fixed loop diameters	20	Fixed diameters of 15–24 mm available. When placed at the pulmonary vein ostium, it can be used to determine pulmonary vein–atrium conduction
HD Mesh (Bard EP, Lowell, MA, USA)	Mesh "basket" catheter with variable diameter	32	May be inserted in pulmonary vein ostium to identify pulmonary vein potentials and determine pulmonary vein–atrium conduction
Constellation (Boston Scientific, San Jose, CA, USA)	Mesh "basket" with fixed basket diameter of 31–75 mm available	64	May be inserted in pulmonary vein ostium to identify pulmonary vein potentials and determine pulmonary vein–atrium conduction. Compatible with Boston Scientific Astronomer system to localize ablation catheter relative to basket catheter electrodes

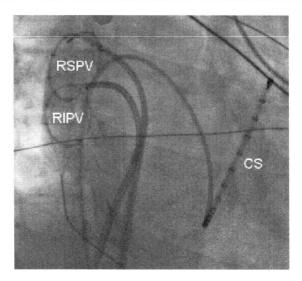

Fig. 5. Fluoroscopic image of two circumferential "lasso" catheters placed in the right superior pulmonary vein (RSPV) and right inferior pulmonary vein (RIPV) during pulmonary vein isolation using the "double lasso" technique. The decapolar catheter placed in the coronary sinus (CS) is also seen.

at the ostium of the pulmonary vein where both left atrial and pulmonary vein signals are recorded. Ablation is then performed in the ostium on the left atrial side of the lasso catheter until pulmonary vein potentials are no longer seen on the catheter (Fig. 5). Pulmonary vein exit block can then be judged by pacing the electrodes of the lasso catheter to confirm pulmonary vein–left atrium electrical disconnection *(37)*. Some operators use a "double lasso" technique, in which three transseptal sheaths are placed and two lasso catheters are placed in ipsilateral pulmonary veins to provide more accurate fluoroscopic guidance of ablation around the veins (Fig. 4).

Several multielectrode "basket" catheters are available, which provide the ability to record pulmonary vein and left atrial signals simultaneously (Table 5). These catheters are passed through an introducer sheath in a retracted profile and then expanded in the left atrium. They can be guided into the ostium of each pulmonary vein to guide ablation similar to the lasso catheter method described above. These catheters provide the added advantages of increased stability in the pulmonary vein ostium and simultaneous recording on either side of the ablation lines in the pulmonary vein isolation technique *(70)*. The Astronomer system (Boston Scientific, San Jose, CA, USA) is a limited three-dimensional mapping system that uses AC current to locate the ablation catheter relative to specific poles on a 64-electrode basket catheter, allowing more precise guidance of circumferential ablations to specific basket electrode poles *(70)*. This system can be used to guide both the pulmonary vein isolation technique and the left atrial circumferential ablation technique *(71)*. Disadvantages of basket catheters include their cost and decreased maneuverability, which can make positioning in the pulmonary vein ostia (particularly in lower pulmonary vein ostia) technically challenging.

3.2.10. ABLATION CATHETERS

Atrial fibrillation ablation procedures require ablation catheters which combine maneuverability and the capacity to create effective lesions in the left atrium. Radiofrequency (RF) energy is most commonly used for ablation, and there are a variety of catheters designed to deliver RF ablations to the endocardium (Table 6). RF ablation involves the application of alternating electrical current to the myocardium, which results in tissue heating and subsequent tissue destruction when adequate temperatures are reached. A small area of tissue adjacent to the catheter tip is heated by resistive heating, and deeper tissues are heated by conductive heating. Increasing power results in deeper lesions and higher surface temperatures. One of the limitations of RF ablation is that high tissue temperatures may be reached adjacent to the catheter, resulting in char formation on the catheter and sudden tissue heating to boiling at 100°C, which may lead to myocardial perforation. During RF ablation, catheter tip temperature is monitored, but studies have shown that the catheter tip–tissue interface temperature underestimates peak tissue temperature due to cooling of the catheter tip by blood flow. Therefore, additional variables such as impedance and electrogram morphology are monitored during ablation to assess effective tissue destruction. Standard catheter tip sizes used for ablation of AF are 4 and 8 mm. A larger tip size distributes RF energy to a larger area of myocardium and produces larger lesions with each ablation *(72)*. Due to the extensive ablations required for both the pulmonary vein isolation method and the left atrial circumferential ablation method, an 8-mm catheter may be most effective *(73)*.

Recently, the limitation of high surface temperatures at the catheter–myocardium interface has been addressed by saline-irrigated catheter systems. These catheters allow saline to be pumped via a lumen to cool the catheter tip during ablation. Externally irrigated systems pump saline out of small holes in the catheter tip, while internally irrigated systems cool the catheter tip from the internal lumen and allow saline to flow out of a separate lumen. Cooling the catheter tip reduces char formation and catheter–myocardial interface temperatures, allowing more uniform tissue heating and significantly deeper ablation lesions *(74)*. Small studies have suggested that while lesion size is comparable between internally and externally irrigated systems, char and thrombus formation is more common with internally irrigated systems *(75)*. These systems have recently been used safely in ablation of atrial fibrillation *(76, 77)*. A potential disadvantage of irrigated ablation catheters is the potential to form large lesions quickly, which may lead to significant tissue damage. Careful monitoring of impedance and the

Table 6
Selected ablation catheters

Catheter	Ablation method	Catheter tip	Comments
Celsius (Biosense Webster, Diamond Bar, CA, USA)	Radiofrequency	4-, 5-, and 8-mm tips	8 mm most commonly used for AF ablation; Bidirectional curve available only for 4- and 5-mm tips; Nonmapping catheter
Stinger (Bard EP, Lowell, MA, USA)	Radiofrequency	4-, 5-, and 8-mm tips	8 mm most commonly used for AF ablation; Bidirectional curve
Blazer II (Boston Scientific, San Jose, CA, USA)	Radiofrequency	4-, 5-, and 8-mm tips	8-mm standard curve most commonly used for AF ablation; Bidirectional curve
Livewire TC (St. Jude Medical, Minnetonka, MN, USA)	Radiofrequency	4- and 8-mm tips	8 mm most commonly used for AF ablation; Bidirectional curve
Safire (St. Jude Medical, Minnetonka, MN, USA)	Radiofrequency	4- and 8-mm tips	8 mm most commonly used for AF ablation; Bidirectional curve; Autolocking steering mechanism
Navistar (Biosense Webster, Diamond Bar, CA, USA)	Radiofrequency	4- and 8-mm tips	Required for use with CARTO system; 8 mm most commonly used for AF ablation; Unidirectional curve
Navistar Thermocool (Biosense Webster, Diamond Bar, CA, USA)	Externally irrigated radiofrequency	3.5-mm tip	External saline irrigation increases lesion size; Compatible with the CARTO system; Also available as nonmapping Celsius Thermocool; Saline irrigation at 2 cm^3/min during mapping and 17 cm^3/min during ablation (and to 30 cm^3/min when ablation power increased to 31–50 W)

Device (Manufacturer)	Technology	Tip/Size	Comments
Chilli II (Boston Scientific, San Jose, CA, USA)	Closed irrigation radiofrequency	4 mm	Increased depth of lesion using irrigated tip Closed system does not require excess saline administration to patient
Freezor (CryoCath Technologies, Montreal, Quebec, Canada)	Cryoablation	4-, 6-, 8-mm tips	Reduced risk of pulmonary vein stenosis Longer procedure times
Cryoblator (Cryocor, San Diego, CA USA)	Cryoablation	6.5-mm tip	Reduced risk of pulmonary vein stenosis Longer procedure times
Arctic Front (CryoCath Technologies, Montreal, Quebec, Canada)	Cryoablation	23- and 28-mm-diameter balloons	Balloon placed in the PV ostium allows cryoablation at the PV–left atrium interface Not approved in the United States, only available in Europe

effect on local electrograms is essential to avoid complications. In addition, externally irrigated catheters require a saline flow rate of 17–30 cm^3/min, which may represent a significant volume load to patients with HF during a prolonged AF ablation. These patients must be carefully monitored and administered parenteral diuretics during the procedure as needed.

Alternative ablation technologies for use in AF ablations were used in 14% of procedures in a one worldwide survey of AF ablation *(36)*. Cryoablation is an established technology for endocardial ablation that allows the creation of reversible and irreversible lesions using a catheter system that circulates liquid nitrous oxide to the catheter tip. Evaporative cooling allows the tip to be cooled to –30°C for the creation of temporary lesions and to –75°C in order to produce a permanent lesion. Atrial fibrillation ablation can be performed with a standard tip cryoablation catheter (Freezor, Cryocath Technologies, Montreal, Quebec, Canada and CryoBlator, CryocCor, San Diego, CA, USA), which has shown reasonable success rates but longer procedure times in published studies *(78)*. A circular expandable catheter (CryoCath Arctic Circler) designed to be placed at the pulmonary vein ostium has shown promise in investigative reports *(79, 80)*. A similar catheter (CryoCath Arctic Front balloon) designed specifically for pulmonary vein isolation employs a balloon which is placed in the pulmonary vein ostium and then cooled to create a circumferential lesion. This system has been shown to produce transmural freezing in animal studies and is currently marketed in Europe *(81)*. Potential advantages of these systems are increased efficiency of pulmonary vein isolation and decreased incidence of pulmonary vein stenosis. The need for dedicated equipment and the difficulty in achieving transmural lesions with cryoablation are potential disadvantages, however.

Another ablation technology which has undergone significant study for the ablation of AF is focused ultrasound. Ultrasound energy directed from the catheter tip can cause effective tissue destruction with a specified depth of penetration. Focused ultrasound balloon catheters are currently being developed for use in AF ablation. In early animal studies, this design was able to cause effective lesions at the PV–atrial junction *(82)*. In published human studies of this device, pulmonary vein isolation was able to be achieved, but the recurrence rate of AF was 61% and there were several severe complications such as stroke and pulmonary vein stenosis among the small study group *(83)*. Another balloon catheter currently undergoing clinical trial [ProRhythm, Inc., Ronkonkoma, NY (formerly Transurgical, Inc.)] emits a high-intensity focused ultrasound, directed toward the left atrium outside the PV in an attempt to minimize PV stenosis. Early animal studies of this catheter demonstrated the ability to create circumferential ablations within the left atrium outside the PV ostium, often with a single ablation *(84)*. Other ablation technologies, including the use of laser and microwave technology, are currently under investigation but are not approved for use in atrial fibrillation ablation and are therefore not in general use.

4. CONCLUSION

Atrial fibrillation is highly prevalent in patients with HF, and catheter ablation of AF has been rapidly growing in popularity. The procedure is technically complex and requires a variety of cardiovascular devices for successful completion. The different ablation strategies in common use and the wide variety of devices available for mapping and ablation make the exact performance of this procedure unique in each electrophysiology laboratory. It is an area of intensive research, and there has been rapid development of new devices for both mapping and ablation. The procedural success rates are moderate. Hopefully, as ablation tools and methodologies continue to evolve, the procedure will become even safer and more effective.

REFERENCES

1. Go AS, Hylek EM, Phillips KA, et al. Prevalence of diagnosed atrial fibrillation in adults: national implications for rhythm management and stroke prevention: the AnTicoagulation and Risk Factors in Atrial Fibrillation (ATRIA) Study. JAMA 2001;285: 2370–5.
2. Effect of metoprolol CR/XL in chronic heart failure: Metoprolol CR/XL Randomised Intervention Trial in Congestive Heart Failure (MERIT-HF). Lancet 1999;353: 2001–7.
3. The SOLVD Investigators. Effect of enalapril on mortality and the development of heart failure in asymptomatic patients with reduced left ventricular ejection fractions. N Engl J Med 1992;327:685–91.
4. Olsson LG, Swedberg K, Ducharme A, et al. Atrial fibrillation and risk of clinical events in chronic heart failure with and without left ventricular systolic dysfunction: results from the Candesartan in Heart failure-Assessment of Reduction in Mortality and morbidity (CHARM) program. J Am Coll Cardiol 2006;47:1997–2004.
5. Dries DL, Exner DV, Gersh BJ, Domanski MJ, Waclawiw MA, Stevenson LW. Atrial fibrillation is associated with an increased risk for mortality and heart failure progression in patients with asymptomatic and symptomatic left ventricular systolic dysfunction: a retrospective analysis of the SOLVD trials. Studies of Left Ventricular Dysfunction. J Am Coll Cardiol 1998;32:695–703.
6. Fonarow GC, Adams KF, Jr., Abraham WT, Yancy CW, Boscardin WJ. Risk stratification for in-hospital mortality in acutely decompensated heart failure: classification and regression tree analysis. JAMA 2005;293:572–80.
7. The CONSENSUS Trial Study Group. Effects of enalapril on mortality in severe congestive heart failure. Results of the Cooperative North Scandinavian Enalapril Survival Study (CONSENSUS). N Engl J Med 1987;316:1429–35.
8. Maisel WH, Stevenson LW. Atrial fibrillation in heart failure: epidemiology, pathophysiology, and rationale for therapy. Am J Cardiol 2003;91:2D–8D.
9. van Veldhuisen DJ, Aass H, El Allaf D, et al. Presence and development of atrial fibrillation in chronic heart failure. Experiences from the MERIT-HF Study. Eur J Heart Fail 2006;8:539–46.
10. Mathew J, Hunsberger S, Fleg J, Mc Sherry F, Williford W, Yusuf S. Incidence, predictive factors, and prognostic significance of supraventricular tachyarrhythmias in congestive heart failure. Chest 2000;118:914–22.
11. Benjamin EJ, Wolf PA, D'Agostino RB, Silbershatz H, Kannel WB, Levy D. Impact of atrial fibrillation on the risk of death: the Framingham Heart Study. Circulation 1998;98:946–52.

12. Wyse DG, Waldo AL, DiMarco JP, et al. A comparison of rate control and rhythm control in patients with atrial fibrillation. N Engl J Med 2002;347:1825–33.

13. Van Gelder IC, Hagens VE, Bosker HA, et al. A comparison of rate control and rhythm control in patients with recurrent persistent atrial fibrillation. N Engl J Med 2002;347:1834–40.

14. Jenkins LS, Brodsky M, Schron E, et al. Quality of life in atrial fibrillation: the Atrial Fibrillation Follow-up Investigation of Rhythm Management (AFFIRM) study. Am Heart J 2005;149:112–20.

15. Roy D, Talajic M, Nattel S, Wyse DG, Dorian P, Lee KL, et al. Rhythm control versus rate control for atrial fibrillation and heart failure. N Engl J Med 2008;358: 2667–77.

16. Fuster V, Ryden LE, Cannom DS, et al. ACC/AHA/ESC 2006 Guidelines for the Management of Patients with Atrial Fibrillation: a report of the American College of Cardiology/American Heart Association Task Force on Practice Guidelines and the European Society of Cardiology Committee for Practice Guidelines (Writing Committee to Revise the 2001 Guidelines for the Management of Patients with Atrial Fibrillation): developed in collaboration with the European Heart Rhythm Association and the Heart Rhythm Society. Circulation 2006;114:e257–354.

17. Bardy GH, Lee KL, Mark DB, et al. Amiodarone or an implantable cardioverter-defibrillator for congestive heart failure. N Engl J Med 2005;352:225–37.

18. Torp-Pedersen C, Moller M, Bloch-Thomsen PE, et al. Dofetilide in patients with congestive heart failure and left ventricular dysfunction. Danish Investigations of Arrhythmia and Mortality on Dofetilide Study Group. N Engl J Med 1999;341:857–65.

19. Doval HC, Nul DR, Grancelli HO, Perrone SV, Bortman GR, Curiel R. Randomised trial of low-dose amiodarone in severe congestive heart failure. Grupo de Estudio de la Sobrevida en la Insuficiencia Cardiaca en Argentina (GESICA). Lancet 1994;344: 493–8.

20. Singh BN, Singh SN, Reda DJ, et al. Amiodarone versus sotalol for atrial fibrillation. N Engl J Med 2005;352:1861–72.

21. Weerasooriya R, Davis M, Powell A, et al. The Australian Intervention Randomized Control of Rate in Atrial Fibrillation Trial (AIRCRAFT). J Am Coll Cardiol 2003;41:1697–702.

22. Puggioni E, Brignole M, Gammage M, et al. Acute comparative effect of right and left ventricular pacing in patients with permanent atrial fibrillation. J Am Coll Cardiol 2004;43:234–8.

23. Haissaguerre M, Jais P, Shah DC, et al. Spontaneous initiation of atrial fibrillation by ectopic beats originating in the pulmonary veins. N Engl J Med 1998;339:659–66.

24. Robbins IM, Colvin EV, Doyle TP, et al. Pulmonary vein stenosis after catheter ablation of atrial fibrillation. Circulation 1998;98:1769–75.

25. Verma A, Marrouche NF, Natale A. Pulmonary vein antrum isolation: intracardiac echocardiography-guided technique. J Cardiovasc Electrophysiol 2004;15:1335–40.

26. Oral H, Scharf C, Chugh A, et al. Catheter ablation for paroxysmal atrial fibrillation: segmental pulmonary vein ostial ablation versus left atrial ablation. Circulation 2003;108:2355–60.

27. Pappone C, Rosanio S, Oreto G, et al. Circumferential radiofrequency ablation of pulmonary vein ostia: a new anatomic approach for curing atrial fibrillation. Circulation 2000;102:2619–28.

28. Karch MR, Zrenner B, Deisenhofer I, et al. Freedom from atrial tachyarrhythmias after catheter ablation of atrial fibrillation: a randomized comparison between 2 current ablation strategies. Circulation 2005;111:2875–80.

29. Arruda M, Natale A. The adjunctive role of nonpulmonary venous ablation in the cure of atrial fibrillation. J Cardiovasc Electrophysiol 2006;17:S37–43.

30. Takahashi Y, Jais P, Hocini M, et al. Shortening of fibrillatory cycle length in the pulmonary vein during vagal excitation. J Am Coll Cardiol 2006;47:774–80.

31. Nademanee K, McKenzie J, Kosar E, et al. A new approach for catheter ablation of atrial fibrillation: mapping of the electrophysiologic substrate. J Am Coll Cardiol 2004;43:2044–53.

32. Calkins H, Brugada J, Packer DL, Cappato R, Chen S-A, Crijns HJG, et al. HRS/EHRA/ECAS Expert consensus statement on catheter and surgical ablation of atrial fibrillation: recommendations for personnel, policy, procedures, and follow-up. Europace 2007;9:335–379.

33. Oral H, Pappone C, Chugh A, et al. Circumferential pulmonary-vein ablation for chronic atrial fibrillation. N Engl J Med 2006;354:934–41.

34. Wazni OM, Marrouche NF, Martin DO, et al. Radiofrequency ablation vs antiarrhythmic drugs as first-line treatment of symptomatic atrial fibrillation: a randomized trial. JAMA 2005;293:2634–40.

35. Jais P, Chauchemez B, Macle L, Daoud E, Khairy P, Subbiah R, et al. Catheter ablation versus antiarrhythmia drugs for atrial fibrillation. Circulation 2008;118:2488–90.

36. Cappato R, Calkins H, Chen SA, et al. Worldwide survey on the methods, efficacy, and safety of catheter ablation for human atrial fibrillation. Circulation 2005;111:1100–5.

37. Essebag V, Baldessin F, Reynolds MR, et al. Non-inducibility post-pulmonary vein isolation achieving exit block predicts freedom from atrial fibrillation. Eur Heart J 2005;26:2550–5.

38. Hsu LF, Jais P, Sanders P, et al. Catheter ablation for atrial fibrillation in congestive heart failure. N Engl J Med 2004;351:2373–83.

39. Khan MN, Jais P, Cummings J, Di Biase L, Sanders P, Martin DO, et al. Pulmonary-vein isolation for atrial fibrillation in patients with heart failure. N Engl J Med 2008;359:1778–85.

40. Daoud EG, Kalbfleisch SJ, Hummel JD. Intracardiac echocardiography to guide transseptal left heart catheterization for radiofrequency catheter ablation. J Cardiovasc Electrophysiol 1999;10:358–63.

41. Ren JF, Schwartzman D, Callans D, Marchlinski FE, Gottlieb CD, Chaudhry FA. Imaging technique and clinical utility for electrophysiologic procedures of lower frequency (9 MHz) intracardiac echocardiography. Am J Cardiol 1998;82:1557–60, A8.

42. Bruce CJ, Packer DL, Seward JB. Intracardiac Doppler hemodynamics and flow: new vector, phased-array ultrasound-tipped catheter. Am J Cardiol 1999;83:1509–12, A9.

43. Jongbloed MR, Schalij MJ, Zeppenfeld K, Oemrawsingh PV, van der Wall EE, Bax JJ. Clinical applications of intracardiac echocardiography in interventional procedures. Heart 2005;91:981–90.

44. Schwartzman D, Nosbisch J, Housel D. Echocardiographically guided left atrial ablation: characterization of a new technique. Heart Rhythm 2006;3:930–8.

45. Morton JB, Sanders P, Byrne MJ, et al. Phased-array intracardiac echocardiography to guide radiofrequency ablation in the left atrium and at the pulmonary vein ostium. J Cardiovasc Electrophysiol 2001;12:343–8.

46. Saad EB, Cole CR, Marrouche NF, et al. Use of intracardiac echocardiography for prediction of chronic pulmonary vein stenosis after ablation of atrial fibrillation. J Cardiovasc Electrophysiol 2002;13:986–9.

47. Wood MA, Wittkamp M, Henry D, et al. A comparison of pulmonary vein ostial anatomy by computerized tomography, echocardiography, and venography in patients with atrial fibrillation having radiofrequency catheter ablation. Am J Cardiol 2004;93:49–53.

48. Marrouche NF, Martin DO, Wazni O, et al. Phased-array intracardiac echocardiography monitoring during pulmonary vein isolation in patients with atrial fibrillation: impact on outcome and complications. Circulation 2003;107:2710–6.

49. Brockenbrough EC, Braunwald E, Ross J, Jr. Transseptal left heart catheterization. A review of 450 studies and description of an improved technic. Circulation 1962;25: 15–21.

50. Mullins CE. Transseptal left heart catheterization: experience with a new technique in 520 pediatric and adult patients. Pediatr Cardiol 1983;4:239–45.

51. Kottkamp H, Burkhardt H, Krauss B, et al. Electromagnetic versus fluoroscopic mapping of the inferior isthmus for ablation of typical atrial flutter: a prospective randomized study. Circulation 2000;102:2082–6.

52. Gepstein L, Hayam G, Ben-Haim SA. A novel method for nonfluoroscopic catheter-based electroanatomical mapping of the heart. In vitro and in vivo accuracy results. Circulation 1997;95:1611–22.

53. Pappone C, Oreto G, Lamberti F, et al. Catheter ablation of paroxysmal atrial fibrillation using a 3D mapping system. Circulation 1999;100:1203–8.

54. Reddy VY, Malchano ZJ, Holmvang G, et al. Integration of cardiac magnetic resonance imaging with three-dimensional electroanatomic mapping to guide left ventricular catheter manipulation: feasibility in a porcine model of healed myocardial infarction. J Am Coll Cardiol 2004;44:2202–13.

55. Earley MJ, Showkathali R, Alzetani M, et al. Radiofrequency ablation of arrhythmias guided by non-fluoroscopic catheter location: a prospective randomized trial. Eur Heart J 2006;27:1223–9.

56. Rotter M, Takahashi Y, Sanders P, et al. Reduction of fluoroscopy exposure and procedure duration during ablation of atrial fibrillation using a novel anatomical navigation system. Eur Heart J 2005;26:1415–21.

57. Hindricks G, Kottkamp H. Simultaneous noncontact mapping of the left atrium in patients with paroxysmal atrial fibrillation. Circulation 2001;104:297–303.

58. Gornick CC, Adler SW, Pederson B, Hauck J, Budd J, Schweitzer J. Validation of a new noncontact catheter system for electroanatomic mapping of left ventricular endocardium. Circulation 1999;99:829–35.

59. Wittkampf FH, Wever EF, Derksen R, et al. LocaLisa: new technique for real-time 3-dimensional localization of regular intracardiac electrodes. Circulation 1999;99: 1312–17.

60. Macle L, Jais P, Scavee C, et al. Pulmonary vein disconnection using the LocaLisa three-dimensional nonfluoroscopic catheter imaging system. J Cardiovasc Electrophysiol 2003;14:693–7.

61. Weerasooriya R, Macle L, Jais P, Hocini M, Haissaguerre M. Pulmonary vein ablation using the LocaLisa nonfluoroscopic mapping system. J Cardiovasc Electrophysiol 2003;14:112.

62. de Groot NM, Bootsma M, van der Velde ET, Schalij MJ. Three-dimensional catheter positioning during radiofrequency ablation in patients: first application of a real-time position management system. J Cardiovasc Electrophysiol 2000;11: 1183–92.

63. Schreieck J, Ndrepepa G, Zrenner B, et al. Radiofrequency ablation of cardiac arrhythmias using a three-dimensional real-time position management and mapping system. Pacing Clin Electrophysiol 2002;25:1699–707.

64. Faddis MN, Blume W, Finney J, et al. Novel, magnetically guided catheter for endocardial mapping and radiofrequency catheter ablation. Circulation 2002;106: 2980–5.

65. Ernst S, Ouyang F, Linder C, et al. Initial experience with remote catheter ablation using a novel magnetic navigation system: magnetic remote catheter ablation. Circulation 2004;109:1472–5.

66. Ernst S, Hachiya H, Chun JK, Ouyang F. Remote catheter ablation of parahisian accessory pathways using a novel magnetic navigation system – a report of two cases. J Cardiovasc Electrophysiol 2005;16:659–62.

67. Pappone C, Vicedomini G, Manguso F, et al. Robotic magnetic navigation for atrial fibrillation ablation. J Am Coll Cardiol 2006;47:1390–400.
68. Reddy VY, Neuzil P, Malchano ZJ, Vijaykumar R, Cury R, Abbara S, et al. View-synchronized robotic image-guided therapy for atrial fibrillation ablation: experimental validation and clinical feasibility. Circulation 2007;115:2705–14.
69. Saliba W, Reddy VY, Wazni O, Cummings JE, Burkhardt JD, Haissaguerre M, et al. Atrial fibrillation ablation using a robotic catheter remote control system. J Am Coll Cardiol 2008;51:2407–11.
70. Arentz T, von Rosenthal J, Blum T, et al. Feasibility and safety of pulmonary vein isolation using a new mapping and navigation system in patients with refractory atrial fibrillation. Circulation 2003;108:2484–90.
71. Arentz T, Von Rosenthal J, Weber R, et al. Effects of circumferential ostial radiofrequency lesions on pulmonary vein activation recorded with a multipolar basket catheter. J Cardiovasc Electrophysiol 2005;16:302–8.
72. Tsai CF, Tai CT, Yu WC, et al. Is 8-mm more effective than 4-mm tip electrode catheter for ablation of typical atrial flutter? Circulation 1999;100:768–71.
73. Marrouche NF, Dresing T, Cole C, et al. Circular mapping and ablation of the pulmonary vein for treatment of atrial fibrillation: impact of different catheter technologies. J Am Coll Cardiol 2002;40:464–74.
74. Nakagawa H, Yamanashi WS, Pitha JV, et al. Comparison of in vivo tissue temperature profile and lesion geometry for radiofrequency ablation with a saline-irrigated electrode versus temperature control in a canine thigh muscle preparation. Circulation 1995;91:2264–73.
75. Yokoyama K, Nakagawa H, Wittkampf FH, Pitha JV, Lazzara R, Jackman WM. Comparison of electrode cooling between internal and open irrigation in radiofrequency ablation lesion depth and incidence of thrombus and steam pop. Circulation 2006;113:11–9.
76. Macle L, Jais P, Weerasooriya R, et al. Irrigated-tip catheter ablation of pulmonary veins for treatment of atrial fibrillation. J Cardiovasc Electrophysiol 2002;13:1067–73.
77. Horlitz M, Schley P, Shin DI, et al. Circumferential pulmonary vein ablation for treatment of atrial fibrillation using an irrigated-tip catheter. Am J Cardiol 2004;94:945–7.
78. Tse HF, Reek S, Timmermans C, et al. Pulmonary vein isolation using transvenous catheter cryoablation for treatment of atrial fibrillation without risk of pulmonary vein stenosis. J Am Coll Cardiol 2003;42:752–8.
79. Wong T, Markides V, Peters NS, Wright AR, Davies DW. Percutaneous isolation of multiple pulmonary veins using an expandable circular cryoablation catheter. Pacing Clin Electrophysiol 2004;27:551–4.
80. Rostock T, Weiss C, Ventura R, Willems S. Pulmonary vein isolation during atrial fibrillation using a circumferential cryoablation catheter. Pacing Clin Electrophysiol 2004;27:1024–5.
81. Garan A, Al-Ahmad A, Mihalik T, et al. Cryoablation of the pulmonary veins using a novel balloon catheter. J Interv Card Electrophysiol 2006;15:79–81.
82. Lesh MD, Diederich C, Guerra PG, Goseki Y, Sparks PB. An anatomic approach to prevention of atrial fibrillation: pulmonary vein isolation with through-the-balloon ultrasound ablation (TTB-USA). Thorac Cardiovasc Surg 1999;47(Suppl 3):347–51.
83. Saliba W, Wilber D, Packer D, et al. Circumferential ultrasound ablation for pulmonary vein isolation: analysis of acute and chronic failures. J Cardiovasc Electrophysiol 2002;13:957–61.
84. Meininger GR, Calkins H, Lickfett L, et al. Initial experience with a novel focused ultrasound ablation system for ring ablation outside the pulmonary vein. J Interv Card Electrophysiol 2003;8:141–8.

10 Percutaneous Treatment of Coronary Artery Disease

Roger J. Laham, MD

CONTENTS

Abstract

More than 2 million percutaneous cardiac interventional procedures are performed annually worldwide to treat coronary artery disease. Many of these patients have reduced ejection fraction and/or heart failure symptoms. This chapter provides a technical and clinical perspective on balloon angioplasty and stenting with bare-metal and drug-eluting stents. Techniques for managing complex patients, including therapeutic angiogenesis, spinal cord stimulation, and enhanced external counterpulsation, are also reviewed.

Key Words: Coronary artery disease; Balloon angioplasty; Stent; Heart failure; Percutaneous cardiac intervention.

1. A HISTORICAL PERSPECTIVE

In September 1977 in Zurich, Switzerland, a young pioneer named Andreas Gruentzig inserted a catheter into a patient's coronary artery and inflated a balloon, successfully opening a blockage and restoring blood flow

From: *Contemporary Cardiology: Device Therapy in Heart Failure*
Edited by: W.H. Maisel, DOI 10.1007/978-1-59745-424-7_10
© Humana Press, a part of Springer Science+Business Media, LLC 2010

to the subtended territory, heralding an era that would make percutaneous coronary intervention and its derivatives the procedure of choice for treating patients with coronary artery disease. Although currently performed percutaneous coronary interventions (PCI) bear little resemblance to the initial crude techniques used then, they are all based on the same principle of dilating a coronary stenosis while minimizing acute and long-term adverse events. Currently, more than 2 million PCI procedures are performed annually worldwide and PCI procedures have surpassed coronary artery bypass surgery both in numbers performed and in patient and physician preference.

2. BALLOON ANGIOPLASTY

Although plain old balloon angioplasty (POBA) is infrequently used as a stand-alone procedure in most patients undergoing PCI, it is befitting to describe what started it all. Balloon dilatation (bare or carrying a stent) is carried out in the majority of PCI. The balloon is inflated to compress the plaque against the arterial wall and create a localized dissection commonly involving the intima, thus leading to an acute gain in luminal diameter (Fig. 1). This is followed by elastic recoil leading to acute loss in luminal diameter, followed over the ensuing months by late loss in luminal diameter resulting from both remodeling of the arterial wall and formation of the neointima (1–5). The neointima results from smooth muscle cell proliferation and migration and matrix deposition (1–5). Several techniques and adjunctive therapeutic agents (such as aspirin and glycoprotein IIb/IIIa inhibitors) were developed to increase the procedural success rate above 95% and reduce the acute complications of POBA to 3–4%. However,

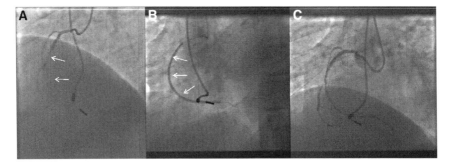

Fig. 1. Balloon angioplasty: A 70-year-old patient presented with congestive heart failure, EF <30%, and a large inferior and inferoposterior reversible defect on nuclear perfusion imaging. (**a**) Coronary angiography showed a chronically occluded RCA (*arrows*). (**b**) Several wires were used to cross the occlusion and a long balloon inflation was used to dilate the RCA (*arrows*). (**c**) Final angiography showed a patent RCA with a 30% residual stenosis and typical balloon angioplasty result with acute recoil. Stenting was not used since patient had a bleeding diathesis and could not tolerate dual-antiplatelet therapy.

they did little to prevent the primary long-term complication, restenosis, which occurred as frequently as 30–40% of the time and even more commonly in certain subsets of patients with diabetes and renal failure and of lesions in proximal LAD location and small vessels (6–17). This led to the development of several devices, including directional atherectomy, laser balloon angioplasty, excimer laser atherectomy, rotational atherectomy, and cutting balloon angioplasty, that promised higher acute success rates and lower restenosis rates, a promise that was never fully achieved relegating these devices to niche applications enabling more complex PCI (15–21). Several trials tested adjunctive therapy for the prevention of restenosis including steroids, angiotensin-converting enzyme inhibitors, methotrexate, calcium channel blockers, fish oil supplementation, gene therapy, antioxidants, HMGcoA reductase inhibitors with only marginal, if any, benefits (22–37).

3. STENTING

The development of stents revolutionized the treatment of coronary artery disease. Intracoronary stent implantation increased the procedural success rate to >98%, reduced acute complications including abrupt closure, and significantly reduced long-term restenosis rates in most patient subgroups (Fig. 2). The addition of aspirin and ticlopidine or clopidogrel reduced the acute and subacute thrombosis rates following stenting to <1% (38–42). The STRESS and BENESTENT studies were seminal investigations in establishing the safety and efficacy of coronary stenting compared to balloon angioplasty. The STRESS study randomly assigned 410 patients with symptomatic coronary disease to elective placement of a Palmaz-Schatz stent or to standard balloon angioplasty. Coronary angiography was performed at

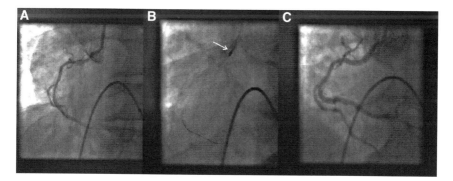

Fig. 2. An 86-year-old man presented with progressive angina. (**a**) Baseline RCA angiography showed a heavily calcified proximal RCA with a severe stenosis. (**b**) Rotational atherectomy was performed with 1.25 and 1.75 mm Burrs (Burr shown, *arrow*). (**c**) After stenting, full stent expansion and no residual stenoses were obtained.

baseline, immediately after the procedure, and 6 months later. Patients who underwent stenting had a higher rate of procedural success than those who underwent standard balloon angioplasty (96.1% vs. 89.6%, $P = 0.011$) and a larger acute lumen. At 6 months, the patients with stented lesions continued to have a larger luminal diameter (1.74±0.60 mm vs. 1.56±0.65 mm, $P = 0.007$) and a lower rate of restenosis (31.6% vs. 42.1%, $P = 0.046$) than those treated with balloon angioplasty (*41*). The BENESTENT study randomized 520 patients with stable angina and a single coronary artery lesion to either stent implantation or standard balloon angioplasty. At 6 months, 52 patients in the stent group (20%) and 76 patients in the angioplasty group (30%) reached a primary clinical end point, mainly due to a reduced need for a repeat revascularization in the stent group (relative risk, 0.58; 95% confidence interval, 0.40–0.85; $P = 0.005$). The restenosis rate was 22% in the stent arm and 32% in the balloon group ($P = 0.02$) (*42*). The excellent procedural success rate and lower rate of restenosis propelled stenting to the procedure of choice when feasible in PCI. Second- and third-generation stents improved deliverability and procedural success and studies showed its cost-effectiveness compared to balloon angioplasty and CABG (*38, 43–49*). Stenting, however, reduced but did not eliminate restenosis and was associated with a significant risk of acute or subacute stent thrombosis, a catastrophic complication that often results in Q-wave myocardial infarction. This risk was significantly reduced to <1% by using two antiplatelet agents [aspirin + thienopyridine (ticlopidine or clopidogrel)], the latter being used for 4 weeks after the procedure (*39*). The predictability of stenting and its lower restenosis rate enabled cardiologists to tackle more complex lesions and multivessel stenting. Several studies compared stenting to CABG and demonstrated similar survival, myocardial infarction, and stroke rates, but a higher rate of repeat revascularization in the stent group (*50–57*). Thus the adoption of stents became widespread with greater than 80% of interventions being performed using stenting. However, restenosis remained the Achilles' heel of PCI and in-stent restenosis became a growing problem worldwide. Brachytherapy was developed for the treatment of in-stent restenosis, inhibiting neointima formation after angioplasty and significantly reducing restenosis rates with late-stent thrombosis necessitating long-term dual-antiplatelet therapy (*58–63*).

4. DRUG-ELUTING STENTS

Although stenting revolutionized the treatment of coronary artery disease, in-stent restenosis remained a major downside limiting their universal use and tempering their impact (Fig. 3). Stents had a clinical restenosis rate of 20–40%, with much higher restenosis rates in the patient subgroups that also had higher restenosis rates with balloon angioplasty, i.e., diabetics, renal insufficiency, female gender, proximal LAD location, small vessels, and long lesions. Restenosis is a complex process resulting from intimal

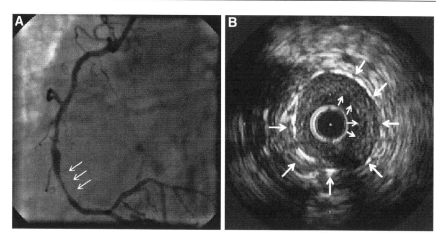

Fig. 3. Bare-metal stent restenosis: A 69-year-old patient presented with recurrent angina s/p stenting of distal RCA. (**a**) Angiography showed diffuse moderate to severe in-stent restenosis (*arrows*). (**b**) IVUS images showed a fully expanded stent (*arrows*) and intimal in-stent restenosis with a thick neointima (*small arrows*).

proliferation and remodeling, with the latter being less important with stenting. Previous attempts have all failed to affect this process since systemic therapy could not achieve therapeutic levels in the injured arterial wall and local delivery devices failed to result in effective local concentrations, distribution, and retention of therapeutic agents secondary to the limited delivery space of the arterial wall (*6, 26–29, 34–36, 64–78*). Intravascular brachytherapy circumvented the delivery issue by directly delivering radiation to the vessel wall resulting in the inhibition of smooth muscle cell migration, proliferation, and matrix formation; however, it was complicated by late-stent thrombosis and geographic miss, a process resulting in restenosis at the edge of the treatment area.

Stents on the other hand provided an ideal drug delivery device which when coated with a polymer that allows sustained release may result in effective tissue concentrations of the therapeutic agent. This was best exemplified by the heparin-coated (Hepacoat) stent coated with base layers of polyethyleneimine and dextran sulfate to which aldehyde-terminated heparin was covalently bonded (*79–81*). Therefore, what was needed was an effective inhibitor of smooth muscle cell proliferation. Numerous agents were considered including rapamycin or sirolimus, actinomycin D, β-estradiol, and paclitaxel. Sirolimus (rapamycin) is a macrocyclic triene antibiotic that has immunosuppressive and antiproliferative properties. Rapamycin is a natural fermentation product produced by *Streptomyces hygroscopicus* and was originally noted to have antifungal properties, resulting in its potential development as an antibiotic. However, recognition of its potent immunosuppressant properties made it unsuitable for use as an antibiotic (*82–85*). Rapamycin was first approved to prevent rejection following organ transplantation and its potential role in preventing accelerated arteriopathy after cardiac transplantation and stent restenosis was recognized only almost a decade later (*86–91*). Rapamycin's cellular actions are mediated by binding to its intracellular receptor, the FK506-binding protein (FKBP12), a member of the immunophilin family of proteins. Rapamycin–FKBP12 has no activity against calcineurin; rather, it inhibits a kinase called the target of rapamycin (TOR), which is a component in a pathway that regulates cell cycle progression, thus inhibiting smooth muscle cell migration and proliferation by blocking cell cycle progression at the G1/S transition (*82, 84, 86–89, 91, 92*).

Paclitaxel (Taxol) on the other hand is a microtubule-stabilizing agent with potent antiproliferative activity. Unlike other antimitotic agents of the colchicine type, it shifts the microtubule equilibrium toward assembly, leading to reduced proliferation, migration, and signal transduction (*93–97*). The possibility of local and sustained delivery with stents led to the rapid preclinical investigation of both sirolimus and paclitaxel demonstrating their ability to reduce restenosis in animal models of vascular injury (*98–105*). The promising results obtained in most preclinical studies propelled the investigation of these drugs in clinical trials.

4.1. Cypher Stent

The first stent to be developed was the Cypher stent (Cordis, JNJ). Sirolimus was blended in a mixture of nonerodable polymers that have been used clinically in bone cements, ocular devices, and drug-releasing intrauterine devices. The first-in-man studies were carried out in 15 patients who received a fast-release (FR) formulation (<15-day drug release) and 15 patients who received a slow-release (SR) formulation (28-day drug release) (*106*). The procedure was successful in all patients. Angiography and intravascular ultrasound was done at baseline and at 4 months and clinical follow-up was obtained at 8 months. There was minimal neointimal hyperplasia in both groups ($11.0\pm3.0\%$ in the SR group and $10.4\pm3.0\%$ in the FR group, $P = $ NS) by ultrasound and quantitative coronary angiography. No angiographic restenosis was observed and no clinical events were seen at 8 months (*106*), with maintained benefit at 2 years (*107, 108*).

This promising early experience led to randomized clinical trials of sirolimus-eluting stents as compared to bare-metal stents, initially studied in RAVEL, a randomized, double-blind trial of 239 patients comparing the slow formulation to bare-metal stents. At 6 months, the degree of neointimal proliferation measured by late luminal loss was significantly lower in the sirolimus stent group than in the standard stent group (-0.01 ± 0.33 mm vs. 0.80 ± 0.53 mm, $P<0.001$). None of the patients in the sirolimus stent group, as compared with 26.6% of those in the standard stent group, had restenosis of 50% or more of the luminal diameter ($P<0.001$). There were no episodes of stent thrombosis (*109–111*). This beneficial effect with low target lesion failure was maintained at 3 years of follow-up (*112*).

The pivotal SIRIUS study confirmed these findings with a randomized, double-blind trial comparing a sirolimus-eluting stent with a standard stent in 1058 patients (26% with diabetes mellitus, mean lesion length of 14.4 mm) at 53 centers in the United States with a de novo lesion in a native coronary artery (*113*). The rate of failure of the target vessel was reduced from 21.0% with a standard stent to 8.6% with a sirolimus-eluting stent (*P*<0.001). This reduction was driven largely by a decrease in the frequency of the need for revascularization of the target lesion (16.6% in the standard stent group vs. 4.1% in the sirolimus stent group, *P*<0.001). The benefit of the sirolimus-eluting stent was maintained in higher risk subgroups such as diabetes mellitus, small vessel diameter, and proximal LAD location.

E-SIRIUS enrolled 352 patients with a single lesion diameter of 2.5–3.0 mm and length 15–32 mm (*114–116*). At 8 months, minimum lumen diameter was significantly higher with sirolimus-eluting stents than with control stents (2.22 mm vs. 1.33 mm, *P*<0.0001), with a significant reduction in binary restenosis with sirolimus-eluting stents compared with control stents (5.9% vs. 42.3%, *P* = 0.0001) (*114–116*). C-SIRIUS enrolled 352 patients with a lesion diameter of 2.5–3.0 mm and lesion length 15–32 mm. At 8 months, minimum lumen diameter was significantly higher with sirolimus-eluting stents than with control stents (2.22 mm vs. 1.33 mm, *P*<0.0001) with lower binary restenosis with sirolimus-eluting stents compared with control stents (5.9% vs. 42.3%, *P* = 0.0001). These benefits were also confirmed and maintained in "real-world" patients in several registries and complex patient and lesion subsets including diffuse disease, in-stent restenosis, bifurcation lesions, diabetes mellitus, saphenous vein grafts, and left main disease (*115, 117–141*). In addition, the cost-effectiveness of sirolimus-eluting stents was demonstrated in multiple analyses (*142, 143*).

4.2. TAXUS Stent

The development of the TAXUS paclitaxel-eluting stent has followed a similar trend and resulted in similar successes. The randomized TAXUS I safety trial (Boston Scientific, MA, paclitaxel-coated NIR stent) demonstrated significant reduction of restenosis lesions at 6 months follow-up (0% vs. 10%) without the excess thrombosis observed in the SCORE trial (which used the Quanam stent), probably secondary to lower dosage (*144, 145*). The TAXUS I trial was a prospective, double-blind, three-center study randomizing 61 patients with de novo or restenotic lesions to receive a TAXUS paclitaxel slow-release stent (*n* = 31) vs. control (*n* = 30) stent (diameter 3.0 or 3.5 mm). No stent thromboses were reported at 1, 6, 9, or 12 months. At 12 months, the major adverse cardiac event (MACE) rate was 3% in the TAXUS group and 10% in the control group. Six-month angiographic restenosis rates were 0% for TAXUS vs. 10% for control patients. There were significant improvements in minimal lumen diameter (2.60±0.49 mm vs. 2.19±0.65 mm), diameter stenosis (13.56±11.77 mm vs. 27.23±16.69 mm), and late lumen loss (0.36±0.48 mm vs. 0.71±0.48 mm) in the TAXUS group (all $P<0.01$). The TAXUS II study was a multicenter, randomized, double-blind trial of 536 patients evaluating slow-release (SR) and moderate-release (MR) formulations of a polymer-based paclitaxel-eluting stent (TAXUS) for revascularization of single, primary lesions in native coronary arteries. Cohort I compared TAXUS-SR with control stents, and Cohort II compared TAXUS-MR with a second control group. At 6 months, the volume of obstructive plaque was significantly lower for TAXUS stents (7.9% SR and 7.8% MR) than for respective controls (23.2 and 20.5%; $P<0.0001$). This corresponded with a reduction in angiographic restenosis from 17.9 to 2.3% in the SR cohort ($P<0.0001$) and from 20.2 to 4.7% in the MR cohort ($P=0.0002$), an effect maintained with direct stenting and at 18 months of follow-up (*146–151*).

This led to the pivotal TAXUS IV trial, which was a study of 1314 patients with single de novo coronary lesions 10–28 mm in length (vessel diameter 2.5–3.75 mm) who were randomized to the slow-release, polymer-based, paclitaxel-eluting TAXUS stent or an identical-appearing bare-metal EXPRESS stent. The TAXUS stent reduced the 12-month rates of target lesion revascularization by 73% (4.4% vs. 15.1%, $P<0.0001$), target vessel revascularization by 62% (7.1% vs. 17.1%, $P<0.0001$), and composite major adverse cardiac events by 49% (10.8% vs. 20.0%, $P<0.0001$). The 1-year rates of cardiac death (1.4% vs. 1.3%), myocardial infarction (3.5% vs. 4.7%), and subacute thrombosis (0.6% vs. 0.8%) were similar between the paclitaxel-eluting and control stents, respectively (*152*). These results were confirmed and extended to "real-world" settings with TAXUS V.

More recently, the Endeavor stent (zotarolimus-eluting, phosphoryl-choline polymer-coated stent, Medtronic, Inc., Minneapolis, MN) and the XIENCE™ V Everolimus Eluting Coronary Stent System (Abbott Vascular, Redwood City, CA) were approved for use in the US cross-trial comparisons, and direct drug-eluting stent comparisons have yielded conflicting results, making it difficult to identify one particular drug-eluting stent as superior to the others (*153–161*).

5. THE CONTROVERSY OF DES

It is important to remember that DES have been approved by the FDA only for patient and lesion subsets that have been evaluated in the pivotal trials. However, by 2004, over 70% of patients who received at least one stent during PCI were treated with a DES (*162*). The ACC/AHA/SCAI Guidelines for PCI assign Class I status to DES "as an alternative to the BMS in subsets of patients in whom trial data suggest efficacy" (*163*). The Cypher stent was approved by the FDA for "improving coronary luminal diameter in patients with symptomatic ischemic disease due to discrete de novo lesions

≤30 mm in length in native coronary arteries with a reference diameter of ≥2.5 to ≤3.5 mm." The TAXUS stent was approved for "improving luminal diameter for the treatment of de novo lesions of length <28 mm in native coronary arteries ≥2.5 to ≤3.75 mm in diameter." Endeavor and Xience V have received similar indications. Given the profound reduction in angiographic and clinical restenosis documented with DES in clinical trials, there should be little debate regarding the efficacy of DES for treatment of lesions in these groups.

However, the history of interventional cardiology is one of rapid dissemination of technology, e.g., bare-metal stents, to "off-label" use. In the case of bare-metal stents, the extension to other lesion and patient subsets such as chronic total occlusion and acute myocardial infarction has been validated in randomized clinical trials. Furthermore, even in the absence of a restenosis benefit, bare-metal stents improved procedural safety compared to balloon angioplasty alone (*164*). The benefit of contemporary DES is entirely attributed to a reduction in target lesion revascularization without any incremental improvement in procedural or long-term safety. Moreover, issues such as the need for prolonged dual-antiplatelet therapy to prevent late-stent thrombosis, hypersensitivity reactions to polymers, and late incomplete strut apposition suggest that this reduction in restenosis must be balanced carefully against any potential safety issues.

Since obstructive coronary artery disease may also be treated by medical therapy, surgical revascularization, balloon angioplasty, or bare-metal stenting, it is imperative that an evidence-based analysis of trial results and registries be performed before recommending the routine use of DES for off-label indications. Finally, with the delayed endothelialization and continued risk of subacute and late-stent thrombosis, these stents are contraindicated in patients who may be noncompliant with dual-antiplatelet therapy or are likely to require premature discontinuation of one or both of the antiplatelet agents. Restenosis can be treated with several strategies and is rarely associated with an increase in mortality or myocardial infarction, in contradistinction to stent thrombosis, which is commonly associated with Q-wave myocardial infarction and high mortality.

6. CORONARY ARTERY DISEASE AND HEART FAILURE

Ischemic heart disease remains the leading cause of heart failure (HF), a problem that has reached epidemic proportion in the United States. Based on the 44-year follow-up of the NHLBI's Framingham Heart Study, HF incidence approaches 10 per 1000 population after age 65 with 22% of male and 46% of female patients with myocardial infarction becoming disabled with heart failure. Hospital discharges for HF rose from 377,000 in 1979 to 995,000 in 2001 (*165*).

Patients with systolic heart failure from ischemic heart disease have higher mortality and morbidity and poorer outcomes with PCI, CABG, or medical therapy. There is always the hope that patients with heart failure have hibernating myocardium with viable but underperfused myocardial distributions that may spring back to life with myocardial revascularization, whether percutaneous or surgical. Despite being technically challenging and carrying a higher periprocedural risk, the performance of revascularization in patients who have ischemic heart failure can provide substantial clinical benefits. Older studies have demonstrated a benefit of CABG over PCI among patients who have depressed ejection fraction undergoing revascularization; however, these studies were conducted during the balloon angioplasty era and before the widespread use of drug-eluting stents that have dramatically reduced the need for repeat revascularization. In addition, the use of intra-aortic balloon catheters and other cardiac support devices may extend the use of PCI and lower rates of periprocedural complications among this high-risk population (Fig. 4) (*166*).

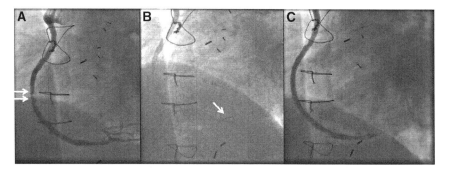

Fig. 4. A 56-year-old man s/p CABG presented with unstable angina. Baseline angiography (**a**) showed a critical stenosis in the saphenous vein graft to the RCA. A filter wire was deployed for distal protection (**b**, *arrow*), which allowed stenting with an excellent result (**c**).

In one study, 220 patients (20% women) with severe LV dysfunction (LV ejection fraction ≤35%) underwent revascularization with either coronary stent implantation or CABG. One hundred and twenty-eight patients received DES and 92 patients underwent surgery. The 30-day mortality was significantly greater in patients undergoing CABG than those receiving DES. At 2-year follow-up, however, both groups had the same survival probability from death (83% in both groups) (*167*). Finally, in the Global Registry of Acute Coronary Events (GRACE), a multinational cohort study, 44,372 patients with an ACS were enrolled and followed up in 113 hospitals in 14 countries between July 1, 1999, and December 31, 2006. Pharmacological reperfusion declined in patients with STEMI by 22%, whereas primary PCI increased by 37%. In patients with non-STEMI, rates of PCI increased markedly by 18%. Not surprisingly, the rates of heart failure and pulmonary edema declined in both populations (9% in STEMI and 6.9% in NSTEMI). Thus, early intervention seems to reduce the risk of CHF (*168*).

7. NO-OPTION PATIENTS

An increasing number of patients are no longer candidates for percutaneous or surgical revascularization or have exhausted or failed these modalities. In a study of 500 patients at the Cleveland Clinic, 59 patients (12%) were considered ineligible for PCI/CABG, a study commonly cited to describe this patient population (*169–171*). However, wide regional and institutional variability in treatment patterns of coronary disease including more or less aggressive revascularization practices contributes to different estimates of the magnitude of the problem, ranging from 5 to 21% of patients with coronary artery disease.

The development of various procedures such as endovascular cardiopulmonary bypass and assist devices (*172*), rotational atherectomy for calcified undilatable lesions (*173*, *174*), distal protection for vein graft interventions (*175–177*), chronic total occlusion wires and devices (*178*) has enabled the treatment of many patients previously deemed to be "no-option." If all these options are exhausted, then patients are deemed truly without any options and alternative treatment strategies are needed.

Therapeutic angiogenesis may provide a treatment strategy for these patients by providing new venues for blood flow. Angiogenesis is a complex process that involves stimulation of endothelial cell proliferation and migration, stimulation of extracellular matrix breakdown, attraction of pericytes and macrophages, stimulation of smooth muscle cell proliferation and migration, formation and "sealing" of new vascular structures, and deposition of new matrix (*179–190*). It is likely that a coordinated action of several mitogens and cascades is needed to achieve this process.

A number of growth factors have been evaluated for their angiogenic potential including fibroblast growth factors, vascular endothelial growth factors, hepatocyte growth/scatter factor (HGF/SF), chemokines such as IL-8 and MCP-1, growth factors involved in maturation of vascular tree such as angiopoietins and platelet-derived growth factor (PDGF) as well as transcription factors that stimulate expression of angiogenic cytokines and their receptors such as hypoxia-induced factor (HIF)-1α. As with any biologic therapy, the necessary steps are understanding the biology, developing therapeutic agents and vectors, site-specific delivery of therapeutic agents, and developing outcome measures to measure the benefits of the therapeutic intervention.

This problem is confounded by a very powerful placebo effect in this patient population, necessitating blinded studies and more powerful imaging and outcome measures to detect the small benefits expected with such therapies. To date, clinical angiogenesis remains experimental and unproven (*186*, *191–195*).

It is also important to discuss treatment modalities that could be offered to these "no-option" patients with angina: spinal cord stimulation and extracorporeal counterpulsation.

7.1. Spinal Cord Stimulation (SCS)

Spinal cord stimulation has been proposed as a treatment strategy that may be effective in end-stage ischemic heart disease patients with intractable angina. The efficacy of spinal cord stimulation on the relief of otherwise intractable angina pectoris was studied in a 2-month-long randomized study with 1-year follow-up by quality-of-life parameters, cardiac parameters, and complications. Twenty-four patients were randomized to either an actively treated group A (12 patients received the device within a 2 weeks' period) or a control group B (10 patients had an implantation after the study period). Spinal cord stimulation improved both quality-of-life and cardiac parameters. The latter included a trend toward reduction in ischemia after implantation of the device in both treadmill exercise and 24-h ambulatory Holter recordings, with a concomitant improvement in exercise capacity (*196*). Indices of ischemia were studied with and without SCS in 10 patients with otherwise intractable angina and evidence of myocardial ischemia on 48-h ambulatory electrocardiographic (ECG) recording. During SCS the total ischemic burden of the entire group was significantly reduced from a median of 27.9 mm × min (range 1.9–278.2) before SCS to 0 mm × min (range 0–70.2) with SCS ($P<0.03$) (*197*).

The efficacy of spinal cord stimulation as a treatment for chronic intractable angina pectoris was further studied for 6 weeks in 13 treated patients and 12 control patients with chronic angina. Assessments were exercise capacity and ischemia, daily frequency of anginal attacks and nitrate tablet consumption, and quality of life. Compared with control, exercise duration ($P=0.03$) and time to angina ($P=0.01$) increased; and anginal attacks and sublingual nitrate consumption ($P=0.01$) and ischemic episodes on 48-h electrocardiogram ($P=0.04$) decreased. ST segment depression on the exercise electrocardiogram decreased at comparable workload ($P=0.01$). Perceived quality of life increased ($P=0.03$), and pain decreased ($P=0.01$) (*198*). Nineteen consecutive patients implanted for spinal cord stimulation were studied. Annual admission rate after revascularization was 0.97/patient per year, compared with 0.27/patient per year after spinal cord stimulation ($P=0.02$). Mean time in hospital/patient per year after revascularization was 8.3 days vs. 2.5 days after spinal cord stimulation ($P=0.04$) (*199*). A major unanswered question regarding SCS is whether the effect of SCS is predominantly the result of a placebo effect and whether it is indeed a revascularization strategy or does it provide only symptomatic relief without any effects on survival, myocardial infarction, need for repeat revascularization, or left ventricular function. These questions may be answered by ongoing and/or proposed studies.

7.2. Enhanced External Counterpulsation (EECP)

EECP is an approved device for use in patients with disabling, chronic angina as well as heart failure. The device comprises inflatable cuffs that encompass the calf, thigh, and upper thigh and squeeze sequentially from low to high during diastole and then rapidly and simultaneously deflate at the onset of systole, with ECG gating. The arterial hemodynamics generated by EECP may simulate intra-aortic balloon pump counterpulsation with the generation of a retrograde arterial wave pulse. The usual course of treatment is 35 one-hour sessions. This treatment modality has flourished on the fringes of main stream academic cardiology with most patients treated in the office setting and has been supported by several registries and randomized clinical trials (200–205). The International EECP Patient Registry (IEPR) was started in 1998 and fashioned on the basis of the NHLBI angioplasty registry in order to study the outcome of patients undergoing EECP (205). This study investigated the long-term outcomes of EECP in relieving angina and improving the quality of life in a large cohort of patients with chronic angina pectoris. Seventy-three percent had a reduction by ≥ 1 angina class at the end of treatment, and 50% reported an improvement in quality-of-life assessment. However, there has been only one randomized, placebo-controlled trial to study the effect and safety of EECP (206) in patients with chronic angina. One hundred and thirty-nine patients were enrolled and had differing pressures applied to the cuffs raising serious concerns about adequate blinding. Both groups had improvement in exercise duration, with the active group exercising for a longer duration (not statistically significant). The active group did show a statistically significant improvement in time to ST segment depression. These effects were less impressive than have been found for patients in the registry (206). Available data are not robust enough to support widespread use; however, it remains an alternative yet unproven treatment strategy for "no-option" patients.

8. CONCLUSIONS

Coronary artery disease is a frequent cause of reduced ejection fraction and heart failure symptoms. The field of percutaneous coronary interventions has undergone remarkable advances in the past three decades and many patients can now benefit from revascularization. Success rates have increased, while the rate of restenosis has declined. Other treatment modalities may become more common as the number of patients with severe, non-revascularizable CAD increases.

REFERENCES

1. Karas SP, Santoian EC, Gravanis MB. Restenosis following coronary angioplasty. *Clin Cardiol.* Oct 1991;14(10):791–801.
2. Lange RA, Flores ED, Hillis LD. Restenosis after coronary balloon angioplasty. *Annu Rev Med.* 1991;42:127–132.
3. King JF, Manley JC, al-Wathiqui MH. Restenosis after angioplasty: mechanisms and clinical experience. *Cardiol Clin.* Nov 1989;7(4):853–864.
4. Liu MW, Roubin GS, King SB, 3rd. Restenosis after coronary angioplasty. Potential biologic determinants and role of intimal hyperplasia. *Circulation.* Jun 1989;79(6):1374–1387.

5. Nikkari ST, Clowes AW. Restenosis after vascular reconstruction. *Ann Med.* Apr 1994;26(2):95–100.
6. Ferns GA, Avades TY. The mechanisms of coronary restenosis: insights from experimental models. *Int J Exp Pathol.* 2000;81(2):63–88.
7. Yutani C, Imakita M, Ishibashi-Ueda H, et al. Coronary atherosclerosis and interventions: pathological sequences and restenosis. *Pathol Int.* Apr 1999;49(4):273–290.
8. Schiele F, Vuillemenot A, Meneveau N, et al. Effects of increasing balloon pressure on mechanism and results of balloon angioplasty for treatment of restenosis after Palmaz-Schatz stent implantation: an angiographic and intravascular ultrasound study. *Catheter Cardiovasc Interv.* Mar 1999;46(3):314–321.
9. Angerio AD, Fink DA. New strategies in the prevention of restenosis. *Crit Care Nurs Q.* May 2001;24(1):62–68.
10. Mauri L, Bonan R, Weiner BH, et al. Cutting balloon angioplasty for the prevention of restenosis: results of the Cutting Balloon Global Randomized Trial. *Am J Cardiol.* Nov 15, 2002;90(10):1079–1083.
11. Popma JJ, Satler LF, Pichard AD, et al. Vascular complications after balloon and new device angioplasty. *Circulation.* Oct 1993;88(4 Pt 1):1569–1578.
12. Wong CS, Leon MB, Popma JJ. New device angioplasty: the impact on restenosis. *Coron Artery Dis.* Mar 1993;4(3):243–253.
13. Popma JJ, Coller BS, Ohman EM, et al. Antithrombotic therapy in patients undergoing coronary angioplasty. *Chest.* Oct 1995;108(4 Suppl):486S–501S.
14. Leclerc G, Isner JM, Kearney M, et al. Evidence implicating nonmuscle myosin in restenosis. Use of in situ hybridization to analyze human vascular lesions obtained by directional atherectomy. *Circulation.* Feb 1992;85(2):543–553.
15. Kuntz RE, Safian RD, Levine MJ, et al. Novel approach to the analysis of restenosis after the use of three new coronary devices. *J Am Coll Cardiol.* Jun 1992;19(7):1493–1499.
16. Kuntz RE, Hinohara T, Safian RD, et al. Restenosis after directional coronary atherectomy. Effects of luminal diameter and deep wall excision. *Circulation.* Nov 1992;86(5):1394–1399.
17. Kuntz RE, Safian RD, Carrozza JP, et al. The importance of acute luminal diameter in determining restenosis after coronary atherectomy or stenting. *Circulation.* Dec 1992;86(6):1827–1835.
18. Safian RD, Gelbfish JS, Erny RE, et al. Coronary atherectomy. Clinical, angiographic, and histological findings and observations regarding potential mechanisms. *Circulation.* Jly 1990;82(1):69–79.
19. Reis GJ, Pomerantz RM, Jenkins RD, et al. Laser balloon angioplasty: clinical, angiographic and histologic results. *J Am Coll Cardiol.* Jly 1991;18(1):193–202.
20. Simons M, Leclerc G, Safian RD, et al. Relation between activated smooth-muscle cells in coronary-artery lesions and restenosis after atherectomy. *N Engl J Med.* Mar 4, 1993;328(9):608–613.
21. Baim DS. New devices for coronary revascularization. *Hosp Pract (Off Ed).* Oct 15, 1993;28(10):41–48, 51–52.
22. Whitworth HB, Roubin GS, Hollman J, et al. Effect of nifedipine on recurrent stenosis after percutaneous transluminal coronary angioplasty. *J Am Coll Cardiol.* Dec 1986;8(6):1271–1276.
23. Meier B. Restenosis after coronary angioplasty: review of the literature. *Eur Heart J.* Mar 1988;9(Suppl C):1–6.
24. Schwartz L, Bourassa MG, Lesperance J, et al. Aspirin and dipyridamole in the prevention of restenosis after percutaneous transluminal coronary angioplasty. *N Engl J Med.* Jun 30, 1988;318(26):1714–1719.
25. Schwartz L, Lesperance J, Bourassa MG, et al. The role of antiplatelet agents in modifying the extent of restenosis following percutaneous transluminal coronary angioplasty. *Am Heart J.* Feb 1990;119(2 Pt 1):232–236.

26. Brozovich FV, Morganroth J, Gottlieb NB, et al. Effect of angiotensin converting enzyme inhibition on the incidence of restenosis after percutaneous transluminal coronary angioplasty. *Cathet Cardiovasc Diagn.* Aug 1991;23(4):263–267.

27. Hattori R, Kodama K, Takatsu F, et al. Randomized trial of a selective inhibitor of thromboxane A2 synthetase, (E)-7-phenyl-7-(3-pyridyl)-6-heptenoic acid (CV-4151), for prevention of restenosis after coronary angioplasty. *Jpn Circ J.* Apr 1991;55(4):324–329.

28. Bairati I, Roy L, Meyer F. Double-blind, randomized, controlled trial of fish oil supplements in prevention of recurrence of stenosis after coronary angioplasty. *Circulation.* Mar 1992;85(3):950–956.

29. Kaul U, Sanghvi S, Bahl VK, et al. Fish oil supplements for prevention of restenosis after coronary angioplasty. *Int J Cardiol.* Apr 1992;35(1):87–93.

30. Chapman GD, Lim CS, Gammon RS, et al. Gene transfer into coronary arteries of intact animals with a percutaneous balloon catheter. *Circ Res.* Jly 1992;71(1):27–33.

31. Violaris AG, Angelini GD. Heparin in coronary artery disease: new uses for an old drug. *Br J Hosp Med.* Jan 6–19, 1993;49(1):37–39, 42–43.

32. Yamaguchi H, Lee YJ, Daida H, et al. Effectiveness of LDL-apheresis in preventing restenosis after percutaneous transluminal coronary angioplasty (PTCA): LDL-apheresis angioplasty restenosis trial (L-ART). *Chem Phys Lipids.* Jan 1994; 67–68:399–403.

33. Ragosta M, Gimple LW, Gertz SD, et al. Specific factor Xa inhibition reduces restenosis after balloon angioplasty of atherosclerotic femoral arteries in rabbits. *Circulation.* Mar 1994;89(3):1262–1271.

34. Wang DW, Zhao HY. Prevention of atherosclerotic arterial stenosis and restenosis after angioplasty with *Andrographis paniculata* nees and fish oil. Experimental studies of effects and mechanisms. *Chin Med J (Engl).* Jun 1994;107(6):464–470.

35. Consigny PM, Miller KT. Drug delivery into the arterial wall: a time-course study with use of a lipophilic dye. *J Vasc Interv Radiol.* Sept–Oct 1994;5(5):731–737.

36. Lincoff AM, Topol EJ, Ellis SG. Local drug delivery for the prevention of restenosis. Fact, fancy, and future. *Circulation.* Oct 1994;90(4):2070–2084.

37. Landau C, Pirwitz MJ, Willard MA, et al. Adenoviral mediated gene transfer to atherosclerotic arteries after balloon angioplasty. *Am Heart J.* Jun 1995;129(6): 1051–1057.

38. Cutlip DE, Leon MB, Ho KK, et al. Acute and nine-month clinical outcomes after "suboptimal" coronary stenting: results from the STent Anti-thrombotic Regimen Study (STARS) registry. *J Am Coll Cardiol.* Sept 1999;34(3):698–706.

39. Leon MB, Baim DS, Popma JJ, et al. A clinical trial comparing three antithrombotic-drug regimens after coronary-artery stenting. Stent Anticoagulation Restenosis Study Investigators. *N Engl J Med.* Dec 3, 1998;339(23):1665–1671.

40. Carrozza JP, Baim DS. Thrombotic and hemorrhagic complications of stenting coronary arteries: incidence, management, and prevention. *J Thromb Thrombolysis.* 1995;1(3):289–297.

41. Fischman DL, Leon MB, Baim DS, et al. A randomized comparison of coronary-stent placement and balloon angioplasty in the treatment of coronary artery disease. Stent Restenosis Study Investigators. *N Engl J Med.* Aug 25, 1994;331(8):496–501.

42. Serruys PW, de Jaegere P, Kiemeneij F, et al. A comparison of balloon-expandable-stent implantation with balloon angioplasty in patients with coronary artery disease. Benestent Study Group. *N Engl J Med.* Aug 25, 1994;331(8):489–495.

43. Cohen DJ, Baim DS. Coronary stenting: costly or cost-effective? *J Invasive Cardiol.* 1995;7(Suppl A):36A–42A.

44. Cohen DJ, Breall JA, Ho KK, et al. Economics of elective coronary revascularization. Comparison of costs and charges for conventional angioplasty, directional atherectomy, stenting and bypass surgery. *J Am Coll Cardiol.* Oct 1993;22(4):1052–1059.

45. Cohen DJ, Breall JA, Ho KK, et al. Evaluating the potential cost-effectiveness of stenting as a treatment for symptomatic single-vessel coronary disease. Use of a decision-analytic model. *Circulation.* Apr 1994;89(4):1859–1874.

46. Baim DS. New technologies in interventional cardiology. *Curr Opin Cardiol.* Jly 1993;8(4):637–644.

47. Baim DS. ASCENT Trial N evaluation of the ACS multi-link stent. *J Invasive Cardiol.* Apr 1998;10(Suppl B):53B–54B.

48. Kereiakes D, Linnemeier TJ, Baim DS, et al. Usefulness of stent length in predicting in-stent restenosis (the MULTI-LINK stent trials). *Am J Cardiol.* Aug 1, 2000;86(3): 336–341.

49. Fitzgerald PJ, Oshima A, Hayase M, et al. Final results of the Can Routine Ultrasound Influence Stent Expansion (CRUISE) study. *Circulation.* Aug 1, 2000;102(5):523–530.

50. Laham RJ, Ho KK, Baim DS, et al. Multivessel Palmaz-Schatz stenting: early results and one-year outcome. *J Am Coll Cardiol.* 1997;30(1):180–185.

51. Caines AE, Massad MG, Kpodonu J, et al. Outcomes of coronary artery bypass grafting versus percutaneous coronary intervention and medical therapy for multivessel disease with and without left ventricular dysfunction. *Cardiology.* 2004;101(1–3):21–28.

52. Legrand VM, Serruys PW, Unger F, et al. Three-year outcome after coronary stenting versus bypass surgery for the treatment of multivessel disease. *Circulation.* Mar 9, 2004;109(9):1114–1120.

53. Yock CA, Boothroyd DB, Owens DK, et al. Cost-effectiveness of bypass surgery versus stenting in patients with multivessel coronary artery disease. *Am J Med.* Oct 1, 2003;115(5):382–389.

54. The ARTS (Arterial Revascularization Therapies Study). Background, goals and methods. *Int J Cardiovasc Intervent.* 1999;2(1):41–50.

55. Grube E, Gerckens U, Muller R, et al. Drug eluting stents: initial experiences. *Z Kardiol.* 2002;91(Suppl 3):44–48.

56. Ekstein S, Elami A, Merin G, et al. Balloon angioplasty versus bypass grafting in the era of coronary stenting. *Isr Med Assoc J.* Aug 2002;4(8):583–589.

57. de Feyter PJ, Serruys PW, Unger F, et al. Bypass surgery versus stenting for the treatment of multivessel disease in patients with unstable angina compared with stable angina. *Circulation.* May 21, 2002;105(20):2367–2372.

58. Popma JJ, Suntharalingam M, Lansky AJ, et al. Randomized trial of 90Sr/90Y beta-radiation versus placebo control for treatment of in-stent restenosis. *Circulation.* Aug 27, 2002;106(9):1090–1096.

59. Lansky AJ, Dangas G, Mehran R, et al. Quantitative angiographic methods for appropriate end-point analysis, edge-effect evaluation, and prediction of recurrent restenosis after coronary brachytherapy with gamma irradiation. *J Am Coll Cardiol.* Jan 16, 2002;39(2):274–280.

60. Waksman R, Bhargava B, White L, et al. Intracoronary beta-radiation therapy inhibits recurrence of in-stent restenosis. *Circulation.* Apr 25, 2000;101(16):1895–1898.

61. Ajani AE, Waksman R, Sharma AK, et al. Three-year follow-up after intracoronary gamma radiation therapy for in-stent restenosis. Original WRIST. Washington Radiation for In-Stent Restenosis Trial. *Cardiovasc Radiat Med.* Oct–Dec 2001;2(4): 200–204.

62. Teirstein P, Reilly JP. Late stent thrombosis in brachytherapy: the role of long-term antiplatelet therapy. *J Invasive Cardiol.* Mar 2002;14(3):109–114.

63. Teirstein PS, Massullo V, Jani S, et al. Three-year clinical and angiographic follow-up after intracoronary radiation: results of a randomized clinical trial. *Circulation.* Feb 1, 2000;101(4):360–365.

64. Shi Y, Fard A, Galeo A, et al. Transcatheter delivery of c-myc antisense oligomers reduces neointimal formation in a porcine model of coronary artery balloon injury. *Circulation.* 1994;90(2):944–951.

65. Gottsauner-Wolf M, Jang Y, Penn MS, et al. Quantitative evaluation of local drug delivery using the InfusaSleeve catheter. *Cathet Cardiovasc Diagn.* 1997;42(1):102–108.
66. Kornowski R, Hong MK, Tio FO, et al. A randomized animal study evaluating the efficacies of locally delivered heparin and urokinase for reducing in-stent restenosis. *Coron Artery Dis.* May 1997;8(5):293–298.
67. Hong MK, Kent KM, Mehran R, et al. Continuous subcutaneous angiopeptin treatment significantly reduces neointimal hyperplasia in a porcine coronary in-stent restenosis model. *Circulation.* Jan 21, 1997;95(2):449–454.
68. Kim WH, Hong MK, Kornowski R, et al. Saline infusion via local drug delivery catheters is associated with increased neointimal hyperplasia in a porcine coronary in-stent restenosis model. *Coron Artery Dis.* Dec 1999;10(8):629–632.
69. Wilensky RL, Tanguay JF, Ito S, et al. Heparin infusion prior to stenting (HIPS) trial: final results of a prospective, randomized, controlled trial evaluating the effects of local vascular delivery on intimal hyperplasia. *Am Heart J.* Jun 2000;139(6):1061–1070.
70. Kipshidze N, Moses J, Shankar LR, et al. Perspectives on antisense therapy for the prevention of restenosis. *Curr Opin Mol Ther.* Jun 2001;3(3):265–277.
71. Regar E, Sianos G, Serruys PW. Stent development and local drug delivery. *Br Med Bull.* 2001;59:227–248.
72. de Maat MP, Jukema JW, Ye S, et al. Effect of the stromelysin-1 promoter on efficacy of pravastatin in coronary atherosclerosis and restenosis. *Am J Cardiol.* 1999;83(6):852–856.
73. Engelmann C, Panis Y, Bolard J, et al. Liposomal encapsulation of ganciclovir enhances the efficacy of herpes simplex virus type 1 thymidine kinase suicide gene therapy against hepatic tumors in rats. *Hum Gene Ther.* 1999;10(9):1545–1551.
74. Fortunato JE, Mauceri HJ, Kocharyan H, et al. Gene therapy enhances the antiproliferative effect of radiation in intimal hyperplasia. *J Surg Res.* 2000;89(2):155–162.
75. Nikol S, Hofling B. Gene therapy for restenosis: progress or frustration? *J Invasive Cardiol.* 1998;10(8):506–514.
76. Natarajan R, Pei H, Gu JL, et al. Evidence for 12-lipoxygenase induction in the vessel wall following balloon injury. *Cardiovasc Res.* 1999;41(2):489–499.
77. Takahashi A, Taniguchi T, Ishikawa Y, et al. Tranilast inhibits vascular smooth muscle cell growth and intimal hyperplasia by induction of p21(waf1/cip1/sdi1) and p53. *Circ Res.* 1999;84(5):543–550.
78. Todaka T, Yokoyama C, Yanamoto H, et al. Gene transfer of human prostacyclin synthase prevents neointimal formation after carotid balloon injury in rats. *Stroke.* 1999;30(2):419–426.
79. Serruys PW, Emanuelsson H, van der Giessen W, et al. Heparin-coated Palmaz-Schatz stents in human coronary arteries. Early outcome of the Benestent-II Pilot Study. *Circulation.* Feb 1, 1996;93(3):412–422.
80. Serruys PW, Kay IP. Benestent II, a remake of benestent I? Or a step towards the era of stentoplasty? *Eur Heart J.* Jun 1999;20(11):779–781.
81. Serruys P. A progress report from BENESTENT II: Heparin coating, restenosis and cost-effectiveness. *J Invasive Cardiol.* 1996;8(Suppl E):22E–24E.
82. Marx SO, Marks AR. Bench to bedside: the development of rapamycin and its application to stent restenosis. *Circulation.* Aug 21, 2001;104(8):852–855.
83. Marks AR. Attacking heart disease with novel molecular tools. *Bull N Y Acad Med.* Summer 1996;73(1):25–36.
84. Sousa JE, Costa MA, Abizaid AC, et al. Sustained suppression of neointimal proliferation by sirolimus-eluting stents: one-year angiographic and intravascular ultrasound follow-up. *Circulation.* Oct 23, 2001;104(17):2007–2011.
85. Rensing BJ, Vos J, Smits PC, et al. Coronary restenosis elimination with a sirolimus eluting stent: first European human experience with 6-month angiographic and intravascular ultrasonic follow-up. *Eur Heart J.* Nov 2001;22(22):2125–2130.

86. Kahan BD. Sirolimus: a ten-year perspective. *Transplant Proc.* Jan–Feb 2004;36(1):71–75.
87. Mayer C, Zhao J, Yuan X, et al. mTOR-dependent activation of the transcription factor TIF-IA links rRNA synthesis to nutrient availability. *Genes Dev.* Feb 15, 2004;18(4):423–434.
88. Dutcher JP. Mammalian target of rapamycin (mTOR) inhibitors. *Curr Oncol Rep.* Mar 2004;6(2):111–115.
89. Wendel HG, De Stanchina E, Fridman JS, et al. Survival signalling by Akt and eIF4E in oncogenesis and cancer therapy. *Nature.* Mar 18, 2004;428(6980):332–337.
90. Huang CC, Lee CC, Hsu KS. An investigation into signal transduction mechanisms involved in insulin-induced long-term depression in the CA1 region of the hippocampus. *J Neurochem.* Apr 2004;89(1):217–231.
91. Bruns CJ, Koehl GE, Guba M, et al. Rapamycin-induced endothelial cell death and tumor vessel thrombosis potentiate cytotoxic therapy against pancreatic cancer. *Clin Cancer Res.* Mar 15, 2004;10(6):2109–2119.
92. Suzuki T, Kopia G, Hayashi S, et al. Stent-based delivery of sirolimus reduces neointimal formation in a porcine coronary model. *Circulation.* Sept 4, 2001;104(10):1188–1193.
93. Sollott SJ, Cheng L, Pauly RR, et al. Taxol inhibits neointimal smooth muscle cell accumulation after angioplasty in the rat. *J Clin Invest.* Apr 1995;95(4):1869–1876.
94. Axel DI, Kunert W, Goggelmann C, et al. Paclitaxel inhibits arterial smooth muscle cell proliferation and migration in vitro and in vivo using local drug delivery. *Circulation.* Jly 15, 1997;96(2):636–645.
95. Herdeg C, Oberhoff M, Karsch KR. Antiproliferative stent coatings: Taxol and related compounds. *Semin Interv Cardiol.* Sept–Dec 1998;3(3–4):197–199.
96. Suh H, Jeong B, Rathi R, et al. Regulation of smooth muscle cell proliferation using paclitaxel-loaded poly(ethylene oxide)-poly(lactide/glycolide) nanospheres. *J Biomed Mater Res.* Nov 1998;42(2):331–338.
97. Herdeg C, Oberhoff M, Baumbach A, et al. Local paclitaxel delivery for the prevention of restenosis: biological effects and efficacy in vivo. *J Am Coll Cardiol.* Jun 2000;35(7):1969–1976.
98. Halkin A, Stone GW. Polymer-based paclitaxel-eluting stents in percutaneous coronary intervention: a review of the TAXUS trials. *J Interv Cardiol.* Oct 2004;17(5):271–282.
99. Scheller B, Speck U, Abramjuk C, et al. Paclitaxel balloon coating, a novel method for prevention and therapy of restenosis. *Circulation.* Aug 17, 2004;110(7):810–814.
100. Oberhoff M, Kunert W, Herdeg C, et al. Inhibition of smooth muscle cell proliferation after local drug delivery of the antimitotic drug paclitaxel using a porous balloon catheter. *Basic Res Cardiol.* May–Jun 2001;96(3):275–282.
101. Burke SE, Lubbers NL, Chen YW, et al. Neointimal formation after balloon-induced vascular injury in Yucatan minipigs is reduced by oral rapamycin. *J Cardiovasc Pharmacol.* Jun 1999;33(6):829–835.
102. Gallo R, Padurean A, Jayaraman T, et al. Inhibition of intimal thickening after balloon angioplasty in porcine coronary arteries by targeting regulators of the cell cycle. *Circulation.* Apr 27, 1999;99(16):2164–2170.
103. Dell CP. Antiproliferative naphthopyrans: biological activity, mechanistic studies and therapeutic potential. *Curr Med Chem.* Jun 1998;5(3):179–194.
104. Poon M, Marx SO, Gallo R, et al. Rapamycin inhibits vascular smooth muscle cell migration. *J Clin Invest.* Nov 15, 1996;98(10):2277–2283.
105. Oberhoff M, Herdeg C, Baumbach A, et al. Stent-based antirestenotic coatings (sirolimus/paclitaxel). *Catheter Cardiovasc Interv.* Mar 2002;55(3):404–408.
106. Sousa JE, Costa MA, Abizaid A, et al. Lack of neointimal proliferation after implantation of sirolimus-coated stents in human coronary arteries: a quantitative coronary angiography and three-dimensional intravascular ultrasound study. *Circulation.* Jan 16, 2001;103(2):192–195.

107. Sousa JE, Costa MA, Sousa AG, et al. Two-year angiographic and intravascular ultrasound follow-up after implantation of sirolimus-eluting stents in human coronary arteries. *Circulation.* Jan 28, 2003;107(3):381–383.

108. Regar E, Serruys PW, Bode C, et al. Angiographic findings of the multicenter Randomized Study with the Sirolimus-Eluting Bx Velocity Balloon-Expandable Stent (RAVEL): sirolimus-eluting stents inhibit restenosis irrespective of the vessel size. *Circulation.* Oct 8, 2002;106(15):1949–1956.

109. Morice MC, Serruys PW, Sousa JE, et al. A randomized comparison of a sirolimus-eluting stent with a standard stent for coronary revascularization. *N Engl J Med.* Jun 6, 2002;346(23):1773–1780.

110. Degertekin M, Serruys PW, Foley DP, et al. Persistent inhibition of neointimal hyperplasia after sirolimus-eluting stent implantation: long-term (up to 2 years) clinical, angiographic, and intravascular ultrasound follow-up. *Circulation.* Sept 24, 2002;106(13):1610–1613.

111. Tanabe K, Gijsen FJ, Degertekin M, et al. Images in Cardiovascular Medicine. True three-dimensional reconstructed images showing lumen enlargement after sirolimus-eluting stent implantation. *Circulation.* Nov 26, 2002;106(22):e179–e180.

112. Fajadet J, Morice MC, Bode C, et al. Maintenance of long-term clinical benefit with sirolimus-eluting coronary stents: three-year results of the RAVEL trial. *Circulation.* Mar 1, 2005;111(8):1040–1044.

113. Moses JW, Leon MB, Popma JJ, et al. Sirolimus-eluting stents versus standard stents in patients with stenosis in a native coronary artery. *N Engl J Med.* Oct 2, 2003;349(14):1315–1323.

114. Schofer J. Lessons from the E-SIRIUS trial. *Ital Heart J.* Jan 2004;5(1):1–2.

115. Schluter M, Schofer J, Gershlick AH, et al. Direct stenting of native de novo coronary artery lesions with the sirolimus-eluting stent: a post hoc subanalysis of the pooled E- and C-SIRIUS trials. *J Am Coll Cardiol.* Jan 4, 2005;45(1):10–13.

116. Schofer J, Schluter M, Gershlick AH, et al. Sirolimus-eluting stents for treatment of patients with long atherosclerotic lesions in small coronary arteries: double-blind, randomised controlled trial (E-SIRIUS). *Lancet.* Oct 4, 2003;362(9390):1093–1099.

117. Lemos PA, Lee CH, Degertekin M, et al. Early outcome after sirolimus-eluting stent implantation in patients with acute coronary syndromes: insights from the Rapamycin-Eluting Stent Evaluated At Rotterdam Cardiology Hospital (RESEARCH) registry. *J Am Coll Cardiol.* Jun 4, 2003;41(11):2093–2099.

118. Lemos PA, Serruys PW, van Domburg RT, et al. Unrestricted utilization of sirolimus-eluting stents compared with conventional bare stent implantation in the "real world": the Rapamycin-Eluting Stent Evaluated At Rotterdam Cardiology Hospital (RESEARCH) registry. *Circulation.* Jan 20, 2004;109(2):190–195.

119. Lemos PA, Hoye A, Goedhart D, et al. Clinical, angiographic, and procedural predictors of angiographic restenosis after sirolimus-eluting stent implantation in complex patients: an evaluation from the Rapamycin-Eluting Stent Evaluated At Rotterdam Cardiology Hospital (RESEARCH) study. *Circulation.* Mar 23, 2004;109(11):1366–1370.

120. Lemos PA, Arampatzis CA, Saia F, et al. Treatment of very small vessels with 2.25-mm diameter sirolimus-eluting stents (from the RESEARCH registry). *Am J Cardiol.* Mar 1, 2004;93(5):633–636.

121. Pedersen SS, Lemos PA, van Vooren PR, et al. Type D personality predicts death or myocardial infarction after bare metal stent or sirolimus-eluting stent implantation: a Rapamycin-Eluting Stent Evaluated at Rotterdam Cardiology Hospital (RESEARCH) registry substudy. *J Am Coll Cardiol.* Sept 1, 2004;44(5):997–1001.

122. Park SJ, Kim YH, Lee BK, et al. Sirolimus-eluting stent implantation for unprotected left main coronary artery stenosis: comparison with bare metal stent implantation. *J Am Coll Cardiol.* Feb 1, 2005;45(3):351–356.

123. Nakamura S, Muthusamy TS, Bae JH, et al. Impact of sirolimus-eluting stent on the outcome of patients with chronic total occlusions. *Am J Cardiol.* Jan 15, 2005;95(2):161–166.
124. Lemos PA, Arampatzis CA, Hoye A, et al. Impact of baseline renal function on mortality after percutaneous coronary intervention with sirolimus-eluting stents or bare metal stents. *Am J Cardiol.* Jan 15, 2005;95(2):167–172.
125. Khattab AA, Hamm CW, Senges J, et al. Sirolimus-eluting stent treatment for isolated proximal left anterior descending artery stenoses. Results from the prospective multicenter German Cypher Registry. *Z Kardiol.* Mar 2005;94(3):187–192.
126. Iakovou I, Stankovic G, Montorfano M, et al. Is overdilatation of 3.0 mm sirolimus-eluting stent associated with a higher restenosis rate? *Catheter Cardiovasc Interv.* Feb 2005;64(2):129–133.
127. Iofina E, Haager PK, Radke PW, et al. Sirolimus- and paclitaxel-eluting stents in comparison with balloon angioplasty for treatment of in-stent restenosis. *Catheter Cardiovasc Interv.* Jan 2005;64(1):28–34.
128. Kastrati A, Mehilli J, von Beckerath N, et al. Sirolimus-eluting stent or paclitaxel-eluting stent vs balloon angioplasty for prevention of recurrences in patients with coronary in-stent restenosis: a randomized controlled trial. *JAMA.* Jan 12, 2005;293(2):165–171.
129. Ge L, Tsagalou E, Iakovou I, et al. In-hospital and nine-month outcome of treatment of coronary bifurcational lesions with sirolimus-eluting stent. *Am J Cardiol.* Mar 15, 2005;95(6):757–760.
130. Duda SH, Bosiers M, Lammer J, et al. Sirolimus-eluting versus bare nitinol stent for obstructive superficial femoral artery disease: The SIROCCO II Trial. *J Vasc Interv Radiol.* Mar 2005;16(3):331–338.
131. Aziz S, Ramsdale DR. Commentary: Sirolimus-eluting stents for the treatment of atherosclerotic ostial lesions. *J Invasive Cardiol.* Jan 2005;17(1):13.
132. Chieffo A, Stankovic G, Bonizzoni E, et al. Early and mid-term results of drug-eluting stent implantation in unprotected left main. *Circulation.* Feb 15, 2005;111(6):791–795.
133. Werner GS, Emig U, Krack A, et al. Sirolimus-eluting stents for the prevention of restenosis in a worst-case scenario of diffuse and recurrent in-stent restenosis. *Catheter Cardiovasc Interv.* Nov 2004;63(3):259–264.
134. Vijayakumar M, Lemos PA, Hoye A, et al. Effectiveness of sirolimus-eluting stent implantation for the treatment of coronary artery disease in octogenarians. *Am J Cardiol.* Oct 1, 2004;94(7):909–913.
135. Serruys PW, Lemos PA, van Hout BA. Sirolimus eluting stent implantation for patients with multivessel disease: rationale for the Arterial Revascularisation Therapies Study part II (ARTS II). *Heart.* Sept 2004;90(9):995–998.
136. Sarembock IJ. Stent restenosis and the use of drug-eluting stents in patients with diabetes mellitus. *Curr Diab Rep.* Feb 2004;4(1):13–19.
137. Saia F, Lemos PA, Arampatzis CA, et al. Clinical and angiographic outcomes after overdilatation of undersized sirolimus-eluting stents with largely oversized balloons: an observational study. *Catheter Cardiovasc Interv.* Apr 2004;61(4):455–460.
138. Saia F, Lemos PA, Arampatzis CA, et al. Routine sirolimus eluting stent implantation for unselected in-stent restenosis: insights from the rapamycin eluting stent evaluated at Rotterdam Cardiology Hospital (RESEARCH) registry. *Heart.* Oct 2004;90(10):1183–1188.
139. Ormiston JA, Currie E, Webster MW, et al. Drug-eluting stents for coronary bifurcations: insights into the crush technique. *Catheter Cardiovasc Interv.* Nov 2004;63(3):332–336.
140. Melikian N, Airoldi F, Di Mario C. Coronary bifurcation stenting. Current techniques, outcome and possible future developments. *Minerva Cardioangiol.* Oct 2004;52(5):365–378.

141. Goy JJ, Stauffer JC, Siegenthaler M, et al. A prospective randomized comparison between paclitaxel and sirolimus stents in the real world of interventional cardiology: the TAXi trial. *J Am Coll Cardiol.* Jan 18, 2005;45(2):308–311.

142. Cohen DJ, Bakhai A, Shi C, et al. Cost-effectiveness of sirolimus-eluting stents for treatment of complex coronary stenoses: results from the Sirolimus-eluting balloon expandable stent in the treatment of patients with de novo native coronary artery lesions (SIRIUS) trial. *Circulation.* Aug 3, 2004;110(5):508–514.

143. Shrive FM, Manns BJ, Galbraith PD, et al. Economic evaluation of sirolimus-eluting stents. *CMAJ.* Feb 1, 2005;172(3):345–351.

144. Grube E, Bullesfeld L. Initial experience with paclitaxel-coated stents. *J Interv Cardiol.* Dec 2002;15(6):471–475.

145. Grube E, Silber S, Hauptmann KE, et al. TAXUS I: six- and twelve-month results from a randomized, double-blind trial on a slow-release paclitaxel-eluting stent for de novo coronary lesions. *Circulation.* Jan 7, 2003;107(1):38–42.

146. Colombo A, Drzewiecki J, Banning A, et al. Randomized study to assess the effectiveness of slow- and moderate-release polymer-based paclitaxel-eluting stents for coronary artery lesions. *Circulation.* Aug 19, 2003;108(7):788–794.

147. Silber S, Hamburger J, Grube E, et al. Direct stenting with TAXUS stents seems to be as safe and effective as with predilatation. A post hoc analysis of TAXUS II. *Herz.* Mar 2004;29(2):171–180.

148. Fox R. American Heart Association 2001 scientific sessions: late-breaking science-drug-eluting stents. *Circulation.* Nov 20, 2001;104(21):E9052.

149. Farb A, Heller PF, Shroff S, et al. Pathological analysis of local delivery of paclitaxel via a polymer-coated stent. *Circulation.* Jly 24, 2001;104(4):473–479.

150. Liistro F, Stankovic G, Di Mario C, et al. First clinical experience with a paclitaxel derivate-eluting polymer stent system implantation for in-stent restenosis: immediate and long-term clinical and angiographic outcome. *Circulation.* Apr 23, 2002;105(16):1883–1886.

151. Bullesfeld L, Gerckens U, Muller R, et al. Long-term evaluation of paclitaxel-coated stents for treatment of native coronary lesions. First results of both the clinical and angiographic 18 month follow-up of TAXUS I. *Z Kardiol.* Oct 2003;92(10):825–832.

152. Stone GW, Ellis SG, Cox DA, et al. One-year clinical results with the slow-release, polymer-based, paclitaxel-eluting TAXUS stent: the TAXUS-IV trial. *Circulation.* Apr 27, 2004;109(16):1942–1947.

153. Perin EC. Choosing a drug-eluting stent: a comparison between CYPHER and TAXUS. *Rev Cardiovasc Med.* 2005;6(Suppl 1):S13–S21.

154. Fajadet J, Wijns W, Laarman GJ, et al. Randomized, double-blind, multicenter study of the Endeavor zotarolimus-eluting phosphorylcholine-encapsulated stent for treatment of native coronary artery lesions: clinical and angiographic results of the ENDEAVOR II trial. *Circulation.* Aug 22, 2006;114(8):798–806.

155. Fajadet J, Wijns W, Laarman GJ, et al. Randomized, double-blind, multicenter study of the Endeavor zotarolimus-eluting phosphorylcholine-encapsulated stent for treatment of native coronary artery lesions. Clinical and angiographic results of the ENDEAVOR II Trial. *Minerva Cardioangiol.* Feb 2007;55(1):1–18.

156. Jain AK, Meredith IT, Lotan C, et al. Real-world safety and efficacy of the endeavor zotarolimus-eluting stent: early data from the E-Five Registry. *Am J Cardiol.* Oct 22, 2007;100(8B):77 M–83 M.

157. Kandzari DE, Leon MB, Popma JJ, et al. Comparison of zotarolimus-eluting and sirolimus-eluting stents in patients with native coronary artery disease: a randomized controlled trial. *J Am Coll Cardiol.* Dec 19, 2006;48(12):2440–2447.

158. Mehta RH, Leon MB, Sketch MH, Jr. The relation between clinical features, angiographic findings, and the target lesion revascularization rate in patients receiving the endeavor zotarolimus-eluting stent for treatment of native coronary artery disease: an

analysis of ENDEAVOR I, ENDEAVOR II, ENDEAVOR II Continued Access Registry, and ENDEAVOR III. *Am J Cardiol.* Oct 22, 2007;100(8B):62 M–70 M.

159. Meredith IT, Ormiston J, Whitbourn R, et al. Four-year clinical follow-up after implantation of the endeavor zotarolimus-eluting stent: ENDEAVOR I, the first-in-human study. *Am J Cardiol.* Oct 22, 2007;100(8B):56 M–61 M.

160. Sakurai R, Bonneau HN, Honda Y, et al. Intravascular ultrasound findings in ENDEAVOR II and ENDEAVOR III. *Am J Cardiol.* Oct 22, 2007;100(8B):71 M–76 M.

161. Cohen H, Williams D, Holmes D, et al. Use of drug-eluting stents in contemporary intervention: a comparison of bare metal stent use in the National Heart, Lung, and Blood Institute Dynamic Registry. *J Am Coll Cardiol.* 2005;45:63A.

162. Torguson R, Waksman R. Overview of the 2007 Food and Drug Administration Circulatory System Devices Panel Meeting on the Xience V Everolimus-Eluting Coronary Stent. *Am J Cardiol.* 2008;102:1624–1630.

163. Smith SC, Jr., Feldman TE, Hirshfeld JW, Jr., et al. ACC/AHA/SCAI 2005 guideline update for percutaneous coronary intervention: a report of the American College of Cardiology/American Heart Association Task Force on Practice Guidelines (ACC/AHA/SCAI Writing Committee to Update 2001 Guidelines for Percutaneous Coronary Intervention). *Circulation.* Feb 21, 2006;113(7):e166–e286.

164. Hannan EL, Racz MJ, Arani DT, et al. A comparison of short- and long-term outcomes for balloon angioplasty and coronary stent placement. *J Am Coll Cardiol.* Aug 2000;36(2):395–403.

165. AHA. AHA statistics. *AHA Website.* 2004;2004.

166. Kirtane AJ, Moses JW. Revascularization in heart failure: the role of percutaneous coronary intervention. *Heart Fail Clin.* Apr 2007;3(2):229–235.

167. Gioia G, Matthai W, Gillin K, et al. Revascularization in severe left ventricular dysfunction: outcome comparison of drug-eluting stent implantation versus coronary artery by-pass grafting. *Catheter Cardiovasc Interv.* Jly 1, 2007;70(1):26–33.

168. Fox KA, Steg PG, Eagle KA, et al. Decline in rates of death and heart failure in acute coronary syndromes, 1999–2006. *JAMA.* May 2, 2007;297(17):1892–1900.

169. Mukherjee D, Bhatt DL, Roe MT, et al. Direct myocardial revascularization and angiogenesis – how many patients might be eligible? *Am J Cardiol.* Sept 1, 1999;84(5):598–600, A598.

170. Hennebry TA, Saucedo JF. "No-option" patients: a nightmare today, a future with hope. *J Interv Cardiol.* Apr 1, 2004;17(2):93–94.

171. Rosinberg A, Khan TA, Sellke FW, et al. Therapeutic angiogenesis for myocardial ischemia. *Expert Rev Cardiovasc Ther.* Mar 2004;2(2):271–283.

172. Reichenspurner H, Boehm DH, Welz A, et al. Minimally invasive coronary artery bypass grafting: port-access approach versus off-pump techniques. *Ann Thorac Surg.* Sept 1998;66(3):1036–1040.

173. Medina A, de Lezo JS, Melian F, et al. Successful stent ablation with rotational atherectomy. *Catheter Cardiovasc Interv.* Dec 2003;60(4):501–504.

174. Mauri L, Reisman M, Buchbinder M, et al. Comparison of rotational atherectomy with conventional balloon angioplasty in the prevention of restenosis of small coronary arteries: results of the Dilatation vs Ablation Revascularization Trial Targeting Restenosis (DART). *Am Heart J.* May 2003;145(5):847–854.

175. Lev E, Teplitsky I, Fuchs S, et al. Clinical experiences using the FilterWire EX for distal embolic protection during complex percutaneous coronary interventions. *Int J Cardiovasc Intervent.* 2004;6(1):28–32.

176. Stone GW, Rogers C, Hermiller J, et al. Randomized comparison of distal protection with a filter-based catheter and a balloon occlusion and aspiration system during percutaneous intervention of diseased saphenous vein aorto-coronary bypass grafts. *Circulation.* Aug 5, 2003;108(5):548–553.

177. Baim DS, Wahr D, George B, et al. Randomized trial of a distal embolic protection device during percutaneous intervention of saphenous vein aorto-coronary bypass grafts. *Circulation*. Mar 19, 2002;105(11):1285–1290.

178. Tadros P. Successful revascularization of a long chronic total occlusion of the right coronary artery utilizing the frontrunner X39 CTO catheter system. *J Invasive Cardiol*. Nov 2003;15(11):3.

179. Laham RJ, Simons M, Tofukuji M, et al. Modulation of myocardial perfusion and vascular reactivity by pericardial basic fibroblast growth factor: insight into ischemia-induced reduction in endothelium-dependent vasodilatation. *J Thorac Cardiovasc Surg*. 1998;116(6):1022–1028.

180. Laham RJ, Simons M, Sellke F. Gene transfer for angiogenesis in coronary artery disease. *Annu Rev Med*. 2001;52:485–502.

181. Laham RJ, Simons M, Pearlman JD, et al. Magnetic resonance imaging demonstrates improved regional systolic wall motion and thickening and myocardial perfusion of myocardial territories treated by laser myocardial revascularization. *J Am Coll Cardiol*. Jan 2, 2002;39(1):1–8.

182. Laham RJ, Simons M. Basic fibroblast growth factor protein for coronary artery disease. In: Leon MB, Kornowski R, Epstein SE, eds. *Handbook of Myocardial Revascularization and Angiogenesis*. New York: Martin Dunitz Ltd; 1999:175–187.

183. Laham RJ, Simons M. Growth factor therapy in ischemic heart disease. In: Rubanyi G, ed. *Angiogenesis in Health and Disease*. New York: Marcel Decker; 2000:451–475.

184. Laham RJ, Rezaee M, Post M, et al. Intracoronary and intravenous administration of basic fibroblast growth factor: myocardial and tissue distribution. *Drug Metab Dispos*. 1999;27(7):821–826.

185. Laham RJ, Mannam A, Post MJ, et al. Gene transfer to induce angiogenesis in myocardial and limb ischaemia. *Expert Opin Biol Ther*. Nov 2001;1(6):985–994.

186. Laham RJ, Oettgen P. Bone marrow transplantation for the heart: fact or fiction? *Lancet*. Jan 4, 2003;361(9351):11–12.

187. Laham RJ, Post M, Sellke FW, et al. Therapeutic angiogenesis using local perivascular and pericardial delivery. *Curr Interv Cardiol Rep*. 2000;2(3):213–217.

188. Laham RJ, Chronos NA, Pike M, et al. Intracoronary basic fibroblast growth factor (FGF-2) in patients with severe ischemic heart disease: results of a phase I open-label dose escalation study. *J Am Coll Cardiol*. 2000;36(7):2132–2139.

189. Laham R, Sellke F, Pearlman J. Magnetic resonance blood-arrival maps provides accurate assessment of myocardial perfusion and collaterization in therapeutic angiogenesis. *Circulation*. 1998;98:I-373.

190. Laham R, Rezaee M, Post M, et al. Intrapericardial delivery of fibroblast growth factor-2 induces neovascularization in a porcine model of chronic myocardial ischemia. *J Pharmacol Exp Ther*. 2000;292:795–802.

191. Rana JS, Mannam A, Donnell-Fink L, et al. Longevity of the placebo effect in the therapeutic angiogenesis and laser myocardial revascularization trials in patients with coronary heart disease. *Am J Cardiol*. Jun 15, 2005;95(12):1456–1459.

192. Laham RJ. *Angiogenesis and Direct Myocardial Revascularization*. Totowa, NJ: Humana Press; 2005.

193. Sellke F, Laham RJ, Voisine P, et al. Therapeutic angiogenesis for the treatment of coronary artery disease: can we improve the results. *J Jpn Coll Angiol*. 2005;45: 221–232.

194. Leon MB, Kornowski R, Downey WE, et al. A blinded, randomized, placebo-controlled trial of percutaneous laser myocardial revascularization to improve angina symptoms in patients with severe coronary disease. *J Am Coll Cardiol*. Nov 15, 2005;46(10):1812–1819.

195. Lee SU, Wykrzykowska JJ, Laham RJ. Angiogenesis: bench to bedside, have we learned anything? *Toxicol Pathol*. 2006;34(1):3–10.

196. de Jongste MJ, Staal MJ. Preliminary results of a randomized study on the clinical efficacy of spinal cord stimulation for refractory severe angina pectoris. *Acta Neurochir Suppl (Wien).* 1993;58:161–164.
197. de Jongste MJ, Haaksma J, Hautvast RW, et al. Effects of spinal cord stimulation on myocardial ischaemia during daily life in patients with severe coronary artery disease. A prospective ambulatory electrocardiographic study. *Br Heart J.* May 1994;71(5):413–418.
198. Hautvast RW, DeJongste MJ, Staal MJ, et al. Spinal cord stimulation in chronic intractable angina pectoris: a randomized, controlled efficacy study. *Am Heart J.* Dec 1998;136(6):1114–1120.
199. Murray S, Carson KG, Ewings PD, et al. Spinal cord stimulation significantly decreases the need for acute hospital admission for chest pain in patients with refractory angina pectoris. *Heart.* Jly 1999;82(1):89–92.
200. Linnemeier G, Rutter MK, Barsness G, et al. Enhanced External Counterpulsation for the relief of angina in patients with diabetes: safety, efficacy and 1-year clinical outcomes. *Am Heart J.* Sept 2003;146(3):453–458.
201. Linnemeier G, Michaels AD, Soran O, et al. Enhanced external counterpulsation in the management of angina in the elderly. *Am J Geriatr Cardiol.* Mar–Apr 2003;12(2):90–94; quiz 94–96.
202. Humphreys DR. Treating angina with EECP therapy. *Nurse Pract.* Feb 2003;28(2):7.
203. Blazing MA, Crawford LE. Enhanced External Counterpulsation (EECP): enough evidence to support this and the next wave? *Am Heart J.* Sept 2003;146(3):383–384.
204. Michaels AD, Accad M, Ports TA, et al. Left ventricular systolic unloading and augmentation of intracoronary pressure and Doppler flow during enhanced external counterpulsation. *Circulation.* Sept 3, 2002;106(10):1237–1242.
205. Michaels AD, Linnemeier G, Soran O, et al. Two-year outcomes after enhanced external counterpulsation for stable angina pectoris (from the International EECP Patient Registry [IEPR]). *Am J Cardiol.* Feb 15, 2004;93(4):461–464.
206. Arora RR, Chou TM, Jain D, et al. The multicenter study of enhanced external counterpulsation (MUST-EECP): effect of EECP on exercise-induced myocardial ischemia and anginal episodes. *J Am Coll Cardiol.* Jun 1999;33(7):1833–1840.

11 Percutaneous Management of Peripheral Arterial Disease

Mobeen A. Sheikh, MD and
Lawrence A. Garcia, MD

CONTENTS

INTRODUCTION
LOWER EXTREMITY
RENAL ARTERY
CAROTID ARTERY
CONCLUSION
REFERENCES

Abstract

Peripheral arterial disease (PAD) affects tens of millions of patients, with the prevalence of the disease directly proportional to age. PAD is a marker for high cardiovascular risk, and many PAD patients have impaired left ventricular function and heart failure. Symptomatic PAD can have effective and durable outcomes with either an endovascular or a surgical intervention. This chapter reviews the clinical approach to PAD as well as the devices available to treat it.

Key Words: Peripheral arterial disease; Heart failure; Coronary artery disease; Medical devices.

1. INTRODUCTION

The term peripheral arterial disease (PAD) is usually synonymous with noncoronary, extracranial occlusive vascular disease. Peripheral arterial disease affects an estimated 40 million Americans, of whom 10 million are symptomatic *(1)*. The prevalence of this disease is directly proportional to

From: *Contemporary Cardiology: Device Therapy in Heart Failure*
Edited by: W.H. Maisel, DOI 10.1007/978-1-59745-424-7_11
© Humana Press, a part of Springer Science+Business Media, LLC 2010

age, with more than 10% of patients over the age of 60 years affected, and PAD is a marker for high-risk patients with a 5-year rate of cardiovascular morbidity and overall mortality as high as 50% (2). Additionally it has been shown that among patients presenting with PAD, as many as two-thirds have objective evidence of significant coronary artery disease (3). Many of these patients have impaired left ventricular function and heart failure. As atherosclerosis is a systemic disease, it remains the major cause of arterial obstructive disease throughout the arterial tree.

Symptomatic PAD can have effective and durable outcomes with either an endovascular or a surgical intervention. The concept of percutaneous intervention for atherosclerotic disease of the lower extremities is not a new one. Dotter and Judkins in 1964 first introduced the technique of catheter-based angioplasty by advancing progressively larger diameter dilatation catheters over a guidewire in peripheral arteries (4) and in 1975 Andreas Gruentzig first developed and then attempted balloon angioplasty in an iliac artery.

In the past decade, endovascular approaches to treat patients with occlusive atherosclerotic peripheral arterial disease have seen a tremendous increase in growth far exceeding that of coronary interventional procedures. This growth rate is due to improved technology and advancements in device systems, improved risk–benefit ratio compared to surgical repair, aggressive endovascular techniques (such as subintimal recanalization of total occlusions), less morbidity and mortality with an endovascular approach, as well as an increase in patient preferences for the less-invasive endovascular approach compared with a surgical revascularization.

The basis of all endovascular therapies is predicated on percutaneous transluminal angioplasty (PTA). Additional options for adjunctive therapy include stenting, atherectomy (laser or mechanical), and cryoplasty (cooling balloon PTA) occupying a role in certain vascular beds and patient subsets. The techniques and outcomes of endovascular therapy will be discussed by vascular bed in this chapter.

2. LOWER EXTREMITY

The severity of lower extremity PAD symptoms runs a spectrum ranging from asymptomatic to intermittent claudication to rest pain and ultimately tissue or limb loss. The term intermittent claudication (IC) refers to exertional pain/discomfort or heaviness that usually occurs in the calves after ambulation and is almost always immediately relieved by rest. However, it is important to note that claudication in its most classic form appears in a minority of patients. Other patients with vascular obstructive disease in proximal/inflow vessels may present with pain in the buttock and thigh region and can often lead to alternative diagnoses such as spinal stenosis or degenerative arthritis.

The term critical limb ischemia (CLI) is reserved for patients with rest pain and/or frank or near tissue loss. Patients with lifestyle-limiting claudication that have failed to respond to pharmacotherapy in addition to an exercise program or those with critical limb ischemia are considered to be candidates for revascularization.

The most dramatic presentation of PAD is acute limb ischemia. Clinically, the presentation of the patient classically is with a painful, pulseless, pale, poikilothermic, paresthetic limb (also known as the 5 Ps). Endovascular management in such cases is primarily catheter-directed thrombolysis followed by adjunctive balloon angioplasty or other adjunctive therapy or technology such as stent placement.

The preferred mode of revascularization (endovascular versus surgical) must be individualized based upon a host of patient, lesion, and operator-dependent characteristics. In general, an endovascular approach to PAD is associated with lower adverse event rates when compared to open surgical revascularization. This generalization is especially true in the case of shorter segment obstructions such as in the superficial femoral artery (SFA) or larger vessel diameter involvement such as in the aorta. As important as this differentiation in approach is, there is still a paucity of randomized trials comparing endovascular and surgical interventions across many anatomic locations. In consideration of certain anatomical and functional characteristics, the lower extremity may be divided into the following arterial segments: aortoiliac, femoropopliteal, and infrapopliteal (also referred to as infrageniculate or tibioperoneal).

This division of the lower extremity into the above-listed arterial segments highlights important differences in terms of indications, techniques/devices, and overall outcomes from an endovascular standpoint and will be discussed in more detail below.

2.1. Aortoiliac Disease

Patients with aortoiliac occlusive disease may present with a variety of symptoms including simple claudication, buttock/thigh claudication, pelvic pain, and/or erectile dysfunction in men (the combination of the latter three symptoms is termed Leriche syndrome). Therapy to this vascular segment has benefited most from the development of endovascular technology since the surgical bypass equivalent traditionally required an intra-abdominal procedure such as an aortofemoral bypass. This surgical procedure has been shown to be associated with significant perioperative mortality in the 2–4% range and complication rates as high as 13% (5). An endovascular approach has been shown to have similar patency rates to surgical revascularization as shown in the Dutch Iliac stent study with 2-year clinical success rate as high as 78% (6).

In many cases and patient presentations, the aortoiliac anatomic locations remains best suited for an endovascular approach. Furthermore, in patients with more severe, multilevel lower extremity PAD obstructions, the aortoiliac level marks a key level for treatment as it represents a principal "inflow" to the leg. The technical success rates of iliac interventions has been listed as greater than 90% *(7–10)* in most series and are more durable than interventions performed in the more distal femoropopliteal segment. The strategies employed for patients with distal aortic, ostial common iliac, and common femoral artery involvement can be different. The Transatlantic Intersociety Consensus (TASC) Working Group have published a morphological classification of lesion types involving the iliac arteries *(11)* (Table 1), which suggests the type of endovascular or surgical revascularization for the specific lesion subset. For example, the consensus recommends an endovascular approach for shorter and more focal lesions, and a surgical approach for TASC D (total occlusions or longer lesions of over 10 cm) lesions. However, given the improved technologies and devices, these recommendations have never been fully implemented and the TASC document was republished in 2007 *(12)*.

Table 1
Transatlantic Intersociety Consensus (TASC) working group classification
of iliac lesions

A	Single stenosis of common or external iliac artery <3 cm long (unilateral or bilateral)
B	Single stenosis 3–10 cm long, not extending into common femoral artery
	Two stenoses of common iliac or external iliac artery <5 cm long not involving the common femoral artery
	Unilateral common iliac artery occlusion
C	Bilateral stenosis of common iliac artery and/or external iliac artery 5–10 cm long not involving the common femoral artery
	Unilateral external iliac artery occlusion not involving the common femoral artery
	Unilateral external iliac artery stenosis extending into the common femoral artery
	Bilateral common iliac artery occlusion
D	Diffuse stenosis of the entire common iliac artery, external iliac artery, and common femoral artery >10 cm long
	Unilateral occlusion of the common iliac artery and external iliac artery
	Bilateral external iliac artery occlusion
	Iliac stenosis adjacent to aortic or iliac aneurysm

There are various technical considerations to be made when performing interventions in the aortoiliac segment. Of particular importance is the obliteration of any pressure gradient across the lesion *(6)*. The common iliac artery has excellent results with PTA alone and patency rates as high as 80% at 1 year if the pressure gradient is less than 10 mmHg at the completion of the intervention *(6)*. Initially used as a bailout for suboptimal results of PTA such as dissection, significant recoil, and residual pressure gradient, stents are now used as primary therapy in most iliac artery endovascular interventions, particularly in longer more complex lesions and total occlusions.

There are primarily two types of stent designs: balloon-expandable and self-expanding. Each has its own special characteristics that make them suitable for particular vascular segments. Balloon-expandable stents are best used in lesions that involve the ostium since they allow precise placement and because their high radial force resists recoil. Because of these characteristics, balloon-expandable stents have become the stent of choice for an ostial common iliac lesion. Self-expanding stents are more conformable and flexible. These characteristics allow for ease of tracking and placement in more tortuous vessels. However, self-expanding stents do not exert much radial strength or much resistance to recoil. Consequently these stents are better suited for nonostial locations such as distal common and proximal external iliac arteries, given the tortuosity of these vessels; the stents are usually oversized to allow for optimal vessel apposition.

Patients with significant bilateral iliac disease or long occlusions, classified as type D lesions as per the TASC criteria to include significant involvement of the common femoral arterial segment, may still be better treated by bypass surgery with a combined common femoral artery endarterectomy.

Given the success and long-term patency rates of endovascular therapies for aortoiliac disease, for many patients, it has become the treatment of choice.

2.2. Femoropopliteal

This section deals with the infrainguinal portion of the arterial supply to the lower extremity: the common femoral, profunda femoral, superficial femoral, and popliteal arteries. The superficial femoral artery (SFA), which constitutes the longest segment of this category, not only is affected by atherosclerosis more frequently than the iliac artery but also more often has occlusive and calcified rather than stenotic disease. Additionally, the SFA experiences unique external forces such as extension, flexion, compression, and torsion whilst coursing through the muscular portion of the thigh. These unique anatomical and functional characteristics of the SFA contribute significantly to the challenges faced in its revascularization strategies.

Although there exists no endovascular "gold standard," historically, surgical revascularization with a femoral to a popliteal bypass (with a venous conduit and an above-the-knee distal anastomosis) was standard treatment of severe femoropopliteal atherosclerotic disease. This graft has an assisted patency rate as high as 81% at 4 years *(13)* and serves as the historical benchmark to which all endovascular procedures are compared. Once again there is a lack of large randomized control trials comparing the different treatment modalities used in the endovascular management of SFA disease. While the durability of a surgical bypass of this segment is good, the perioperative mortality rate and wound complication rate for this procedure range from 1.3 to 6% and 17 to 44%, respectively *(14)*.

Most data are in registry, nonrandomized formats. A more contemporary trial (BASIL) published in 2005 *(15)* was one of the first to demonstrate that in patients presenting with critical limb ischemia suitable for either approach, surgery or endovascular intervention resulted in similar rates of amputation-free survival, while an angioplasty first approach was more cost effective when compared with surgical revascularization. Other data have shown benefits though not long-term durability of lower extremity revascularization with a variety of devices, technologies, or adjunctive pharmacotherapies (for example, the BLASTER trial which examined the possible benefit of concurrent abciximab use in SFA stenting *(16)*, the PARIS trial which examined the role of intravascular radiation therapy after SFA angioplasty *(17)*, the SIROCCO trial that looked into the use of drug-eluting stents to minimize restenosis rates *(18)*, and the VascuCoil trial that examined the use of IntraCoil self-expanding peripheral stent as a primary stenting strategy *(19)*).

PTA alone represents a good option for patients with focal or short segment involvement of the SFA *(20–24)*. However, the nature of disease in the SFA is more commonly diffuse and in many cases restenosis rates may be as high as 60–70% *(22, 23, 25–27)* at 1 year with PTA alone. Because of these restenosis rates, it seemed intuitive that stents would provide more durable patencies. However, stents have not met tremendous success in this anatomic location. Because of the arterial "gymnastics" the SFA undergoes in its normal activities, no stent to date has had a patency rate exceeding 70% in any large trial. Early studies with a stainless steel self-expanding stent *(28)* did not produce the desired superiority over PTA. More recent studies have focused on self-expanding nitinol (nickel and titanium alloy) stents. Although, none has shown better long-term patency rates, they have shown improved patency compared with PTA alone *(29, 30)*. Because of this lack of patency, current recommendation from the TASC and the American College of Cardiology (ACC)/American Heart Association (AHA) do not recommend primary stenting of the SFA and support its use only in case of suboptimal angioplasty results. A more recent study has shown the superiority of primary stenting versus PTA for long lesions (average treated length 132 mm) of the SFA at 1 year *(31)* and thus may mark a change to primary stenting versus a bailout indication.

Since restenosis is the major hurdle in SFA stenting, drug-eluting stents (DES) were also studied in the SFA in the hope to replicate the data on restenosis from the coronaries. To this end, SIRROCO I *(32)* and II *(32)* were trials that compared a bare-metal versus drug-coated self-expanding nitinol stents in 83 patients, which demonstrated the binary restenosis rates at 6 months to be encouraging, but at 9 months the binary restenosis rates in the DES arm were no better than the bare-metal stent group. Because of this, currently, DES has not had a role in SFA treatment. Additional DES trials will further evaluate this question.

Another issue brought to light during these studies was the potential breach in the structural integrity of nitinol stents in the form of stent strut fractures. The reports of stent fracture rates are variable and in SIROCCO I they were reported to occur in 8% of cases. It is still not completely understood, however, to what extent these stent fractures contribute to restenosis, with the vast majority of cases remaining asymptomatic and underdiagnosed. However, other trials have shown that stent strut fractures do occur and do so at sometimes alarming rates *(30)*. These fractures have not been fully characterized but may have some impact on restenosis.

Because restenosis poses such a major challenge in the SFA, there has also been a very robust development of adjunctive technologies in this segment.

Bioresorbable stents are stents that are metallic alloys made to be bioresorbable such that after placement they begin to dissolve and over time no longer are present as an endoprosthesis. Although minimal data are available for these stents, interest remains high in developing methods for drug delivery without the downsides of permanent endoprostheses *(33)*.

Crypoplasty is performed with a special balloon catheter that simultaneously dilates and cools the plaque. The physiologic premise is that cooling induces apoptosis (programmed cell death) of the smooth muscle cells and thus limits smooth muscle proliferation and the resultant restenosis. Limited data on 100 patients from the CHILL registry trial suggest 1-year patency rates of 85% when this technique is utilized on SFA lesions shorter than 10 cm (average lesion length of 7–8 cm) *(34)*. The patency rates have remained good at 3 years of follow-up (albeit in a small number of patients).

Laser atherectomy is performed with an excimer-laser catheter (CliRpath Extreme, Spectranetics Corp., USA). The laser ablates the atheromatous tissue through an energy transfer and microcavitary bubble in front of the laser device. Currently, candidates for this technique are patients with critical limb ischemia who have SFA occlusions and have failed conventional endovascular techniques. The CELLO trial is investigating the effectiveness of this technique.

The underlying premise for *excisional atherectomy* is to remove atherosclerotic plaque; however, unlike PTA, it does not induce barotrauma. It is a useful device in cases where one wishes to avoid stenting (such as the common femoral, popliteal, and profunda femoral artery). The SilverHawk (FoxHollow Technologies, Rosemont, CA, USA) atherectomy catheter is the latest iteration of a directional atherectomy device. Recent reports suggest that use of this device in de novo lesions of the SFA resulted in 73 and 89% primary and secondary clinical patency rates, respectively, at 18 months *(35)*. The multicenter TALON (Treating peripherAls with SiLverHawk: Outcomes collectioN) registry *(36)* not only had a 6-month and 12-month freedom from target vessel revascularization of 90 and 80%, respectively, but also included arterial segments proximal and distal to the SFA. However, with longer lesions, the primary patency rate declines significantly to 50%. In addition, patency rates are even lower in a critical limb population, although the limb salvage rates are quite acceptable.

Covered stents may be used in the SFA. The concept of one approved covered stent, the Gore Viabahn endoprosthesis (Gore and associates, Flagstaff, AZ, USA), is to replicate a percutaneous bypass by creating a new channel for blood flow rather than simply propping open the diseased vessel with a balloon or a stent. The stent's extreme flexibility is an advantage that enables it to conform to the SFA. There have been several studies with favorable 1-year outcomes with the use of this stent in the SFA *(37, 38)* as well as data suggesting comparable outcomes to above-the-knee surgical bypass in selected patients *(39)*. The ongoing VIBRANT trial, which is randomizing patients to nitinol stents or the Viabahn device, will provide further insight into the utility of this device.

In total, the SFA, despite its key anatomic location for PAD and resultant claudication, remains the most challenging and difficult peripheral location to achieve long-term patency with any device. No trial to date has shown superiority and better durability than femoral–popliteal bypass surgery although PTA alone in this anatomic location appears inferior to primary stenting.

2.3. Infrapopliteal

A percutaneous approach to patients with disease in the infrapopliteal segment has been, in the past, exclusively reserved for those with critical limb ischemia. More commonly, revascularization in this vascular territory may be performed as an adjunctive procedure to interventions on the preceding femoropopliteal segment in an attempt to improve outflow and subsequent durability of the femoropopliteal intervention. For patients with critical limb ischemia, the goal is to provide "in-line" (pulsatile, palpable) flow to the foot for limb salvage.

Traditionally, femoral–tibial bypass grafts with venous conduits are the revascularization strategy for limb preservation in patients with significant obstructive disease in this segment. The surgical patency rates have been far lower than those reported with SFA bypass and are typically ~50% at 4 years *(40)*. There are no rigorous studies examining the patency of this segment as more often the goal of therapy has been limb salvage. When "in-line" flow has been restored, limb salvage rates approach 91% *(41)*. Data on restenosis rates of an endovascular approach in this segment are limited; the clinical goal is primarily relief of rest pain, improved wound healing, and limb salvage.

The tibial vessels are considerably smaller (similar in size to coronary vessels) than the more proximal peripheral arteries and are typically high-resistive conduits. For most devices including PTA, stents *(42)*, laser *(43)*, and directional atherectomy *(44)*, limb salvage rates are similar, reaching 85–90% if in-line flow is restored.

Thus, while the SFA should be considered the most difficult territory for long-term patency with an endovascular approach, the infrapopliteal vessels are small with minimal data on long-term patency. Indeed, additional well-conducted scientific studies are needed to better define the long-term patency and clinical benefits of most peripheral endovascular therapies.

3. RENAL ARTERY

The most common cause of renal artery stenosis (RAS) is atherosclerosis although the principal origin of renal atherosclerotic obstruction is extension of atherosclerotic disease from the aorta. The renal artery is also the most common site of fibromuscular dysplasia (FMD), a nonatherosclerotic narrowing that accounts for approximately 10% of all RAS. The incidence of renal artery stenosis in the general population is uncertain; the incidence in patients undergoing coronary angiography may be as high as 19% *(45)*.

The clinical indications for percutaneous endovascular treatment of atherosclerotic renal artery stenosis are debated. However, most agree that interventions are warranted to prevent progression of stenotic renal artery disease to occlusion, to prevent deterioration of renal function, to prevent recurrent heart failure, and to improve blood pressure control in the refractory hypertensive patient.

In many patients, RAS is very often an overlooked vascular disease. A high clinical suspicion is required to suspect and diagnose renal vascular disease (Table 2). While more than 10% of patients with >60% RAS progress

Table 2
Clinical clues to suggest renovascular disease

- Onset of hypertension before the age of 30 or after the age of 55 years
- Hypertension that was well controlled and has now become more difficult to control
- Malignant or accelerated hypertension
- Resistant hypertension
- Epigastric bruit audible in both systole and diastole
- Atrophic kidney or discrepancy in size between two kidneys
- Azotemia after receiving angiotensin-converting enzyme (ACE) inhibitors
- Azotemia in the elderly patient with atherosclerosis in other vascular beds
- Patients with generalized atherosclerosis
- Recurrent pulmonary edema despite normal left ventricular systolic function

to renal artery occlusion within 2 years *(46)*, the relationship between RAS and renal function is less clear. Indeed, it can be challenging to prospectively identify the patients that will most benefit from renal artery revascularization. Renal artery revascularization is clinically more compelling in a patient with bilateral renal artery stenosis (or the equivalent such as unilateral renal artery stenosis in a patient with a solitary kidney), but the benefits of revascularization are not experienced by all patients and it remains difficult to identify those patients that will improve most. Ongoing studies may help clarify the clinical indications for endovascular renal artery intervention and may help clarify issues related to reimbursement.

Van Jaarsveld et al. compared angioplasty alone (although a small number of patients underwent adjunctive stenting) to aggressive medical therapy for control of hypertension in 100 patients with RAS *(47)*. No benefit of renal artery angioplasty was observed. Unfortunately, there were several important limitations to the study. For one, no hemodynamic pressure gradients were reported. Further, nearly 50% of the medical therapy patients crossed over to angioplasty by 3 months of follow-up. Creatinine clearance was significantly improved in the angioplasty group at 3 months, but there was no statistically significant difference at 12 months.

In contrast, Dorros et al. *(48)* demonstrated that blood pressure control was stable and creatinine/renal function improved over 48 months of follow-up in a nonrandomized cohort of patients. Others have tried to identify non-invasive methods to stratify patients who may benefit from renal artery interventions. Radermacher et al. *(49)* utilized a Doppler-derived resistance index to help predict the clinical response to renal artery intervention. In the study, patients with a higher resistance index did not demonstrate improvements in blood pressure control or renal function following renal artery intervention, suggesting that the resistance index represents a surrogate for the severity of intrinsic renal disease. However, the results of this study have not been reproduced with consistency in any other trials.

Unlike RAS caused by atherosclerosis, FMD typically affects the medial layer of the renal artery. FMD most commonly occurs in the midsegment of the renal artery and spares the ostium. These lesions usually respond well to percutaneous transluminal renal angioplasty (PTRA) alone, with stenting reserved for complications such as flow-limiting dissections and recurrent stenosis. FMD recurrences after PTRA occur more commonly in cases of distal renal artery disease or at bifurcation locations.

Balloon-expandable stents are the preferred stent type for ostial renal artery disease locations. Although there are stents FDA approved for renal artery use (Palmaz and IntraCoil double strut, for example), these are not used commonly today. Most balloon-expandable stents used for renal artery revascularization are FDA approved only for biliary indications. The 1-year restenosis rates vary from 5 to 21% with an average of 11–15% *(50–54)*.

Because renal artery atherosclerosis is typically an extension of aortic atherosclerosis, the lesions tend to be friable and to be prone to atheroemboli during endovascular intervention. Indeed, embolization of atherosclerotic debris during PTRA and/or stenting may paradoxically hasten the deterioration of renal function if sufficient debris is embolized. Hence, the concept of utilizing embolic protection devices during renal artery revascularization has received much interest. However, to date, no studies have been performed to demonstrate the utility of distal embolic protection during renal artery revascularization; therefore, routine use at this time cannot be recommended.

The NIH-sponsored CORAL *(55)* (Cardiovascular Outcomes in Renal Atherosclerotic Lesions) trial is randomizing patients with >60% RAS to either best medical therapy only or endovascular intervention combined with best medical therapy. Because the study will include stented patients both with and without the use of distal protection devices, it should provide an insight into the effectiveness of distal protection devices on long-term renal and cardiovascular outcomes.

In summary, to date, quality-randomized trials comparing renal artery stenosis stenting to best medical therapy are lacking. As such, the best treatment for many asymptomatic or minimally symptomatic patients with renal artery stenosis is unclear.

4. CAROTID ARTERY

Stroke is a leading cause of death worldwide. A number of studies, including the NASCET *(56)*, the ACAS *(57)*, and the ECST *(58)* trials, have demonstrated the effectiveness of open carotid surgical repair for stroke prevention. These trials compared surgical endarterectomy (CEA) with best available medical therapy (limited to aspirin alone) and helped establish CEA as the gold standard for therapy of symptomatic patients with moderate-to-severe carotid stenosis and asymptomatic patients with severe carotid stenosis. The rate of stroke in patients despite best medical therapy was 12% in the asymptomatic group (ACAS) and 23% in the symptomatic group (NASCET) but could be as high as 53% over 1–2 years if treated with aspirin alone.

Endovascular management of carotid artery disease was revolutionized by the development of embolic protection devices (EPD). There are three major variations in these devices based on their mode of protection:

1. Distal occlusion balloon (PercuSurge Guidewire, Medtronic, Inc., Minneapolis, MN)
2. Proximal occlusion balloon (Parodi, ArteriA Medical Science, Inc., San Francisco, CA)
3. Distal filters (Angioguard, Cordis, Diamond Bar, CA; Accunet filter wire, Guidant, Santa Clara, CA; Spider, ev3, Irvine, CA; Emboshield, Abbott Labs, Redwood City, CA)

Early reports of angioplasty performed in the carotid arteries appeared in the literature in the early 1990s coincident with the development of endovascular therapy in other vascular beds. However, the risk of distal embolization and resultant stroke was a major limiting factor; the advent of distal embolic protection devices (EPD) addressed this major hazard of endovascular carotid revascularization. Because carotid revascularization was already established as the gold-standard treatment, carotid artery stenting (CAS) had the onerous task of first proving to be an acceptable risk in patients who were traditionally considered at too high risk for surgery based on a number of clinical and anatomical features (Table 3). These patients historically were excluded from surgical trials.

Table 3
High-risk features of patients enrolled in carotid artery stent trials

Clinical
- Age >80 years
- Congestive heart failure (NYHA class III/IV)
- Severe left ventricular systolic dysfunction (LVEF <30%)
- Recent MI (>24 h and <4 weeks)
- Unstable angina (CCS class III/IV)
- Open heart surgery needed within 6 weeks
- Severe pulmonary disease

Anatomical
- Previous CEA with recurrent stenosis
- High cervical lesions
- Contralateral carotid occlusion
- Radiation therapy to neck
- Prior radical neck surgery

In order to gather outcome data, CAS patients were enrolled in several high-risk registries such as ARCHeR *(59)*. The first randomized control trial of CAS versus CEA was the stenting and angioplasty with protection in patients at high risk for endarterectomy (SAPPHIRE) trial *(60)*; carotid lesions in this study had to be revascularizable by either surgical or endovascular means. For the first time, the primary endpoint in a carotid revascularization trail included not only stroke or death at 30 days and 1 year but also myocardial infarction. Stroke or death endpoints occurred in 5.5 and 8.4% of the stent and surgical groups, respectively (P = 0.36). However, the primary endpoint, a composite of stroke, death, and MI, occurred at 1 year in 12.2% versus 20.1% in the stent and surgery groups, respectively. This trial helped prove that stenting with the use of embolic protection devices was not inferior to carotid endarterectomy in high-surgical-risk patient populations and along with the ARCHeR registry was the basis of FDA approval for CAS in high-risk patients.

The data on low-operative-risk patients are more limited. The CAVATAS *(61)* trial looked at low risk, mostly symptomatic patients, and the results were favorable for carotid angioplasty. This trial, however, did not use embolic protection devices and stenting was performed in only 25% of patients; as a result, the results are minimally applicable to today's practice. More recent trials of low-risk patients conducted in Europe have been halted early due to unfavorable stroke rates in the stenting arm.

Compared to SAPPHIRE, patients in the endovascular versus stenting in patients with symptomatic severe carotid stenosis (EVA-3S) *(62)* study were at lower surgical risk and all were symptomatic; these factors alone, however, do not explain the discrepant results as most strokes were noted to occur on the procedure day, suggesting a relationship to the procedure itself. Complicating interpretation of the studies is that the EVA-3S trial utilized numerous different embolic protection devices, while SAPPHIRE employed a single type. EVA-3S also lacked a clearly defined antiplatelet strategy. The other recently published trial, the stent-protected angioplasty versus carotid endarterectomy in symptomatic patients (SPACE) *(63)* trial, failed to prove the noninferiority of carotid stenting compared to CEA at 30 days; importantly, however, the use of an embolic protection device with stenting was not required.

The Centers for Medicare and Medicaid services (CMS) provide reimbursement for carotid artery stenting if it fulfills the following three criteria:

1. Greater than 70% stenosis (angiographic or duplex derived)
2. Symptoms attributable to the side of stenosis
3. High cardiovascular risk for open surgical repair.

The NIH-sponsored carotid revascularization endarterectomy versus stent trial (CREST) *(63)* is randomizing patients at low risk/acceptable cardiovascular risk for surgery to either open repair or carotid stenting with distal protection. Currently, all FDA-approved devices have also been undergoing further FDA-mandated postapproval studies. One postmarket approval database *(64)* showed that operators who have been fully credentialed and trained to perform CAS can do so with low risk to patients as demonstrated by a low risk of neurologic event. This conclusion was independent of operator experience as long as the operator was fully trained with the device. Importantly, the long-term durability of CAS has been very good with an average restenosis rate of 2.4% at 3 years of follow-up *(65)*. The stroke rates are very low and acceptable for this high-risk patient population.

5. CONCLUSION

Millions of patients have PAD. Reduced cardiac output, as occurs in patients with heart failure, can contribute to impaired distal perfusion. For patients with PAD, endovascular therapy has greatly replaced surgical revascularization for most anatomic locations. However, ease of use, device, and technological advancements has outpaced the development of scientific evidence supporting their widespread use. Safety, however, is generally widely accepted. Long-term patency following an endovascular procedure is region specific with excellent results for the carotid and aortoiliac locations and less-satisfying results in the SFA and renal artery territories. Although the effectiveness of endovascular therapies is less robust in the SFA and infrapopliteal locations, these territories remain key locations of controversy as to the best approach for revascularization and long-term durability.

REFERENCES

1. Hirsch AT, Criqui MH, Treat-Jacobson D, et al. Peripheral arterial disease detection, awareness, and treatment in primary care. JAMA 2001;286(11):1317–24.
2. Weitz JI, Byrne J, Clagett GP, et al. Diagnosis and treatment of chronic arterial insufficiency of the lower extremities: a critical review. Circulation 1996;94(11):3026–49.
3. Hertzer NR, Beven EG, Young JR, et al. Coronary artery disease in peripheral vascular patients. A classification of 1000 coronary angiograms and results of surgical management. Ann Surg 1984;199(2):223–33.
4. Dotter CT, Judkins MP. Transluminal treatment of arteriosclerotic obstruction. Description of a new technic and a preliminary report of its application. Circulation 1964;30:654–70.
5. Brewster D. Direct reconstruction for aortoiliac occlusive disease. In: Rutherford R, ed. Vascular Surgery. Philadelphia, PA: WB Saunders; 1995:766–94.
6. Tetteroo E, Haaring C, van der Graaf Y, van Schaik JP, van Engelen AD, Mali WP. Intraarterial pressure gradients after randomized angioplasty or stenting of iliac artery lesions. Dutch Iliac Stent Trial Study Group. Cardiovasc Intervent Radiol 1996;19(6):411–7.
7. Martin EC, Katzen BT, Benenati JF, et al. Multicenter trial of the Wallstent in the iliac and femoral arteries. J Vasc Interv Radiol 1995;6(6):843–9.
8. Vorwerk D, Gunther RW, Schurmann K, Wendt G. Aortic and iliac stenoses: follow-up results of stent placement after insufficient balloon angioplasty in 118 cases. Radiology 1996;198(1):45–8.
9. Murphy TP, Webb MS, Lambiase RE, et al. Percutaneous revascularization of complex iliac artery stenoses and occlusions with use of Wallstents: three-year experience. J Vasc Interv Radiol 1996;7(1):21–7.
10. Henry M, Amor M, Ethevenot G, et al. Palmaz stent placement in iliac and femoropopliteal arteries: primary and secondary patency in 310 patients with 2–4-year follow-up. Radiology 1995;197(1):167–74.
11. Dormandy JA, Rutherford RB. Management of peripheral arterial disease (PAD). TASC Working Group. TransAtlantic Inter-Society Consensus (TASC). J Vasc Surg 2000;31(1 Pt 2):S1–296.
12. Norgren L, Hiatt WR, Dormandy JA, Nehler MR, Harris KA, Fowkes FG. Inter-Society Consensus for the Management of Peripheral Arterial Disease (TASC II). J Vasc Surg 2007;45(Suppl S):S5–67.
13. Dorrucci V. Treatment of superficial femoral artery occlusive disease. J Cardiovasc Surg (Torino) 2004;45(3):193–201.
14. Lee ES, Santilli SM, Olson MM, Kuskowski MA, Lee JT. Wound infection after infrainguinal bypass operations: multivariate analysis of putative risk factors. Surg Infect (Larchmt) 2000;1(4):257–63.
15. Adam DJ, Beard JD, Cleveland T, et al. Bypass versus angioplasty in severe ischaemia of the leg (BASIL): multicentre, randomised controlled trial. Lancet 2005;366(9501):1925–34.

16. Ansel GM, Silver MJ, Botti CF, Jr., et al. Functional and clinical outcomes of nitinol stenting with and without abciximab for complex superficial femoral artery disease: a randomized trial. Catheter Cardiovasc Interv 2006;67(2):288–97.

17. Waksman R, Laird JR, Jurkovitz CT, et al. Intravascular radiation therapy after balloon angioplasty of narrowed femoropopliteal arteries to prevent restenosis: results of the PARIS feasibility clinical trial. J Vasc Interv Radiol 2001;12(8):915–21.

18. Duda SH, Bosiers M, Lammer J, et al. Drug-eluting and bare nitinol stents for the treatment of atherosclerotic lesions in the superficial femoral artery: long-term results from the SIROCCO trial. J Endovasc Ther 2006;13(6):701–10.

19. Greenberg D, Rosenfield K, Garcia LA, et al. In-hospital costs of self-expanding nitinol stent implantation versus balloon angioplasty in the femoropopliteal artery (the Vascu-Coil Trial). J Vasc Interv Radiol 2004;15(10):1065–9.

20. Jeans WD, Armstrong S, Cole SE, Horrocks M, Baird RN. Fate of patients undergoing transluminal angioplasty for lower-limb ischemia. Radiology 1990;177(2):559–64.

21. Capek P, McLean GK, Berkowitz HD. Femoropopliteal angioplasty. Factors influencing long-term success. Circulation 1991;83(2 Suppl):I70–80.

22. Johnston KW. Femoral and popliteal arteries: reanalysis of results of balloon angioplasty. Radiology 1992;183(3):767–71.

23. Matsi PJ, Manninen HI, Vanninen RL, et al. Femoropopliteal angioplasty in patients with claudication: primary and secondary patency in 140 limbs with 1–3-year follow-up. Radiology 1994;191(3):727–33.

24. Murray JG, Apthorp LA, Wilkins RA. Long-segment (> or = 10 cm) femoropopliteal angioplasty: improved technical success and long-term patency. Radiology 1995;195(1):158–62.

25. Hunink MG, Wong JB, Donaldson MC, Meyerovitz MF, de Vries J, Harrington DP. Revascularization for femoropopliteal disease. A decision and cost-effectiveness analysis. JAMA 1995;274(2):165–71.

26. Gallino A, Mahler F, Probst P, Nachbur B. Percutaneous transluminal angioplasty of the arteries of the lower limbs: a 5 year follow-up. Circulation 1984;70(4):619–23.

27. Krepel VM, van Andel GJ, van Erp WF, Breslau PJ. Percutaneous transluminal angioplasty of the femoropopliteal artery: initial and long-term results. Radiology 1985;156(2):325–8.

28. Sapoval MR, Long AL, Raynaud AC, Beyssen BM, Fiessinger JN, Gaux JC. Femoropopliteal stent placement: long-term results. Radiology 1992;184(3):833–9.

29. Schlager O, Dick P, Sabeti S, et al. Long-segment SFA stenting – the dark sides: in-stent restenosis, clinical deterioration, and stent fractures. J Endovasc Ther 2005;12(6):676–84.

30. Scheinert D, Scheinert S, Sax J, et al. Prevalence and clinical impact of stent fractures after femoropopliteal stenting. J Am Coll Cardiol 2005;45(2):312–5.

31. Schillinger M, Sabeti S, Loewe C, et al. Balloon angioplasty versus implantation of nitinol stents in the superficial femoral artery. N Engl J Med 2006;354(18):1879–88.

32. Duda SH, Pusich B, Richter G, et al. Sirolimus-eluting stents for the treatment of obstructive superficial femoral artery disease: six-month results. Circulation 2002;106(12):1505–9.

33. Zilberman M, Eberhart RC. Drug-eluting bioresorbable stents for various applications. Annu Rev Biomed Eng 2006;8:153–80.

34. Biamino JLG. Results of the cryovascular peripheral balloon catheter safety registry. In: Transcatheter Cardiovascular Therapeutics. Washington, DC; 2003.

35. Zeller T, Rastan A, Sixt S, et al. Long-term results after directional atherectomy of femoro-popliteal lesions. J Am Coll Cardiol 2006;48(8):1573–8.

36. Ramaiah V, Gammon R, Kiesz S, et al. Midterm outcomes from the TALON Registry: treating peripherals with SilverHawk: outcomes collection. J Endovasc Ther 2006;13(5):592–602.

37. Fischer M, Schwabe C, Schulte KL. Value of the Hemobahn/Viabahn endoprosthesis in the treatment of long chronic lesions of the superficial femoral artery: 6 years of experience. J Endovasc Ther 2006;13(3):281–90.
38. Bauermeister G. Endovascular stent-grafting in the treatment of superficial femoral artery occlusive disease. J Endovasc Ther 2001;8(3):315–20.
39. Kedora J, Hohmann S, Garrett W, Munschaur C, Theune B, Gable D. Randomized comparison of percutaneous Viabahn stent grafts vs prosthetic femoral–popliteal bypass in the treatment of superficial femoral arterial occlusive disease. J Vasc Surg 2007;45(1):10–6; discussion 6.
40. Pomposelli FB, Jr., Marcaccio EJ, Gibbons GW, et al. Dorsalis pedis arterial bypass: durable limb salvage for foot ischemia in patients with diabetes mellitus. J Vasc Surg 1995;21(3):375–84.
41. Dorros G, Jaff MR, Dorros AM, Mathiak LM, He T. Tibioperoneal (outflow lesion) angioplasty can be used as primary treatment in 235 patients with critical limb ischemia: five-year follow-up. Circulation 2001;104(17):2057–62.
42. Feiring AJ, Wesolowski AA, Lade S. Primary stent-supported angioplasty for treatment of below-knee critical limb ischemia and severe claudication: early and one-year outcomes. J Am Coll Cardiol 2004;44(12):2307–14.
43. Laird JR, Zeller T, Gray BH, et al. Limb salvage following laser-assisted angioplasty for critical limb ischemia: results of the LACI multicenter trial. J Endovasc Ther 2006;13(1):1–11.
44. Kandzari DE, Kiesz RS, Allie D, et al. Procedural and clinical outcomes with catheter-based plaque excision in critical limb ischemia. J Endovasc Ther 2006;13(1): 12–22.
45. Rihal CS, Textor SC, Breen JF, et al. Incidental renal artery stenosis among a prospective cohort of hypertensive patients undergoing coronary angiography. Mayo Clin Proc 2002;77(4):309–16.
46. Zierler RE, Bergelin RO, Isaacson JA, Strandness DE, Jr. Natural history of atherosclerotic renal artery stenosis: a prospective study with duplex ultrasonography. J Vasc Surg 1994;19(2):250–7; discussion 7–8.
47. van Jaarsveld BC, Krijnen P, Pieterman H, et al. The effect of balloon angioplasty on hypertension in atherosclerotic renal-artery stenosis. Dutch Renal Artery Stenosis Intervention Cooperative Study Group. N Engl J Med 2000;342(14):1007–14.
48. Dorros G, Jaff M, Mathiak L, He T. Multicenter Palmaz stent renal artery stenosis revascularization registry report: four-year follow-up of 1,058 successful patients. Catheter Cardiovasc Interv 2002;55(2):182–8.
49. Radermacher J, Chavan A, Bleck J, et al. Use of Doppler ultrasonography to predict the outcome of therapy for renal-artery stenosis. N Engl J Med 2001;344(6):410–7.
50. Lederman RJ, Mendelsohn FO, Santos R, Phillips HR, Stack RS, Crowley JJ. Primary renal artery stenting: characteristics and outcomes after 363 procedures. Am Heart J 2001;142(2):314–23.
51. Burket MW, Cooper CJ, Kennedy DJ, et al. Renal artery angioplasty and stent placement: predictors of a favorable outcome. Am Heart J 2000;139(1 Pt 1):64–71.
52. White CJ, Ramee SR, Collins TJ, Jenkins JS, Escobar A, Shaw D. Renal artery stent placement: utility in lesions difficult to treat with balloon angioplasty. J Am Coll Cardiol 1997;30(6):1445–50.
53. Rocha-Singh KJ, Mishkel GJ, Katholi RE, et al. Clinical predictors of improved long-term blood pressure control after successful stenting of hypertensive patients with obstructive renal artery atherosclerosis. Catheter Cardiovasc Interv 1999;47(2): 167–72.
54. Rodriguez-Lopez JA, Werner A, Ray LI, et al. Renal artery stenosis treated with stent deployment: indications, technique, and outcome for 108 patients. J Vasc Surg 1999;29(4):617–24.

55. Cooper CJ, Murphy TP, Matsumoto A, et al. Stent revascularization for the prevention of cardiovascular and renal events among patients with renal artery stenosis and systolic hypertension: rationale and design of the CORAL trial. Am Heart J 2006;152(1):59–66.

56. North American Symptomatic Carotid Endarterectomy Trial Collaborators. Beneficial effect of carotid endarterectomy in symptomatic patients with high-grade carotid stenosis. N Engl J Med 1991;325(7):445–53.

57. Executive Committee for the Asymptomatic Carotid Atherosclerosis Study. Endarterectomy for asymptomatic carotid artery stenosis. JAMA 1995;273(18):1421–8.

58. European Carotid Surgery Trialists' Collaborative Group. Randomised trial of endarterectomy for recently symptomatic carotid stenosis: final results of the MRC European Carotid Surgery Trial (ECST). Lancet 1998;351(9113):1379–87.

59. Gray WA, Hopkins LN, Yadav S, et al. Protected carotid stenting in high-surgical-risk patients: the ARCHeR results. J Vasc Surg 2006;44(2):258–68.

60. Yadav JS, Wholey MH, Kuntz RE, et al. Protected carotid-artery stenting versus endarterectomy in high-risk patients. N Engl J Med 2004;351(15):1493–501.

61. CAVATAS Investigators. Endovascular versus surgical treatment in patients with carotid stenosis in the Carotid and Vertebral Artery Transluminal Angioplasty Study (CAVATAS): a randomised trial. Lancet 2001;357(9270):1729–37.

62. Mas JL, Chatellier G, Beyssen B, et al. Endarterectomy versus stenting in patients with symptomatic severe carotid stenosis. N Engl J Med 2006;355(16):1660–71.

63. Ringleb PA, Allenberg J, Bruckmann H, et al. 30 day results from the SPACE trial of stent-protected angioplasty versus carotid endarterectomy in symptomatic patients: a randomised non-inferiority trial. Lancet 2006;368(9543):1239–47.

64. Gray WA, Yadav JS, Verta P, et al. The CAPTURE registry: results of carotid stenting with embolic protection in the post approval setting. Catheter Cardiovasc Interv 2007;69(3):341–8.

65. Wholey MH, Al-Mubarek N. Updated review of the global carotid artery stent registry. Catheter Cardiovasc Interv 2003;60(2):259–66.

12 Percutaneous Management of Valvular Heart Disease

Joanna J. Wykrzykowska, MD and Joseph P. Carrozza Jr., MD

CONTENTS

Abstract

Heart failure afflicts nearly five million Americans, with a large proportion of patients over the age 65. While ischemic heart disease accounts for most cases, 6–9% of all cases of heart failure may be attributed to valvular heart disease. This chapter describes the percutaneous therapies available to treat valvular heart disease and includes both a review of available clinical data and a discussion of past and current device technologies.

Key Words: Valvular heart disease; Mitral regurgitation; Aortic stenosis; Medical device; Heart failure.

From: *Contemporary Cardiology: Device Therapy in Heart Failure*
Edited by: W.H. Maisel, DOI 10.1007/978-1-59745-424-7_12
© Humana Press, a part of Springer Science+Business Media, LLC 2010

1. INTRODUCTION

1.1. Valvular Heart Disease and Heart Failure – Scope of the Problem and Challenges for the Therapy

Heart failure afflicts nearly five million Americans, with a large proportion of patients over the age 65 *(1)*. While ischemic heart disease accounts for most cases, 6–9% of all cases of heart failure may be attributed to valvular heart disease, especially in the developing world where rheumatic heart disease remains a significant problem. Unfavorable remodeling with ventricular dilation is a consequence of end stage heart failure regardless of etiology, resulting in a vicious cycle of mitral and tricuspid annular dilatation, valvular insufficiency, and worsening heart failure. Despite improvements in medical and surgical treatment of valvular heart disease and heart failure, the rate of hospitalization for heart failure remains high and the mortality for symptomatic heart failure is 45% at 1 year *(2)*.

Counteracting improvements in therapy is an aging population with multiple comorbidities limiting the use of proven therapeutics. For example, the use of angiotensin-converting enzyme inhibitors and angiotensin receptor antagonists may be limited in elderly patients with renal insufficiency. Similarly, digoxin reduces rehospitalization rates and improves symptoms, but may have higher incidence of toxicity in the elderly. Advanced age is also associated with increased morbidity and mortality from valvular surgery according to a recent retrospective Society of Thoracic Surgeons database analysis of over 400,000 patients, conferring a twofold risk of mortality *(3)*. Based on that study, aortic valve and mitral valve replacement have an adjusted mortality of 5.5 and 7.7%, respectively. However, patients 70 years and older have mortality of 9.1%, and those with heart failure symptoms have mortality of 8.3%. Many patients with multiple comorbidities such as cerebrovascular disease, obstructive lung disease, renal insufficiency, prior cardiac surgery, and hepatic dysfunction are not considered as candidates for valvular surgery. Thus, these registry data almost certainly underestimate the true risk of surgical morbidity and mortality in very high-risk patients. The increasing prevalence and poor prognosis of patients with heart failure and significant valvular heart disease have become the impetus for development of minimally invasive and endovascular treatments for these disorders.

2. PERCUTANEOUS TREATMENT OF PULMONIC VALVULAR DISEASE

2.1. Balloon Valvotomy

Symptomatic patients with moderate (peak systolic gradient >40 and <80 mmHg) pulmonic valvular stenosis and asymptomatic patients with severe (≥ 80 mmHg) pulmonic stenosis and no significant pulmonary regurgitation may benefit from balloon valvotomy to enlarge the effective pulmonic valve area *(4)*. In one series of 53 adolescent and adult patients, pulmonary systolic pressure decreased from 91 to 38 mmHg following valvotomy. Only mild pulmonic insufficiency was present in seven patients which resolved at follow-up. Patients who have undergone multiple prior surgical or percutaneous interventions have significant degree of pulmonic valve incompetence, or have very dilated pulmonary vessels are not ideal candidates for valvotomy and may require replacement of the valve. The 2008 ACC/AHA Guidelines *(5)* confer a Class Ic recommendation for balloon valvotomy for those adolescents and young adults with exertional dyspnea, angina, syncope, or presyncope and an RV-to-PA peak-to-peak gradient of 30 mmHg at catheterization, or in asymptomatic patients with RV-to-PA peak-to-peak gradient of 40 mmHg. A weaker recommendation (IIb) is given for those asymptomatic patients with RV-to-PA peak-to-peak gradients of 30–40 mmHg, and valvotomy is not recommended for asymptomatic patients whose gradients are less than 30 mmHg.

2.2. Percutaneous Pulmonic Valve Implantation (PPVI)

2.2.1. HISTORICAL PERSPECTIVE AND INITIAL VALVE DESIGN

The first percutaneous valve implantation was performed by Bonhoeffer in 2000 *(6)*. The prosthesis was constructed from a venous valve of a bovine cadaver and sewn into a vascular expandable stent. The stent was crimped onto an 18–22 mm balloon and expanded in the right ventricular outflow tract (RVOT). Implantation was successful in 7 of 11 animals. This was followed by the first human implantation in a 12-year old boy with prior history of congenital heart disease and symptoms of heart failure secondary to pulmonic regurgitation *(7)*. Since then the experience with balloon expandable pulmonary valve implantation has been successful in more than 100 patients *(8)*. The valve design currently used is illustrated in Fig. 1 *(7)*.

2.2.2. INDICATIONS

The procedure is indicated in patients with repaired congenital heart disease such as tetralogy of Fallot, who have symptoms of right ventricular failure and RVOT dysfunction, and would otherwise qualify for surgical re-operation *(9)*. Patients must also have favorable RVOT morphology with diameters of less than 22 mm by MRI (Fig. 2) or echocardiographic assessment.

2.2.3. CLINICAL OUTCOME OF PERCUTANEOUS PULMONARY VALVE IMPLANTATION

The results of pulmonic valve implantation performed in 59 consecutive patients were recently published *(10)*. As measured by cardiac MRI, right

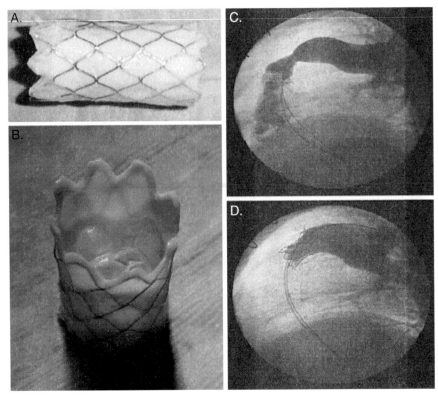

Fig. 1. Percutaneous pulmonary valve implantation. (**a**) Original wind sock pulmonary valve *(6)* and (**b**) current pulmonary stent valve design. (**c**) Pulmonary angiogram showing severe pulmonary regurgitation and (**d**) Pulmonary angiogram after pulmonary stent valve implantation showing resolution of severe pulmonary regurgitation *(8)*.

ventricular systolic pressure decreased from 64 to 50 mmHg, with a significant increase in diastolic pulmonary artery pressure from 9.9 to 13.5 mmHg. Patients with pulmonic regurgitation had an increase in pulmonary artery diastolic pressure immediately post-procedure. A subset of patients underwent MRI assessment at a median follow-up of 6 days post-procedure with significant decrease in right ventricular dimensions and decrease in pulmonic regurgitant fraction. In addition, there was an improvement in NYHA class as well as an increase in exercise capacity, as measured by oxygen consumption, from 26 to 29 ml/kg/min at 6 days. Most importantly, the procedure appeared reasonably safe at 9-months follow-up and the effects on echocardiographic gradients were sustained. There were only three major early procedural complications (two stent migrations of the guidewire and one pulmonary homograft dissection during pre-dilation with significant bleeding). There were seven cases of incomplete valve apposition to the stent wall due to improper suturing of the valve with consequent in-stent

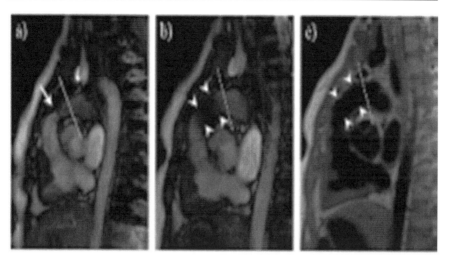

Fig. 2. Cardiac MRI performed to evaluate pulmonary stenosis. (**a**) Pulmonary stenosis (*arrow*) with imaging of right ventricular outflow tract; (**b, c**) Images post-stent implantation *(10)*.

stenosis or so-called "hammock effect" (Fig. 3). There were also seven stent fractures.

These results were also compared with surgical outcomes *(8)*. There was one death in the surgical group (1/93) and none in the interventional group (0/35). The rate of severe complications was 8.5% in the surgical group (re-operation, neurological sequelae) and 5.7% in the percutaneous group (infection and hammock effect with older stent design). There were

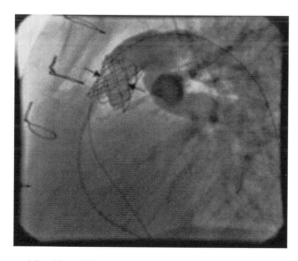

Fig. 3. "Hammock" effect following percutaneous pulmonic valve replacement *(10)*.

no late surgical complications and event-free survival was 100% at 1 year and 95% at 5 years. Six (17%) patients treated percutaneously required re-intervention for restenosis and 86% were free from repeat intervention at 1 year.

2.2.4. LIMITATIONS OF THE APPROACH AND FUTURE DIRECTIONS

While a percutaneous approach may offer promise in patients with RVOT disorders, additional design modifications and long-term follow-up are needed. Also, its application is limited to patients with ideal RVOT geometry. Patients with dilated RVOT requiring simultaneous patching and plasty of the RVOT are not candidates for the percutaneous approach. The two approaches may be combined in the future in hybrid procedures *(11)*. One such approach was tried in an animal model where a balloon expandable conduit is surgically anastomosed and subsequently the valve is inserted and deployed percutaneously *(12)*. Another approach with dilated pulmonary arteries involved surgical banding of the pulmonary artery to decrease its diameter with subsequent percutaneous valve implantation (Fig. 4) *(13)*.

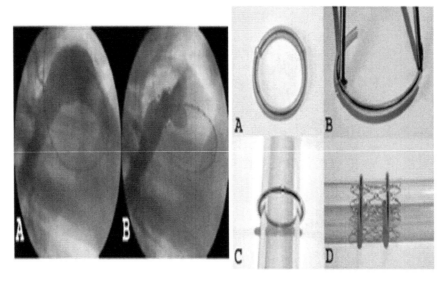

Fig. 4. Hybrid approach to percutaneous pulmonic valve replacement – pulmonary artery banding to decrease the diameter of the outflow tract prior to percutaneous valve implantation *(13)*: *Left*: Angiograms before (**a**) and after (**b**) the pulmonary artery banding, showing the reduction of the diameter and the radiopaque marker of the rings. *Right*: In vitro views of the various phases of the procedure. (**a**) The ring used for the pulmonary artery banding is made of nitinol and has a spontaneous diameter of 18 mm. (**b**) The ring is opened and straightened before its passage around the main pulmonary artery. (**c**) View showing the aspect of the ring around a glass tube. (**d**) View showing the aspect of a stent placed inside the glass tube after placement of two rings.

Patients most ideally suited for such approach could be identified by MRI. In addition, balloon expandable stents could be developed to fit to the dilated RVOT tract *(14)*. Recently, the Edwards–Cribier Percutaneous Heart Valve (PHV) (Edwards Lifesciences, Irvine, CA) was successfully implanted in the pulmonary artery of a 16-year-old boy with a stenotic right ventricle to pulmonary artery homograft *(15)*.

3. PERCUTANEOUS TREATMENT OF AORTIC VALVE DISEASE

3.1. Aortic Stenosis

Aortic stenosis presents with symptoms of chest pain, syncope, or heart failure usually in the 4th or 5th decade of life in patients with bicuspid aortic valves. Tricuspid aortic valves usually do not become severely stenotic (valve area <1 cm^2) until the 7th or even 8th decade of life *(16)*. Of the 150,000 patients undergoing aortic valve replacement annually, a high proportion (up to 40%) are octogenarians with multiple comorbidities in whom surgical aortic valve replacement may be associated with significant morbidity and mortality *(17)*. The mortality increases in the presence of coronary artery disease, severe left ventricular dysfunction, advanced NYHA class, re-operation, or severe obstructive pulmonary disease.

3.2. Indications for Intervention

Development of symptoms (chest pain, syncope, and dyspnea) usually heralds a precipitous decline in survival and provides a firm indication for valve replacement. Initially, patients with preserved left ventricular systolic function may complain of exertional dyspnea secondary to diastolic dysfunction. Left ventricular dysfunction and overt heart failure are late manifestations of aortic stenosis and portend a poor prognosis with increased operative risk. However, even patients with depressed left ventricular ejection fraction and severe aortic stenosis benefit from valve replacement *(18)*. Patients, however, who have prohibitively high surgical risk related to poor pre-operative status are the exception. Before the initial work by Andresen (1992) *(19)* and Cribier (2002) *(20)*, the only option for such patients was palliative balloon valvuloplasty. Medical management of heart failure in patients with severe aortic stenosis does not appear effective, despite some reports of successful use of vasodilators such as nitroprusside *(21)*. The apparent effectiveness of nitroprusside treatment may have been due to selection bias of patients with pseudo aortic stenosis whose symptoms were predominantly due to cardiomyopathy with decreased ejection fraction. The use of this treatment is also limited to a highly selected and monitored intensive care unit setting *(22)*. Judicious use of diuretics may provide short-term palliation of symptoms. Regardless of medical therapy, symptomatic and severe aortic stenosis (defined as AVA <1.0 cm^2, mean gradient >40 mmHg, or peak velocity >4.0 m/s) requires an interventional approach to improve quality of life. AVR is recommended currently for symptomatic patients with severe AS (Class I) or asymptomatic patients with a depressed ejection fraction (Class I), blood pressure decline with exercise testing (Class IIb), or severe calcific disease with rapid progression (IIb) (5). Many patients who meet these criteria have significant comorbidities limiting their surgical candidacy, and for these patients percutaneous approaches may offer symptomatic improvement with a more acceptable risk–benefit profile. Attempts to define these patients more quantitatively, such as with the European System for Cardiac Operative Risk Evaluation (EuroSCORE), have met with mixed results (23). Reliable and consistent metrics for identifying optimal candidates will remain an important component of investigations advancing this field.

3.3. Balloon Aortic Valvuloplasty (BAV)

The technique was first described in 1985 by Cribier. Typically, a retrograde aortic approach via the femoral artery is used (24). After hemodynamic assessment, a stiff guidewire is placed in the left ventricle and a 20–22 mm balloon filled with diluted contrast is positioned across the aortic valve. Following balloon inflation, the gradient is re-measured. An alternative approach is to access the femoral vein and perform the procedure via transseptal approach, potentially decreasing the risk of arterial complications.

While patients improve somewhat symptomatically after balloon valvuloplasty for about 6 months, the rate of complications from this procedure such as stroke, death, aortic injury, and vascular complication is as high as 10–20% (25). In addition, balloon dilatation of a calcified, non-rheumatic aortic valve results in only modest luminal enlargement from annular stretching rather than commissural tearing. Typically, the transvalvular gradient is reduced by approximately 50% and the patient is left with a severely narrowed valve (~0.8–1.0 cm^2). Nevertheless, this may reduce pulmonary venous congestion, augment cardiac output, and provide symptom relief. Renarrowing is almost universal, the palliative effect is short-lived, and the procedure does not alter overall mortality which remains high (26, 27). A more recent retrospective analysis of 212 patients showed somewhat more encouraging results (28). The mortality at 1 year was still 64% but many patients were symptom free for 18 months. The valve area increased on average from 0.6 to 1.2 cm^2 with decrease in mean aortic valve gradient from 44 to 18 mmHg. Vascular complications occurred in 13.5% of the patients. The 2008 ACC/AHA guidelines weakly recommend BAV as a potentially reasonable option (IIb) as a bridge to aortic surgery for unstable patients deemed high risk for AVR, or for palliation of severe symptoms in patients who are not surgical candidates *(5)*. BAV is not recommended to bridge patients with severe AS through *noncardiac* surgery, however.

3.4. *Percutaneous Aortic Valve Replacement*

3.4.1. AORTIC PERCUTANEOUS VALVE DESIGNS AND PRELIMINARY CLINICAL RESULTS

Because balloon aortic valvuloplasty lacks a durable hemodynamic effect and fails to improve prognosis, there remains a need for percutaneous approaches to aortic valve replacement, particularly for patients with heart failure, advanced age, or those with prohibitive surgical risk due to other comorbidities. As the population ages, the prevalence of degenerative aortic stenosis and heart failure will likely increase. This expanding population of patients referred for aortic valve replacement will present significant challenges for traditional surgical approaches to valve replacement. Initial animal studies of percutaneous aortic prostheses were performed in 1992 by Andersen and Pavcnik *(19, 29)*. The initial prototype was a balloon expandable valve stent, the placement of which was difficult due to anatomic considerations. A later design was a self-expanding cage-ball valve. Initial attempts at placement were unsuccessful, and it was not until Cribier's implantation of the balloon-expandable percutaneous heart valve (PHV) in 60 sheep *(30)* and subsequent implantation *(20)* in a patient with cardiogenic shock, that the field of percutaneous aortic valve implantation gathered momentum. The valve was composed of three porcine leaflets separately sewn into a stent mounted on a balloon. A major challenge in the animal model was frequent valve migration due to smoothness and lack of calcifications of the aorta.

The first human implantation was performed via antegrade transseptal approach in a 57-year-old man with multiple comorbidities who presented in cardiogenic shock with left ventricular ejection fraction of 14%. The implantation was successful and the patient improved hemodynamically. Unfortunately, the patient expired within 4 months from other comorbidities. In 2004, eight octogenarians with severe aortic stenosis deemed unacceptably high risk for surgical valve replacement underwent either antegrade (six of eight) or retrograde (two of eight) aortic valve implantation *(31)*. The mean aortic valve area increased from 0.6 to 1.7 cm^2 and the peak gradient decreased from 46 to 8 mmHg. The ejection fraction increased from 48 to 57% 24 h post-procedure. The procedure was performed successfully in all eight patients and five of eight patients were alive at 1 month.

In the antegrade approach, following transseptal catheterization, a pulmonary artery catheter is placed across the interatrial septum and mitral valve and a stiff guidewire is directed across the aortic valve which is snared from the arterial side (Fig. 5) *(32)*. The interatrial septum is dilated and a large (24 French) sheath is advanced to allow delivery and placement of the valve. In the retrograde approach a large sheath is placed in the femoral artery. The valve is predilated using a conventional valvuloplasty balloon

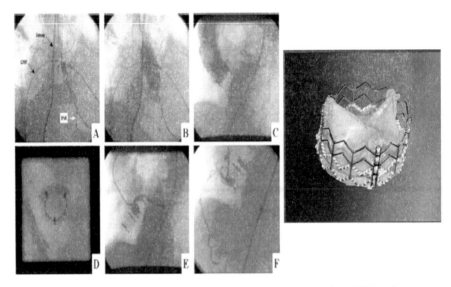

Fig. 5. Antegrade approach to Edwards percutaneous heart valve (PHV) placement; *Left*: (**a**) The percutaneous valve in position across the native calcific aortic valve before delivery. GW, extra-stiff guide wire; PM, pacemaker lead in the right ventricle for brief period of rapid pacing at the time of balloon inflation. Sones catheter is advanced over the guide wire from the left femoral artery. The stent graft is positioned across the native aortic valve. (**b**) Balloon inflation for valve deployment. (**c**) Post-implantation supra-aortic angiogram showing mild aortic regurgitation. (**d**) Right anterior oblique cranial view of the valve showing the circular stent frame pushing away the calcified native valve. Selective left (**e**) and right (**f**) coronary angiogram post-implantation showing patent coronary ostia *(31, 32)*; *Right*: Edwards balloon expandable stent aortic valve (Lifesciences).

(Fig. 6). During stent valve placement, the ventricle is paced at 220 bpm to prevent ejection and migration of the valve during deployment. In the initial cohort in the RECAST trial, 22 of 26 (85%) antegrade implantations were successful. Of the four failures, two were due to valve migration and two were due to hemodynamic instability. Three of seven retrograde procedures were unsuccessful due to inability to cross the valve. An improvement of one or two NYHA classes at 9-months follow-up was observed in >90% of patients in whom the percutaneous heart valve was successfully implanted. In the surviving patients, the aortic valve area improved from 0.7 to 1.6 cm^2. The left ventricular ejection fraction at 1 week increased from 45 to 53% and the improvement was most marked in patients with the most depressed left ventricular function. By 6 months, ten patients had died and 26% had suffered major complications. Problems such as valve migration, aortic insufficiency secondary to paravalvular leaks, occlusion of the coronary ostia, and hemodynamic compromise during delivery dampened some of the initial enthusiasm for this breakthrough technology. The risk of hemo-

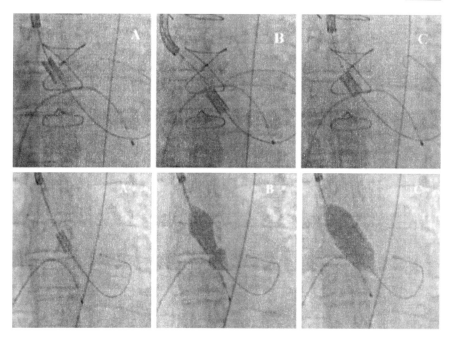

Fig. 6. Retrograde approach to the aortic valve placement angiogram; *Upper panel*: (**a**) The prosthesis could not be advanced through the commissure of the native valve. (**b**) The active deflection catheter facilitates redirection through the valve orifice. (**c**) The prosthesis is carefully positioned adjacent to the calcified native aortic valve; *Lower panels*: (**a**) Balloon-mounted prosthetic valve positioned adjacent to native valve calcification. (**b**) Partial inflation of the deployment balloon. (**c**) Full inflation of the deployment balloon *(33)*.

dynamic compromise due to tethering of the mitral valve can be minimized by employing the retrograde approach. Using a steerable delivery catheter, Webb successfully deployed the percutaneous heart valve in patients via the retrograde approach *(33)*. The issues of migration and paravalvular leaks were addressed by utilizing larger valve sizes. In this series, no valve migrations occurred and the aortic insufficiency did not increase significantly following valve implantation. The major limitation of the retrograde approach is the risk of vascular compromise secondary to placement of large caliber arterial sheaths and to manipulation of diseased, atherosclerotic iliofemoral vessels and aorta.

A second prototype, a self-expanding stent valve (Core Valve, Paris, France) has also been deployed successfully (Fig. 7) *(17)*. The implantation procedure is performed via retrograde approach and offers the theoretical advantage of enhanced conformation to the aorta and valve, thus reducing the chance of a significant paravalvular leak. In the initial report, the left ventricular ejection fraction increased from 45 to 76% and NYHA class decreased from IV to II. CT angiography performed after the proce-

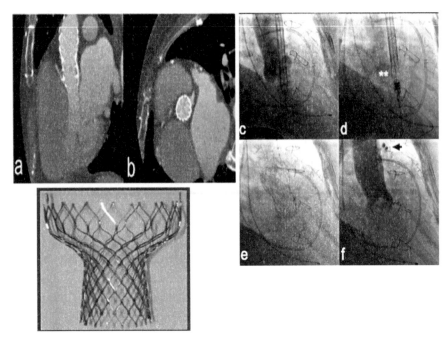

Fig. 7. CoreValve Implantation: (**a, b**) *CT Angiography* 3 days after CoreValve placement; (**c–f**) *Implantation* of the self-expanding aortic valve prosthesis: (**c**) device is positioned within the native valve; (**d**) Pull back of the outer sheath and deployment of the self-expanding prosthesis; (**e**) Fully expanded valve prosthesis; (**f**) Final angiogram with no evidence of aortic regurgitation; (**g**) ex vivo appearance of expanded valve *(17)*.

dure showed appropriate valve positioning and apposition (Fig. 7a and b). Percutaneous placement of an aortic valve typically is performed under general anaesthesia with transesophageal echocardiography guidance.

3.4.2. LIMITATIONS AND FUTURE DIRECTION

The RECAST trial results, while encouraging despite a high-risk patient population, illustrate the myriad of obstacles that must be overcome before the use of this exciting technology can be routinely employed. Refinement of imaging techniques prior to, and during deployment, as well as new valve designs and sizes will allow more precise matching of the prosthetic valve to the annulus of the individual patient. This may result in more accurate placement and better anchoring, reducing the risk of migration, paravalvular leak, and coronary ostial compromise. Vascular trauma remains an important limitation to the retrograde approach. However, advances in technology may permit the construction of a more collapsible valve that can be delivered through sheath sizes as small as 8 French (Fig. 8) *(34)*. Develop-

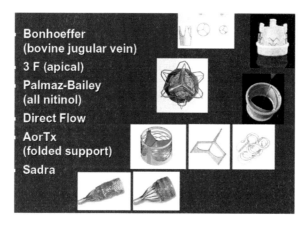

Fig. 8. Novel aortic valve designs *(34)*.

ments may also permit valve placement without cardiopulmonary bypass; Lichtenstein has recently reported a series of seven patients in which the PHV has been successfully deployed via an antegrade approach using direct

Table 1
Selected ongoing trials of percutaneous mitral and aortic valves

Trial name	*Valve*	*Device*	*Study design*
EVEREST II	Mitral	Evalve, Inc. Cardiovascular valve repair system	Prospective, multicenter, randomized
EVEREST High-risk registry	Mitral	Evalve, Inc. Cardiovascular valve repair system	Single arm, non-randomized
PARTNER	Aortic	Edwards SAPIEN transcatheter heart valve	Randomized
PTOLEMY-2	Mitral	PTMA system	Single arm, uncontrolled
RESTOR-MV	Mitral	Coapsys device	Randomized
VIVID	Mitral	i-Coapsys device	Single arm, uncontrolled
An observational, prospective evaluation of the Trifecta™ valve	Aortic	St. Jude Medical Trifecta valve	Single arm, uncontrolled

(Continued)

Table 1
(Continued)

Trial name	Valve	Device	Study design
Catheter-based transapical implantation of the Ventor Embracer™ heart valve prosthesis in patients with severe aortic valve disease	Aortic	Ventor Embracer heart valve	Single arm, uncontrolled

EVEREST, endovascular valve edge-to-edge repair study; PARTNER, placement of aortic transcatheter valve trial; RESTOR-MV, randomized evaluation of a surgical treatment for off-pump repair of the mitral valve; VIVID, valvular and ventricular improvement via iCoapsys Delivery.

apical puncture of the left ventricle through a small incision without cardiopulmonary bypass (35). Walther et al. also demonstrated feasibility of the transapical approach in a study of 59 elderly patients with severe calcific AS and advanced heart failure (NYHA Class III–IV) (36). Implantation was successful in 55 of 59 patients, and echocardiographic assessment demonstrated favorable initial hemodynamics with a mean AV gradient of only 9±6 mmHg. Ongoing clinical trials will continue to explore the technical and clinical outcomes associated with each approach to percutaneous aortic valve replacement. Table 1 highlights selected active investigations.

4. PERCUTANEOUS TREATMENT OF MITRAL VALVE DISEASE

4.1. Mitral Stenosis and Valvuloplasty

Rheumatic mitral stenosis accounts for the overwhelming majority of cases of mitral stenosis (24). Typically, patients present with exertional dyspnea, atrial arrhythmias, and later pulmonary hypertension and right heart failure with edema, ascites, and hepatic congestion. Operative repair is recommended for patients with mean transvalvular gradients >10 mmHg and significant symptoms (Class Ic), or more weakly for patients with milder symptoms or pulmonary hypertension (Class IIa) (5). Based on observations from surgical commissurotomy, catheter-based percutaneous commissurotomy was proposed. In 1982, Inoue performed the first successful percutaneous commissurotomy, heralding the application of catheter-based techniques to treat mitral valve disorders (37). Balloon mitral valvuloplasty (BMV) is indicated in symptomatic patients with a favorable echocardiographic score (38). The transvenous transseptal approach with Inoue technique of balloon commissurotomy is the most popular technique today (4). Although, complications such as death (0–3%), hemopericardium

(0.5–12%), embolism (0.5–5%), or severe mitral regurgitation (2–12%) do occur, their incidence is highly dependent on the operator experience. Patients with favorable results by echocardiography (decreased gradient, increased valve area and absence of severe mitral regurgitation) have good prognosis, but the restenosis rate is 40% at 7 years *(39)*. In a randomized trial of BMV versus open commissurotomy in 60 patients, mitral valve areas improved in both groups, from 0.9 to 2.0 cm². Mitral valve areas were greater in the patients in the BMV group at 3 years (2.4 cm² vs. 1.8 cm²). Restenosis occurred in three patients in the BMV group and four in the surgery group. Three patients (two in the BMV group and one in the surgery group) had severe mitral regurgitation. Seventy-two percent of the patients after BMV and 57% of the surgically treated patients were free of cardiovascular symptoms at 3 years *(40)*. Similar results were achieved in two other randomized trials; thus establishing BMV as a mainstay procedure for mitral stenosis *(41, 42)*.

4.2. *Percutaneous Mitral Valve Repair for Mitral Regurgitation*

4.2.1. PRIMARY VERSUS SECONDARY MITRAL REGURGITATION AND INDICATIONS FOR INTERVENTION

Percutaneous mitral valve repair of mitral regurgitation presents even greater challenges to the interventional cardiologist than percutaneous correction of mitral stenosis due to the multiple different etiologies of mitral regurgitation. Generally, mitral regurgitation may occur due to intrinsic valvulopathies such as myxomatous degeneration, or secondarily following alterations in annular geometry in patients with left ventricular dilation. For the past 10–20 years, there has been a major shift in the surgical approach to mitral regurgitation away from valve replacement to repair. While surgical techniques of mitral valve repair *(43, 44)* or placement of annuloplasty rings with leaflet plasty have also improved mitral valve surgical outcomes *(45)*, the mortality especially in patients with ischemic and dilated cardiomyopathy and depressed ejection fraction may be substantial. In addition, patients with ischemic mitral regurgitation have a high incidence of recurrent mitral regurgitation within 6 months following annuloplasty *(46)*. In patients with primary valvular pathology such as rheumatic heart disease, mitral valve prolapse, or myxomatous degeneration of the leaflets, if surgical intervention occurs prior to irreversible left ventricular dysfunction, symptoms of heart failure can be reversed *(47, 48)*. The 2008 ACC/AHA guidelines confer a Class Ib recommendation on *surgical* intervention for patients with symptomatic acute severe MR; chronic severe MR with NYHA Class II–IV symptoms but without severe LV dysfunction (LVEF <30% or end-diastolic dimension of <55 mm); or asymptomatic patients with chronic severe MR and mild–moderate LV dysfunction (LVEF 30–60% or LVEDD >40 mm). Weaker support is offered for intervention in those patients with asymptomatic chronic severe MR without LV dysfunction, or for those symptomatic patients with chronic severe MR but severe LV dysfunction *(5)*.

These recommendations highlight the ever-increasing patient population with ischemic or dilated cardiomyopathies, reduced left ventricular ejection fraction, and secondary mitral regurgitation in whom the risks of surgery may be significant and the impact on heart failure symptoms may be less predictable. Unfortunately, significant mitral regurgitation is often difficult to medically manage with afterload reduction and diuresis alone, and left ventricular dilation may progress resulting in a vicious cycle of increasing regurgitation and left ventricular decompensation. The presence of ischemic mitral regurgitation increases mortality in patients with coronary artery disease irrespective of their left ventricular function *(49)*.

4.2.2. ANATOMIC CHALLENGES ASSOCIATED WITH MITRAL REGURGITATION AND LEFT VENTRICULAR DILATATION

Mitral valve repair, either surgical or percutaneous, is complicated by the anatomic complexity of the valve, subvalvular apparatus, and annular geometry (Fig. 9a and b). Cardiac MRI and 3D echocardiography demonstrates in both animals and humans with left ventricular dilatation and mitral regurgitation, that the septal to lateral annular distance is increased, but the annulus itself is flattened *(50, 51)*. The current surgical and percutaneous approaches attempt to both decrease the septal to lateral annular distance and to restore the saddle shape of the annulus. In addition to mitral annular dilation, the geometry of the dilated ventricle causes splaying of the papillary muscles away from the annular apparatus and the chordal apparatus tethering. This results in the failure of leaflet coaptation and persistent mitral regurgitation even after annuloplasty *(52, 53)*. Levine proposed cutting some of the strategically positioned chord at the base to prevent tethering (Fig. 9c). The latter problem may continue to limit the success of percutaneous treatments.

4.2.3. APPROACHES TO REPAIR OF PRIMARY VALVULAR PATHOLOGY

4.2.3.1. Edge-to-Edge Repair.
The surgical technique of approximating the anterior and posterior leaflets of the mitral valve with a suture was introduced by Alifieri *(54)*. This technique essentially creates a dual lumen mitral orifice and is most effective when structures other than leaflets are minimally distorted and the annulus is without significant calcification. This technique alone (without annuloplasty) is of limited value in the treatment of mitral regurgitation with left ventricular dilatation. Based on the principles of the Alfieri repair, an analogous catheter-based approach was developed utilizing the MitraClip® (Evalve Inc.; Menlo Park, CA) (Fig. 10) delivered through a 24-French catheter via a transseptal approach under

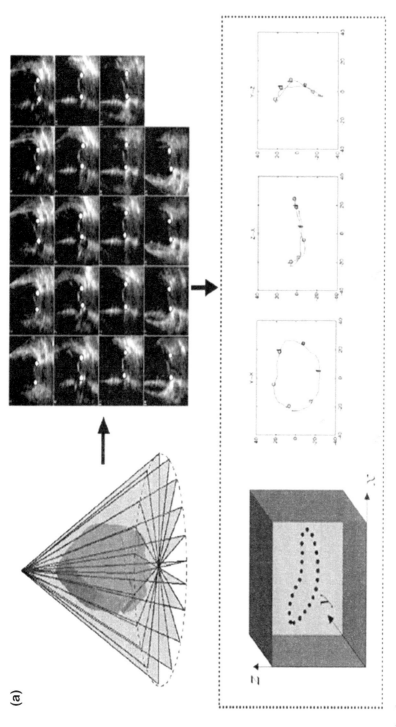

Fig. 9. Anatomy and pathology of the mitral annulus. (**a**) *3-D Echo* – 3-D volumetric image was automatically cropped into 18 equally spaced radial planes: the mitral annulus was manually marked in each cropped plane in mid-systole; from these data, 3-D images of the annulus were reconstructed for the quantitative measurements (51). (**b**) *Magnetic resonance imaging (MRI) of the mitral annulus – Left:*

(b)

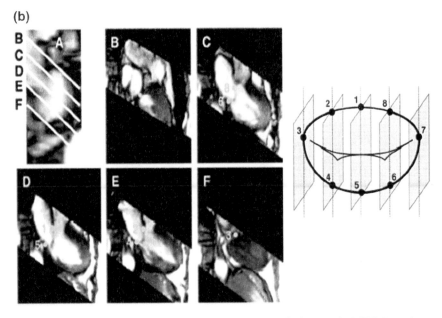

Fig. 9. (continued) Volumetric images from endsystolic long-axis MRI data showing how to obtain 5 anteroposterior planes and 8 points with multiplanar reforma-
tion. By moving and rotating cut planes on a cross-sectional volumetric image at
mitral valvular level (**a**), 5 anteroposterior planes were created from the lines of
intersection. The 8 mitral annular points (numbered *yellow dots*) were obtained on
the reconstructed images of the 5 planes (**b–f**). 3D coordinates of the points were
determined on these images; *Right*: Schematic representation of the mitral annular
points used in the study. Points 2 and 8 correspond with the *right* and *left* trigones,
respectively. Points 3 and 7 correspond with the posterior and anterior commissures,
respectively; for the purpose of 3D reconstruction of MRI, this view is the reverse of
the surgeon's view *(50)*. (**c**) Cordal apparatus anatomy and leaflet tethering – *Left*:
At baseline, leaflet area exceeds that needed to cover the annulus, creating a coapting leaflet surface to prevent mitral regurgitation. *Center*: Inferior infarction distorts
the base of the anterior leaflet, which is tethered by basal chordae to form a bend,
reducing the coapting surface and causing regurgitation. *Right*: Basal chordal cutting
can eliminate this bend, improve coaptation, and reduce MR; the marginal chordae
prevent prolapse. *Bottom panel*: corresponding 2-D Echocardiographic images *(52)*.
Ao = aorta; LA = left atrium; MR = mitral regurgitation.

transesophageal echo guidance. The catheter system grasps the two leaflets
and deploys a clip to create the double-orifice mitral valve.

Recently the EVEREST (Endovascular Valve Edge-to-edge REpair
STudy) I pilot study of 27 patients treated with the Evalve system were
published *(55)*. Procedural success was reported in 24 of 27 patients.
Two patients had clip detachment without other sequelae and five patients
required surgical repair of the mitral valve. Of the 22 patients discharged

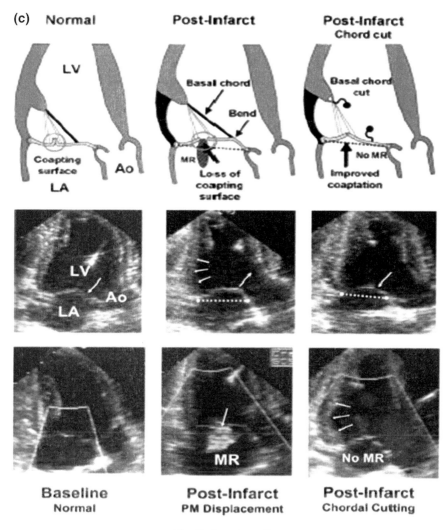

Fig. 9. (continued)

from the hospital with a successfully implanted clip, 18 had reduction in mitral regurgitation to less than 2+, and 13 patients were free of significant mitral regurgitation at 6 months. The average time required for implantation was 3.5 h, with a reduction in procedure time with operator experience. However, the long case times underscore the technical difficulty of the procedure The pivotal EVEREST II trial is a prospective, phase II study of patients with degenerative mitral regurgitation and normal annular dimensions currently randomizing patients to either surgical repair or valve replacement, or endovascular cinching with the E-valve system. The primary composite endpoint is freedom from surgery for valve dysfunction, death, and moderate to severe or severe mitral regurgitation at 12 months. Preliminary data from 70

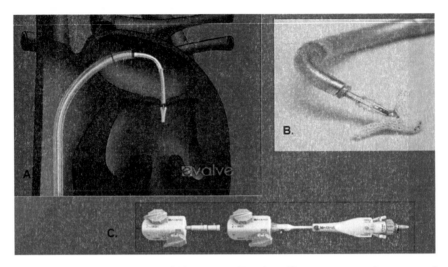

Fig. 10. *E-valve clip* and its delivery: (**a**) E-valve: Transvenous and transseptal approach to clip placement. (**b**) Clip photograph: The clip is covered with polyester fabric. The two arms are opened and closed by control mechanisms on the clip delivery system. The two arms have an opened span of approximately 2 cm and a width of 4 mm. (**c**) Delivery system *(55)*.

patients treated with Evalve in the EVEREST I Registry and EVEREST II roll-in phase have been presented. Successful clip implantation occurred in 90% of patients and 96% of patients were free of major adverse events by 30 days *(34)*.

4.2.3.2. Percutaneous Annuloplasty Approaches. Percutaneous annuloplasty procedures most commonly involve implantation of a rod-like device in the coronary sinus which courses along the atrioventricular groove and posterior annulus opposite from the anterior fibrous trigone. This exploits the natural anatomic relationship of the coronary sinus and posterior annulus. The Viking Percutaneous Mitral Annuloplasty device (Edwards Lifesciences, Irvine, CA) is composed of two self-expanding anchors (stent-like larger proximal anchor in the proximal coronary sinus and smaller distal anchor in the great cardiac vein) joined by a stiffening/shortening rod (Fig. 11). Venous access is obtained, the coronary sinus is cannulated, and a wire is passed through the sinus. Delivery catheter and sheath are then advanced over the wire into the coronary sinus and the great cardiac vein. With fluoroscopic guidance the straightening connecting rod brings the two anchors closer and reduces the septal to lateral dimensions of the mitral annulus. After proper positioning, the sheath is retracted releasing the anchors and deploying the device. This approach was recently tested in five patients *(56)*. Implantation and proper anchor placement was achieved in all five patients without evidence for device migration at 3 months. One

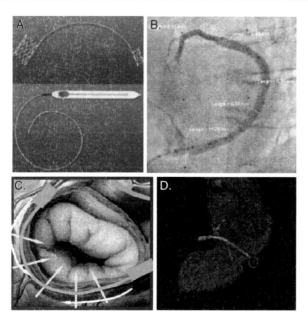

Fig. 11. *Viking Device (56)*: (**a**) *Top*, The Viking percutaneous mitral valve annuloplasty device is constructed of nitinol and consists of a larger proximal anchor, a flexible shortening bridge segment, and a smaller distal anchor. *Bottom*, The delivery system consists of an over-the-wire inner catheter, on which is mounted the compressed implant and an outer restraining sheath. The sheath is retracted with a thumb sliding mechanism that sequentially releases the self-expanding distal and then the proximal anchor. (**b**) Coronary sinus angiography: Distal injection through an angiographic catheter opacifies the coronary sinus. Radiopaque markers allow estimation of vessel length and diameter and selection of an appropriately sized implant. (**c**) Schematic representation of the device placed in the coronary sinus with the distal portion in the great cardiac vein and the proximal portion in the proximal coronary sinus. (**d**) Multidetector-row cardiac-gated CT Scan showing an intact device within the coronary sinus, adjacent to the mitral annulus, 6 months after successful implantation. The anchoring devices in the coronary sinus (*right*) and great cardiac vein (*left*) and the connecting bridge are very visible.

patient died (unrelated to the device) and the other four were alive at 3 months. Coronary angiography did not demonstrate compromise of the left circumflex artery. In the four surviving patients, the left ventricular ejection fraction increased from 42 to 50%. However, there was no significant improvement in the NYHA class. Mitral regurgitation decreased proportionally to the degree of shortening of the distance between two anchors.

Another device design, PTMA™ (Viacor, Wilmington, MA) consists of a flexible catheter placed in the coronary sinus that can accommodate three rods of varying stiffness thereby allowing for adjustment of the annular diameter with the use of different rod combinations (Fig. 12a) *(57, 58)*. Access is obtained via the subclavian vein with a 10-French sheath. The

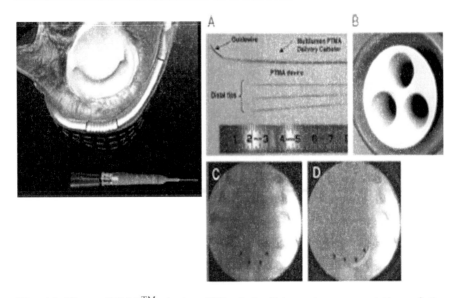

Fig. 12. Viacor PTMA™ device *(58)*: *Left*: Schematic representation of the device; *Right*: Guidewire, multilumen delivery catheter, PTMA devices, and fluoroscopic images during percutaneous mitral annuloplasty. (**a**) Distal portion of guidewire and multilumen delivery catheter with tips of 3 different PTMA devices. (**b**) Magnified cross section of multilumen delivery catheter. If number of devices, up to 3, and stiffness of each device are varied, total stiffness can be magnified, increasing force delivered to posterior mitral annulus. (**c, d**) Fluoroscopic images during PTMA. Guidewire was introduced into CS with its distal end in anterior interventricular vein under fluoroscopic guidance (**c**). Anterior–posterior remodeling of mitral annulus was achieved with annuloplasty device in CS (**d**). Guidewire from *left* image (**c**) is superimposed in white to illustrate geometric change. Note movement of CS and adjacent posterior annulus by annuloplasty device (*arrows*). (**b**) *Left*: Schematics of commissure–commissure (C–C) plane and 3 anteroposterior (A-P) planes (*left*) and geometric measurements of mitral annulus (*left*) and Mitral Valve (MV) (*right*). Moving and rotating cut planes on cross-sectional 3D image at MV level give C–C plane connecting both commissures and 3 A-P planes in medial (M), central (C), and lateral (L) sides of MV. AML indicates anterior mitral leaflet; PML, posterior mitral leaflet; Ao, aorta; LA, left atrium; and MVTht, MV tenting height. *Right*: *3D echocardiographic images of MV during mid systole* in medial (*left*), central (*middle*), and lateral (*right*) A-P planes at baseline (*top*) and after device implantation (*bottom*). MV tenting (*top arrow*) was significantly improved in medial A-P plane by device implantation in CS (*lower arrow*) vs lateral A-P plane. LA indicates left atrium *(58)*.

delivery system with tensioning rods is capped and sutured in the subcutaneous tissue. It theoretically allows for re-accessing the rods and subsequent exchange of stiffening rods to alter the geometry of the annulus depending on the loading conditions and clinical requirements. The disadvantage is that the proximal portion of the delivery catheter is sutured under the skin

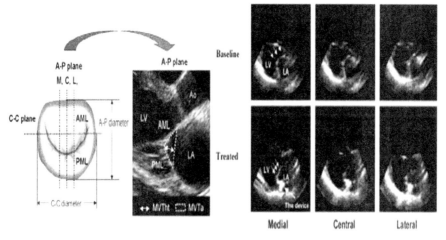

Schematics of C-C plane and 3 A-P planes (left) and geometric measurements of mitral annulus (left) and MV (right).

3D echocardiographic images of MV

Fig. 12. (continued)

increasing the risk of migration and also long-term risk of infection. The device has been tested in an ovine model of mitral regurgitation secondary to dilated cardiomyopathy with encouraging results. Using 3D echocardiography, this approach was evaluated not only for its ability to decrease the septal to lateral annular diameter, but also for its effects on the saddle shape and geometry of the valve (Fig. 12b). The device not only reduced the mitral regurgitant area from 5.4 to 1.3 cm^2, but also reduced "tenting" and valve flattening. Long-term follow-up will be required to assess the permanence of this effect in both animal and human studies. A phase I pilot study is currently enrolling patients.

An important issue with all techniques of mitral annuloplasty employing coronary sinus prostheses for annular geometric alteration is potential compromise of the left circumflex coronary artery. Surgical mitral annuloplasty can cause left circumflex injury and myocardial infarction (59, 60). The risk of this potential complication may be reduced by carefully assessing the coronary anatomy and its relationship to the left circumflex artery with multidetector computer tomography or magnetic resonance imaging. A recent anatomic study also raised the concern of the coronary sinus lying behind the left atrium rather than the mitral annulus resulting in the device potentially constricting the atrium rather than the annulus (61). Lastly, a potential limitation of the coronary sinus approach in patients with ischemic cardiomyopathy is the interference of the device with placement of biventricular pacemaker for resynchronization therapy. Possibly in the future, coronary sinus devices may be fitted with pacing ports to allow for institution of both therapies in this challenging heart failure group.

Most recently, another septal to lateral (S–L) annular cinching device was introduced that takes advantage of the Amplatzer Atrial Septal Occluder (AGA Medical, MN) device placed proximally with a magnet in the great coronary vein (Fig. 13) *(62)*. The interaction between the two decreases the annular diameter and creates a transatrial bridge. This device promises to

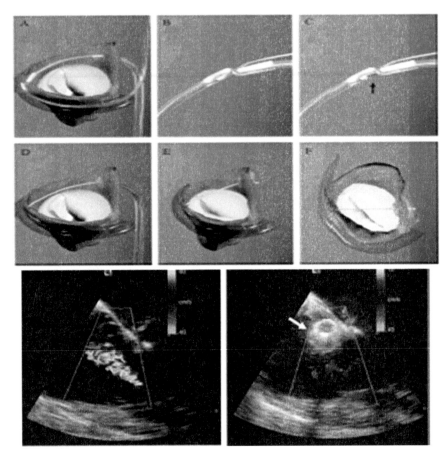

Fig. 13. Percutaneous septal sinus shortening device *(PS3) (62)*: *Top*: PS3 system implantation procedure. (**a**) GCV and LA MagneCaths in position and magnetically linked. (**b**) Close-up of magnetically linked LA and GCV MagneCaths. (**c**) Coring catheter (*arrow*) in position to allow passage of the loop glide wire from the LA to GCV (the loop wire allows the bridge element to be pulled back across the LA). (**d**) The PS3 system in place before tensioning. (**e**) Tensioning the bridge results in precise shortening and elimination of FMR; the final position is secured with a suture lock. (**f**) Superior view of the PS3 system. Because the interatrial septal anchor passes through the fossa ovalis, the angle of the bridge element is 20–30° posterior to a true anteroposterior orientation. *Bottom*: Intracardiac echocardiography before and after PS3 system implantation – the improvement in MR from 3+ (*left*) to trace (*right*) after device implantation. Septal anchor is seen on the *right* (*arrow*).

have greater ability to reduce the S–L diameter and also to circumvent the possibility of left circumflex artery injury.

Selected ongoing trials of percutaneous mitral valve placement are included in Table 1.

5. PERCUTANEOUS ATRIOVENTRICULAR VALVE REPLACEMENT – PRELIMINARY RESULTS

Boudjemine and colleagues recently proposed the concept of percutaneous treatment of atrioventricular valvular disease by introducing the first prototype of an atrioventricular valve replacement *(63)*. The device is made of braided nitinol wire that forms two disks (40 mm for ventricular disk and 18 mm for atrial disk) interconnected by a tubular structure (15 mm) (Fig. 14). The device delivery and deployment is very similar to the deploy-

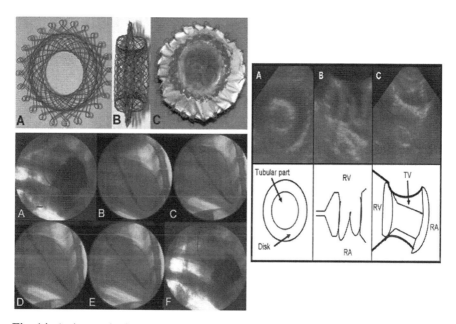

Fig. 14. Atrioventricular valve replacement *(63)*: *Left Top*: En face and lateral views of the *newly designed stent* before its covering (**a** and **b**), after its covering by a polytetrafluoroethylene membrane and the suture of the valve in the central tubular part (**c**). The stent is shown from the ventricular side with a valve in closed position. *Left Bottom: Angiograms* showing the various steps of device deployment. (**a**) Lateral view before valve deployment. (**b**) The delivery system is advanced over a wire placed in the distal pulmonary artery. (**c**) The ventricular disk is progressively opened in the right ventricle. (**d**) The ventricular disk is fully opened and applied to the tricuspid annulus. (**e**) The device is completely deployed. (**f**) Angiogram showing the good function of the implanted valve. *Right*: Echocardiographic and schematic views showing the profile of the device on the long and short axis. RA – right atrium; RV – right ventricle; TV – tricuspid valve.

ment of an atrial septal occluder device. The larger disk is positioned on the right ventricular side and unsheathed, the tubular portion is then deployed and finally the uncovered right atrial disk is unsheathed. Of the eight devices seven were successfully implanted. In the longer-term follow-up cohort of four animals there was only one paravalvular leak due to PTFE membrane tearing and no device erosion or migration.

6. GUIDELINES FOR PERCUTANEOUS VALVE INTERVENTIONS

The 2008 ACC–AHA guidelines outline the indications for intervention for specific valvular lesions, including areas where the available literature supports use of percutaneous options for selected patients (5). Table 2 highlights the recommendations for percutaneous valvotomy. Percutaneous valve placement is not included in the 2008 recommendations as the procedure and the devices are still considered investigational. Clinical practice and future consensus guidelines will likely evolve quickly in response to new emerging data in this rapidly advancing field.

7. FUTURE DIRECTIONS AND CHALLENGES

The increasing prevalence of heart failure in an aging population provides the impetus for development of less invasive approaches for management of concomitant valvular heart disease. Catheter-based devices for treatment of valvular heart disease are in very early stages of development, and the initial results are encouraging. Preliminary results with pulmonary valve replacement in over 100 patients are promising. Percutaneous aortic valve replacement may offer hope to many elderly patients with critical aortic valve disease and comorbidities. Technical challenges related to device delivery and valve stability are significant challenges. Before the device can be offered to healthier individuals, lower profile devices, improved delivery techniques, and consistently reliable placement are needed. Finally, performance and long-term outcome must be measured against the "gold standard" of surgical aortic valve replacement. Mitral valve repair will continue to pose a myriad of challenges due to the differing etiologies of disease. Given the complexity of the mitral valvular apparatus and the protean etiologies of mitral regurgitation, a variety of techniques and devices will need to be developed and tailored to individual patients. It is possible that some patients may require a multifaceted approach incorporating leaflet cinching and annuloplasty. Imaging techniques such as 3D echocardiography and magnetic resonance imaging will be critically important for patient selection and assessment of anatomic success. More importantly, the ultimate role of these procedures will be determined by long-term follow-up of clinical endpoints such as mortality and need for repeat intervention. Surgical valve repair and replacement remains the standard against which emerging catheter-based therapies must be measured. Inevitably, surgical approaches

Table 2
ACC/AHA guidelines for percutaneous balloon valvotomy (BV)

Valvular lesion	Recommendation class	Level of evidence	Patient population
Aortic stenosis	IIb	C	1. Aortic BV might be reasonable as a bridge to surgery in hemodynamically unstable adult patients with AS who are at high risk for AVR
	III	B	2. Aortic BV might be reasonable for palliation in adult patients with AS in whom AVR cannot be performed because of serious comorbid conditions Aortic BV is not recommended as an alternative to AVR in adult patients with AS; certain younger adults without valve calcification may be an exception
Mitral stenosis	I	A	Percutaneous mitral BV is effective for symptomatic patients (NYHA functional Class II–IV), with moderate or severe MS and valve morphology favorable for percutaneous mitral BV in the absence of LA thrombus or moderate to severe MR
	I	C	Percutaneous mitral BV is effective for asymptomatic patients with moderate or severe MS and valve morphology that is favorable for percutaneous mitral BV who have pulmonary hypertension (PA systolic pressure >50 mmHg at rest or >60 mmHg with exercise) in the absence of LA thrombus or moderate to severe MR
	IIa	C	Percutaneous mitral BV is reasonable for patients with moderate or severe MS who have a nonpliable calcified valve, are in NYHA functional Class III–IV, and are either noncandidates for surgery or are at high risk for surgery

(Continued)

Table 2
(Continued)

Valvular lesion	Recommendation class	Level of evidence	Patient population
	IIb	C	1. Percutaneous mitral BV may be considered for asymptomatic patients with moderate or severe MS and valve morphology favorable for percutaneous mitral BV who have new onset of AF in the absence of LA thrombus or moderate to severe MR 2. Percutaneous mitral BV may be considered for symptomatic patients (NYHA functional Class II–IV) with MV area greater than 1.5 cm^2 if there is evidence of hemodynamically significant MS based on pulmonary artery systolic pressure >60 mmHg, pulmonary artery wedge pressure $\geq$25 mmHg, or mean MV gradient >15 mmHg during exercise 3. Percutaneous mitral BV may be considered as an alternative to surgery for patients with moderate or severe MS who have a nonpliable calcified valve and are in NYHA functional Class III–IV

	III	C	1. Percutaneous mitral BV is not indicated for patients with mild MS
			2. Percutaneous mitral BV should not be performed in patients with moderate to severe MR or LA thrombus
Pulmonary stenosis	I	C	1. BV is recommended in adolescent and young adult patients with pulmonic stenosis who have exertional dyspnea, angina, syncope, or presyncope and an RV-to-PA peak-to-peak gradient greater than 30 mmHg at catheterization
			2. BV is recommended in asymptomatic adolescent and young adult patients with pulmonic stenosis and RV-to-PA peak-to-peak gradient greater than 40 mmHg at catheterization
	IIb	C	BV may be reasonable in asymptomatic adolescent and young adult patients with pulmonic stenosis and an RV-to-PA peak-to-peak gradient of 30–39 mmHg at catheterization
	III	C	BV is not recommended in asymptomatic adolescent and young adult patients with pulmonic stenosis and RV-to-PA peak-to-peak gradient less than 30 mmHg at catheterization

AF, atrial fibrillation; AS, aortic stenosis; AVR, aortic valve replacement; BV, balloon valvotomy; LA, left atrial; MS, mitral stenosis; PA, pulmonary artery.

will undergo evolution and become less invasive. Possibly new opportunities will arise for hybrid surgical and percutaneous approaches to valve repair and replacement such as transapical valve placement thus morphing surgical and endovascular approaches together. The key to the advancement of this field will be collaboration between interventional cardiologists and surgeons and a critical, evidence-based, and open-minded assessment of each new technology with appropriate and thorough evaluation of safety and efficacy. Today many patients with heart failure and either primary or secondary valvular disease often have few options beyond medical management. While the field of percutaneous valve repair and replacement is in its early stages of development, outcomes with first-generation devices offer promise, but remaining technical challenges to widespread implementation should not be minimized.

REFERENCES

1. Jessup M, Brozena S. Heart failure. N Engl J Med 2003;348:2007–18.
2. Konstam MA. Progress in heart failure management? Lessons from the real world. Circulation 2000;102:1076–8.
3. Rankin JS, Hammill BG, Ferguson TB, Jr., et al. Determinants of operative mortality in valvular heart surgery. J Thorac Cardiovasc Surg 2006;131:547–57.
4. Chen CR, Cheng TO, Huang T, et al. Percutaneous balloon valvuloplasty for pulmonic stenosis in adolescents and adults. N Engl J Med 1996;335:21–5.
5. Bonow RO, Carabello BA, Chatterjee K, de Leon AC Jr., Faxon DP, Freed MD, Gaasch WH, Lytle BW, Nishimura RA, O'Gara PT, O'Rourke RA, Otto CM, Shah PM, Shanewise JS. 2008 focused update incorporated into the ACC/AHA 2006 guidelines for the management of patients with valvular heart disease: a report of the American College of Cardiology/American Heart Association Task Force on Practice Guidelines (Writing Committee to Develop Guidelines for the Management of Patients With Valvular Heart Disease). J Am Coll Cardiol 2008;52:e1–142.
6. Bonhoeffer P, Boudjemline Y, Saliba Z, et al. Transcatheter implantation of a bovine valve in pulmonary position: a lamb study. Circulation 2000;102:813–6.
7. Bonhoeffer P, Boudjemline Y, Saliba Z, et al. Percutaneous replacement of pulmonary valve in a right-ventricle to pulmonary-artery prosthetic conduit with valve dysfunction. Lancet 2000;356:1403–5.
8. Coats L, Tsang V, Khambadkone S, et al. The potential impact of percutaneous pulmonary valve stent implantation on right ventricular outflow tract re-intervention. Eur J Cardiothorac Surg 2005;27:536–43.
9. Vliegen HW, van Straten A, de Roos A, et al. Magnetic resonance imaging to assess the hemodynamic effects of pulmonary valve replacement in adults late after repair of tetralogy of fallot. Circulation 2002;106:1703–7.
10. Khambadkone S, Coats L, Taylor A, et al. Percutaneous pulmonary valve implantation in humans: results in 59 consecutive patients. Circulation 2005;112:1189–97.
11. Boudjemline Y, Pineau E, Borenstein N, Behr L, Bonhoeffer P. New insights in minimally invasive valve replacement: description of a cooperative approach for the off-pump replacement of mitral valves. Eur Heart J 2005;26:2013–7.
12. Boudjemline Y, Laborde F, Pineau E, et al. Expandable right ventricular-to-pulmonary artery conduit: an animal study. Pediatr Res 2006;59:773–7.
13. Boudjemline Y, Schievano S, Bonnet C, et al. Off-pump replacement of the pulmonary valve in large right ventricular outflow tracts: a hybrid approach. J Thorac Cardiovasc Surg 2005;129:831–7.

14. Boudjemline Y, Agnoletti G, Bonnet D, Sidi D, Bonhoeffer P. Percutaneous pulmonary valve replacement in a large right ventricular outflow tract: an experimental study. J Am Coll Cardiol 2004;43:1082–7.

15. Garay F, Webb J, Hijazi ZM. Percutaneous replacement of pulmonary valve using the Edwards-Cribier percutaneous heart valve: first report in a human patient. Catheter Cardiovasc Interv 2006;67:659–62.

16. Carabello BA, Crawford FA, Jr. Valvular heart disease. N Engl J Med 1997;337:32–41.

17. Grube E, Laborde JC, Zickmann B, et al. First report on a human percutaneous transluminal implantation of a self-expanding valve prosthesis for interventional treatment of aortic valve stenosis. Catheter Cardiovasc Interv 2005;66:465–9.

18. Quere JP, Monin JL, Levy F, et al. Influence of preoperative left ventricular contractile reserve on postoperative ejection fraction in low-gradient aortic stenosis. Circulation 2006;113:1738–44.

19. Andersen HR, Knudsen LL, Hasenkam JM. Transluminal implantation of artificial heart valves. Description of a new expandable aortic valve and initial results with implantation by catheter technique in closed chest pigs. Eur Heart J 1992;13:704–8.

20. Cribier A, Eltchaninoff H, Bash A, et al. Percutaneous transcatheter implantation of an aortic valve prosthesis for calcific aortic stenosis: first human case description. Circulation 2002;106:3006–8.

21. Khot UN, Novaro GM, Popovic ZB, et al. Nitroprusside in critically ill patients with left ventricular dysfunction and aortic stenosis. N Engl J Med 2003;348:1756–63.

22. Zile MR, Gaasch WH. Heart failure in aortic stenosis – improving diagnosis and treatment. N Engl J Med 2003;348:1735–6.

23. Brown ML, Schaff HV, Sarano ME, Li Z, Sundt TM, Dearani JA, Mullany CH, Orszulak TA. Is the European System for Cardiac Operative Risk Evaluation model valid for estimating the operative risk of patients considered for percutaneous aortic valve replacement? J Thorac Cardiovasc Surg 2008;136:566–71.

24. Vahanian A, Palacios IF. Percutaneous approaches to valvular disease. Circulation 2004;109:1572–9.

25. American Heart Association. Percutaneous balloon aortic valvuloplasty. Acute and 30-day follow-up results in 674 patients from the NHLBI Balloon Valvuloplasty Registry. Circulation 1991;84:2383–97.

26. Otto CM, Mickel MC, Kennedy JW, et al. Three-year outcome after balloon aortic valvuloplasty. Insights into prognosis of valvular aortic stenosis. Circulation 1994;89:642–50.

27. Lieberman EB, Bashore TM, Hermiller JB, et al. Balloon aortic valvuloplasty in adults: failure of procedure to improve long-term survival. J Am Coll Cardiol 1995;26:1522–8.

28. Agarwal A, Kini AS, Attanti S, et al. Results of repeat balloon valvuloplasty for treatment of aortic stenosis in patients aged 59 to 104 years. Am J Cardiol 2005;95:43–7.

29. Pavcnik D, Wright KC, Wallace S. Development and initial experimental evaluation of a prosthetic aortic valve for transcatheter placement. Work in progress. Radiology 1992;183:151–4.

30. Cribier A, Eltchaninoff H, Borenstein N et al. Trans-catheter implantation of balloon-expandable prosthetic heart valves: early results in an animal model. Circulation 2001;104:II-552.

31. Bauer F, Eltchaninoff H, Tron C, et al. Acute improvement in global and regional left ventricular systolic function after percutaneous heart valve implantation in patients with symptomatic aortic stenosis. Circulation 2004;110:1473–6.

32. Cribier A, Eltchaninoff H, Tron C, et al. Early experience with percutaneous transcatheter implantation of heart valve prosthesis for the treatment of end-stage inoperable patients with calcific aortic stenosis. J Am Coll Cardiol 2004;43:698–703.

33. Webb JG, Chandavimol M, Thompson CR, et al. Percutaneous aortic valve implantation retrograde from the femoral artery. Circulation 2006;113:842–50.

34. Leon MB. Interventions in Structural Heart Disease: My Expectations for the Disease: My Expectations for the Next 5–10 years. Catheter Interventions in Congenital Catheter Interventions in Congenital & Structural Heart Disease & Structural Heart Disease 9th International Workshop Frankfurt, Germany 2006.

35. Lichtenstein SV, Cheung A, Ye J, et al. Transapical transcatheter aortic valve implantation in humans: initial clinical experience. Circulation 2006;114:591–6.

36. Walther T, Simon P, Dewey T, et al. Transapical minimally invasive aortic valve implantation: multicenter experience. Circulation 2007;116:I240–5.

37. Feldman T, Herrmann HC, Inoue K. Technique of percutaneous transvenous mitral commissurotomy using the Inoue balloon catheter. Cathet Cardiovasc Diagn 1994;Suppl 2:26–34.

38. Wilkins GT, Weyman AE, Abascal VM, Block PC, Palacios IF. Percutaneous balloon dilatation of the mitral valve: an analysis of echocardiographic variables related to outcome and the mechanism of dilatation. Br Heart J 1988;60:299–308.

39. Palacios IF, Sanchez PL, Harrell LC, Weyman AE, Block PC. Which patients benefit from percutaneous mitral balloon valvuloplasty? Prevalvuloplasty and postvalvuloplasty variables that predict long-term outcome. Circulation 2002;105:1465–71.

40. Reyes VP, Raju BS, Wynne J, et al. Percutaneous balloon valvuloplasty compared with open surgical commissurotomy for mitral stenosis. N Engl J Med 1994;331:961–7.

41. Patel JJ, Shama D, Mitha AS, et al. Balloon valvuloplasty versus closed commissurotomy for pliable mitral stenosis: a prospective hemodynamic study. J Am Coll Cardiol 1991;18:1318–22.

42. Turi ZG, Reyes VP, Raju BS, et al. Percutaneous balloon versus surgical closed commissurotomy for mitral stenosis. A prospective, randomized trial. Circulation 1991;83:1179–85.

43. Maisano F, Schreuder JJ, Oppizzi M, Fiorani B, Fino C, Alfieri O. The double-orifice technique as a standardized approach to treat mitral regurgitation due to severe myxomatous disease: surgical technique. Eur J Cardiothorac Surg 2000;17:201–5.

44. Maisano F, Torracca L, Oppizzi M, et al. The edge-to-edge technique: a simplified method to correct mitral insufficiency. Eur J Cardiothorac Surg 1998;13:240–5; discussion 245–6.

45. Enriquez-Sarano M, Schaff HV, Orszulak TA, Tajik AJ, Bailey KR, Frye RL. Valve repair improves the outcome of surgery for mitral regurgitation. A multivariate analysis. Circulation 1995;91:1022–8.

46. McGee EC, Gillinov AM, Blackstone EH, et al. Recurrent mitral regurgitation after annuloplasty for functional ischemic mitral regurgitation. J Thorac Cardiovasc Surg 2004;128:916–24.

47. Otto CM. Clinical practice. Evaluation and management of chronic mitral regurgitation. N Engl J Med 2001;345:740–6.

48. Otto CM, Salerno CT. Timing of surgery in asymptomatic mitral regurgitation. N Engl J Med 2005;352:928–9.

49. Grigioni F, Enriquez-Sarano M, Zehr KJ, Bailey KR, Tajik AJ. Ischemic mitral regurgitation: long-term outcome and prognostic implications with quantitative Doppler assessment. Circulation 2001;103:1759–64.

50. Kaji S, Nasu M, Yamamuro A, et al. Annular geometry in patients with chronic ischemic mitral regurgitation: three-dimensional magnetic resonance imaging study. Circulation 2005;112:I409–14.

51. Watanabe N, Ogasawara Y, Yamaura Y, et al. Mitral annulus flattens in ischemic mitral regurgitation: geometric differences between inferior and anterior myocardial infarction: a real-time 3-dimensional echocardiographic study. Circulation 2005;112:I458–62.

52. Messas E, Guerrero JL, Handschumacher MD, et al. Paradoxic decrease in ischemic mitral regurgitation with papillary muscle dysfunction: insights from three-

dimensional and contrast echocardiography with strain rate measurement. Circulation 2001;104:1952–7.

53. Messas E, Guerrero JL, Handschumacher MD, et al. Chordal cutting: a new therapeutic approach for ischemic mitral regurgitation. Circulation 2001;104:1958–63.

54. Fucci C, Sandrelli L, Pardini A, Torracca L, Ferrari M, Alfieri O. Improved results with mitral valve repair using new surgical techniques. Eur J Cardiothorac Surg 1995;9:621–6; discussion 626–7.

55. Feldman T, Wasserman HS, Herrmann HC, et al. Percutaneous mitral valve repair using the edge-to-edge technique: six-month results of the EVEREST Phase I Clinical Trial. J Am Coll Cardiol 2005;46:2134–40.

56. Webb JG, Harnek J, Munt BI, et al. Percutaneous transvenous mitral annuloplasty: initial human experience with device implantation in the coronary sinus. Circulation 2006;113:851–5.

57. Liddicoat JR, Mac Neill BD, Gillinov AM, et al. Percutaneous mitral valve repair: a feasibility study in an ovine model of acute ischemic mitral regurgitation. Catheter Cardiovasc Interv 2003;60:410–6.

58. Daimon M, Shiota T, Gillinov AM, et al. Percutaneous mitral valve repair for chronic ischemic mitral regurgitation: a real-time three-dimensional echocardiographic study in an ovine model. Circulation 2005;111:2183–9.

59. Virmani R, Chun PK, Parker J, McAllister HA, Jr. Suture obliteration of the circumflex coronary artery in three patients undergoing mitral valve operation. Role of left dominant or codominant coronary artery. J Thorac Cardiovasc Surg 1982;84:773–8.

60. Wykrzykowska J, Cohen D, Zimetabum P. Mitral annuloplasty causing left circumflex injury and infarction: novel use of intravascular ultrasound to diagnose suture injury. J Invasive Cardiol 2006;18:505–8.

61. Maselli D, Guarracino F, Chiaramonti F, Mangia F, Borelli G, Minzioni G. Percutaneous mitral annuloplasty: an anatomic study of human coronary sinus and its relation with mitral valve annulus and coronary arteries. Circulation 2006;114:377–80.

62. Rogers JH, Macoviak JA, Rahdert DA, Takeda PA, Palacios IF, Low RI. Percutaneous septal sinus shortening: a novel procedure for the treatment of functional mitral regurgitation. Circulation 2006;113:2329–34.

63. Boudjemline Y, Agnoletti G, Bonnet D, et al. Steps toward the percutaneous replacement of atrioventricular valves an experimental study. J Am Coll Cardiol 2005;46:360–5.

13 Ventricular Assist Devices and Total Artificial Hearts

Arie Blitz, MD and James C. Fang, MD

CONTENTS

Abstract

Advanced heart failure (ACC/AHA stage D) affects about 10% of all patients with heart failure secondary to systolic dysfunction, and is defined by persistent symptoms and disease progression despite optimal medical and device therapy. This group of patients has a mortality rate that approaches 50% at 6 months. Heart transplantation, the best currently available solution for the appropriate patient, is unfortunately limited by donor availability. This chapter discusses

From: *Contemporary Cardiology: Device Therapy in Heart Failure*
Edited by: W.H. Maisel, DOI 10.1007/978-1-59745-424-7_13
© Humana Press, a part of Springer Science+Business Media, LLC 2010

alternative device therapy for patients with advanced heart failure, including ventricular assist devices and total artificial hearts.

Key Words: Heart failure; Medical device; Ventricular assist devices; Artificial hearts; Transplant.

1. BACKGROUND

Advanced heart failure (ACC/AHA stage D) affects about 10% of all patients with heart failure secondary to systolic dysfunction *(1)*, and is defined by persistent symptoms and disease progression despite optimal medical and device therapy. This group of patients has a mortality rate that approaches 50% at 6 months. Heart transplantation, the best currently available solution for the appropriate patient, is unfortunately limited by donor availability. Although post-transplant survival is good (85% at 1 year and 50% at 10 years), fewer than 2500 heart transplants are performed in the United States annually, and this number appears to be falling. In 2006, UNOS reports that 1853 heart transplants were performed in the United States, the lowest number in the past 10 years. Yet the number of people with advanced heart failure who could potentially benefit from transplantation may be as great as 50,000. Hence, heart transplantation is an effective treatment on the individual level, but is trivial in its epidemiologic impact. Transplantation is also complicated by other issues. Paradoxically, patients at highest risk of dying from heart failure are often not considered transplant candidates because of their advanced age or comorbidities. Finally, there has historically been a significant mortality due to heart failure while on the transplant waiting list.

Mechanical circulatory support (MCS) serves an important role in advanced heart failure in light of the limitations of cardiac transplantation. Such devices replace or supplement the native cardiac output and consist of ventricular assist devices (VADs) and total artificial hearts (TAHs). There are approximately 30 devices either in use or in preclinical phase. This review will include discussion of the more commonly used devices in the United States. VADs provide a parallel circulation to the heart and can assume most if not all of the function of one ventricle. TAHs completely replace the native heart and assume the function of both ventricles. These devices have a variety of evolving applications including postcardiotomy circulatory support (PCCS), bridge to transplantation (BTT), bridge to recovery (BTR), and destination therapy (DT). Newly evolving concepts are the use of devices as a bridge to bridge or bridge to decision. Overall, MCS is emerging as the standard of care for treating acute and chronic heart failure refractory to medical therapy *(2, 3)*.

The era of MCS was inaugurated by Gibbon in 1953 with his invention of the heart–lung machine and cardiopulmonary bypass (CPB), allowing for contemporary cardiac surgery (Table 1). The early MCS devices consisted of

Table 1
History of mechanical circulatory support

Year	Milestone
1953	Cardiopulmonary bypass
1959	Demonstration of postcardiotomy shock support
1961	Development of intra-aortic counterpulsation
1962	First use roller pump for left ventricular assistance
1964	Artificial Heart Program established by the NHLBI
1966	First postcardiotomy mechanical bridge to recovery with assist pump
1967	First clinical application of IABP for cardiogenic shock
1967	First heart transplantation with human donor heart
1969	First total artificial heart as a bridge to transplantation
1974	Redirection of the Artificial Heart Program toward implantable devices
1978	Report of patients bridged to transplant with an abdominal LVAD
1978	Report of patients bridged to transplant with IABP
1980	NIH requests proposals for left heart assist systems
1982	First total artificial heart for permanent replacement
1984	First successful use of LVAD as bridge to transplant
1994	Heartmate LVAD FDA approved as bridge to transplant
2001	REMATCH trial published
2002	Heartmate XVE FDA approved for destination therapy

roller pumps or centrifugal pumps adapted from the cardiopulmonary bypass circuit. Although these devices could support the heart and circulation perioperatively, they were not practical for more extended periods of time due to blood trauma and the challenges of adapting pump speed for changes in filling pressures. The intra-aortic balloon pump (IABP), a passive form of a MCS, was developed by Moulopoulos in 1961 (4). Adrian Kantrowitz was the first to report survival of a patient with cardiogenic shock after a myocardial infarction on IABP support (5). With the establishment of the Artificial Heart Program by the NIH in 1964, government-sponsored research of MCS helped to propel the technology into the current state of the art. The current generation of active displacement pulsatile pumps is now giving way to second and third generation continuous flow VADs. TAHs developed in a parallel manner. Cooley and Liotta performed the first total artificial heart as a BTT in 1969, but the patient succumbed to complications after transplantation. DeVries implanted the first TAH for permanent replacement, the well-publicized Jarvik 7. The FDA-approved Cardiowest TAH is a descendent of the original Jarvik 7 although other TAHs are in clinical trials.

2. PHYSIOLOGIC CONSIDERATIONS

All MCS devices impart energy to blood that is converted to augmented flow. Energy is imparted either via a rotating shaft, pusher plate, or pneumatic pressure line. The conversion of energy from electricity to blood flow involves some loss of energy, which is reflected in the pump's efficiency. First-generation devices consist exclusively of positive displacement pumps due to the perception that pulsatile perfusion was necessary for normal end-organ function. This paradigm has been challenged by the recent success of second-generation devices – i.e., non-displacement or rotary pumps – that provide continuous relatively nonpulsatile flow over extended periods of time *(6, 7)*. The main advantages of the non-displacement pumps are their more compact size and their greater durability. Third-generation VADs use magnetically levitated systems that eliminate contact and friction between the moving and non-moving parts of the VAD, a critical issue for durability.

Most VADs provide some pulsatility within the patient's vascular system, independent of the method by which the VAD provides flow. Positive displacement pumps initiate a pulse by the intermittent displacement of a blood volume. Positive displacement pumps are preload dependent and are relatively independent of afterload. As long as the afterload can be overcome, flow in a functioning pump is a direct reflection of its preload. Exceptions occur when the patient is very hypertensive or there are technical issues with the outflow graft or anastomosis. In contrast, rotary pumps have no inherent pulsatility, yet circulatory pulsatility may be present. Because the native heart continues to pump, there is a continuously changing pulsatile difference between the LV chamber and the aortic pressure. A continuous flow VAD will consequently alter its flow rate dependent upon the speed of the impeller and the continually changing difference between the proximal pressure (preload) and distal pressure (afterload). Unlike the positive displacement pumps, rotary pumps are highly dependent on *both* preload and afterload. For any given preload, the greater the pressure differential between the left ventricle and the aorta, the greater the instantaneous flow of the device. Furthermore, if the left ventricle is not completely unloaded by the device, flow across the native aortic valve will occur during systole. However, the in vivo pulse pressure of the rotary pumps is attenuated when compared to positive displacement pumps.

For the most part, positive displacement pumps whose inlet is connected to the LV apex result in complete emptying of the heart. Hence, the aortic valve rarely opens and the device's output is tantamount to total cardiac output. In effect, both the native left ventricle and the device chamber are functioning in series (Fig. 1). Because of the negative pressure of the device chamber, the native LV becomes a passive conduit for the VAD *(8)*. By virtue of their preload dependence, the ejection rate of a properly functioning positive displacement pump in its automatic or volume mode is dependent upon the rate of filling of the pump prior to ejection. Device bradycardia reflects slow filling from volume depletion; device tachycardia suggests rapid device filling from volume overload. Slow device filling, or device bradycardia, can also occur when worsening native RV function is unable to push blood

Circuitry of VADs

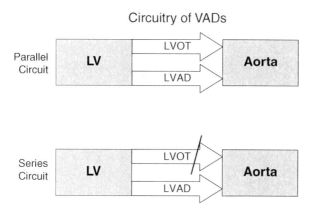

Fig. 1. VAD circulations.

over to the left side or when native LV function competes for filling. Distinguishing among these possibilities can usually be accomplished by echocardiography.

Biventricular support is a more complex phenomenon, since the two VAD circuits function somewhat independently but must provide flow to one another in series. Importantly, the total cardiac output on the left side is greater than that on the right, since some part of the bronchial blood supply returns to the LV via the pulmonary veins. With the TAH, a capacitance chamber must be present to equilibrate the right- and left-sided outputs.

3. THE DEVICES

Choice of MCS device is dependent upon a number of factors but most importantly the anticipated duration of support and the implantation method, i.e., surgical or percutaneous. In general, the more short-term the device, the greater its applicability to acute cardiovascular collapse, as in the case of cardiogenic shock from myocardial infarction or inflammatory diseases and postcardiotomy syndrome (when the device is used to "bridge to decision" and/or "bridge to bridge"). More long-term devices are generally meant to provide elective circulatory support in chronic medically refractory heart failure as a bridge to transplantation, bridge to recovery, or as destination therapy. A select number of devices will be briefly described.

4. SHORT-TERM DEVICES (<1 MONTH OF SUPPORT)

4.1. Tandemheart Percutaneous Ventricular Assist®

The Tandemheart pump (CardiacAssist Inc, Pittsburgh, PA) is a centrifugal pump that is inserted percutaneously via the femoral vessels (Fig. 2). The system consists of a 21 Fr trans-septal inflow cannula inserted via the

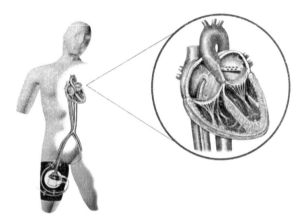

Fig. 2. TandemHeart.

femoral vein, an outflow cannula inserted via the femoral artery, a small centrifugal pump with a hydrodynamic bearing, an upper blood chamber, and a lower mechanical motor chamber. It has a very low prime volume of 10 ml, and it is driven by a three phase, brushless, DC servomotor. A unique lubrication system of heparinized saline provides a hydrodynamic bearing that supports a spinning rotor. The controller drives the pump and supplies the lubricant. Batteries can support the patient up to 1 h for patient transport or in the event of AC power failure. The device can provide up to 5 l/min and can be used up to two weeks. It has FDA clearance and CE Mark-approved status. The most common current applications of the Tandemheart are to provide circulatory support during acute cardiogenic shock and high risk percutaneous interventions such as coronary stenting, valvuloplasty, and arrhythmia ablation.

4.2. Impella Recover®

The Impella Recover systems (Abiomed, Danvers, MA) consist of devices that can be implanted either percutaneously or surgically, and can provide 2.5–5.5 l/min. The systems can be used for left, right, or biventricular support (Fig. 3) and has CE Mark approval. All the Impella devices are driven by a universal mobile console. The control panel can be operated with rechargeable batteries for up to 1 h; a power pack is available for longer periods of support. The catheters are as small as 12 Fr (4.0 mm) and have a maximal weight of 8 g. The percutaneous Impella devices are inserted via the femoral artery and are placed retrograde across the aortic valve with the tip lying in the ventricle. The Impella® RD is the smallest available fully implantable, right ventricular support device and weighs only 17 g. The Impella® RD can deliver up to 5.5 l/min from the right atrium via an outlet graft into the

The Impella Devices

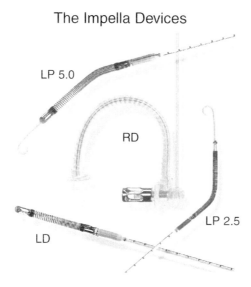

Fig. 3. The Impella systems.

pulmonary artery. It is a small paracardiac pump with a short inlet cage, which is inserted into the right atrium. The outflow graft is ring-enforced and is sewn to the pulmonary artery.

4.3. Abiomed BVS 5000® and AB 5000®

The Abiomed BVS 5000 (Abiomed, Danvers, MA) is a positive displacement extracorporeal assist device meant for short-term (<7–10 days) support (Fig. 4), typically in the postcardiotomy setting. The most recent console manufactured by the company can drive both the BVS 5000 pump as well as the paracorporeal AB 5000 pump (see below). The BVS pump is pneumatically driven, self regulating, and can provide up to 6 l/min. Inflow is most commonly via the right or left atrium, and passive filling occurs under gravity. The outflow graft is sewn to the pulmonary artery or the ascending aorta. The pump can be used for right, left, or biventricular support. Each system consists of two polyurethane valves connected in series. An advantage of the BVS cannula system is the same cannulae can be used for the longer-term (30 days) AB 5000 device, a pneumatically driven pump. Hence, conversions from the BVS to the AB system can be performed at the bedside without requiring a repeat surgical procedure or cardiopulmonary bypass. Another advantage of the BVS system is its simplicity and ease of insertion. It is one of the more commonly used devices in community hospitals for postcardiotomy support which then enables transfer of these patients to a tertiary referral center for further management.

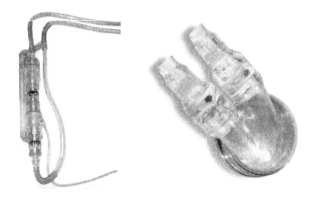

Fig. 4. The Abiomed devices.

4.4. Levitronix CENTriMAG®

The Levitronix CentriMag (Levitronix, Waltham, MA) is a magnetically levitated extracorporeal LVAD (Fig. 5). The device is inserted intraoperatively and can be used for right, left, or biventricular support. It can be connected to conventional cannulae used for cardiopulmonary bypass. Its magnetic levitation system, a feature of third-generation VADs, is unique in that it eliminates mechanical friction, which decreases hemolysis and thromboembolism as well as improving durability. It has CE Mark approval in Europe, but remains investigational in the United States. The centrifugal pump design permits rotation of the impeller at lower speeds than axial flow pumps for comparable flows, thus decreasing blood trauma. The revolutions

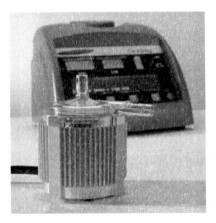
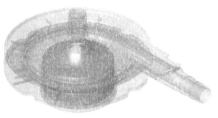

Fig. 5. Levitronix® CentriMag®.

per minute (RPM) range is 1500–5500 and can provide flow up to 9.9 l/min. The system consists of a single-use pump, a motor, and a drive console.

5. LONG-TERM DEVICES (>1 MONTH OF SUPPORT)

5.1. Thoratec® Paracorporeal and Intracorporeal Ventricular Assist Devices (PVAD/IVAD)

The Thoratec PVAD (Thoratec Corporation, Pleasanton, CA), developed at Penn State, was first used clinically for postcardiotomy support in 1982, for bridge to transplant in 1984, and FDA approved in 1995 *(9, 10)* (Fig. 6). Each VAD has an externalized pneumatic pusher-plate pump that rests on the anterior abdominal wall and is connected to the heart via cannulae that traverse the abdominal or chest wall. Inflow cannulation can be either from the atrium or the ventricle. A major advantage of the Thoratec PVAD device is that it can be used to assist either or both ventricles. It is a positive displacement pump that has a stroke volume of 65 ml and two mechanical valves. The pump chamber is composed of a smooth surface segmented flexible polyurethane sac and a rigid polysulfone shell. The rate range for the device is 40–100 bpm, and the output range is 1.3–7.2 l/min *(11)*. Since the PVAD is a paracorporeal device, it can be used in small patients with body surface areas (BSA) as small as 0.73 m^2. Its power source is pneumatic via either the dual drive console (DDC) or the portable TLC-II driver. The exteriorized pump is easier to troubleshoot than other VADs because it is transparent. The Thoratec IVAD is similar to the PVAD, but is an intracorporeal device that was developed from the PVAD. The most notable differences from the PVAD include a smooth polished titanium pump housing for implantability and a reduced weight (339 g versus 417 g) and volume (252 ml versus 318 ml). Delrin occluder disks are built into the inflow and outflow ports. The PVAD and IVAD are the only long-term devices that can be used for biventricular support and accommodate home discharge. Because the IVAD is intracorporeal, its use is limited to larger patients with BSA >1.3 m^2.

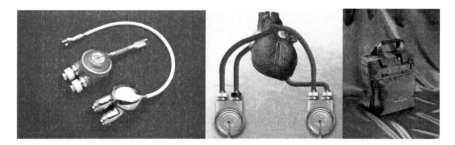

Fig. 6. Thoratec IVAD and PVAD.

5.2. Heartmate® LVAD

The Heartmate LVAD (Thoratec Corporation, Pleasanton, CA) (Fig. 7) is an intracorporeal device designed solely for left ventricular support and can be driven either pneumatically (IP) or electrically (XVE). Although originally approved as a bridge to transplant, it is now also FDA approved for destination therapy. The percutaneous driveline of the device contains both an electric cable and air vent *(12)* and is covered by a polyester woven velour material designed for tissue ingrowth. The pump itself consists of a rigid titanium housing containing a flexible polyurethane diaphragm. On one side of the diaphragm is the blood chamber and on the other is the electric motor. The diaphragm is displaced by rotation of the motor, which is connected to the controller via the driveline. The external housing of the pump is made of a titanium alloy. The interior of the blood chamber is covered by a patented textured internal surface composed of titanium microspheres. This unique surface promotes the formation of a pseudointima from deposition of a fibrin-cellular matrix, rendering the blood chamber minimally thrombogenic *(13, 14)*. Minimal anticoagulation is required for this device; only an aspirin is suggested. The textured surface, however, may lead to systemic immune activation and HLA sensitization, potentially limiting compatible donors for heart transplantation *(15–17)*.

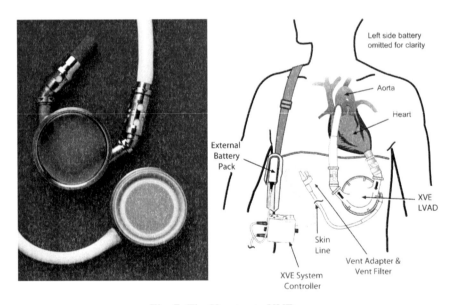

Fig. 7. The Heartmate XVE.

Like the Thoratec VADs, the Heartmate is a positive displacement pump. The pump is implanted intracorporeally in either a preperitoneal or intraperitoneal location and therefore limited to patients with BSA >1.5 m². The inflow valve conduit is attached to the apex of the ventricle, and a woven

Dacron^{TM} graft is anastomosed to the ascending aorta. The maximum stroke volume is 83 ml, the rate range is 50–120 bpm, and it can pump up to 10 (XVE) or 12 (IP) l/min. The weight of the blood pump along with the implantable components is 1255 g. The controller is a microprocessor-based unit and can be operated in either the fixed or automatic modes. In the fixed mode, the rate of the device is set by the clinician and the pump will beat at that set rate regardless of the blood chamber's fill state. In the auto mode, the pump will eject when the blood chamber has reached about 97% capacity (approximately 80 ml) and is therefore preload sensitive. Pneumatic pumping is available for backup purposes when there is electric motor failure. The electrical power can arise from either a portable battery system or a stationary power supply. The batteries (0.65 kg) are 12-V, sealed lead-acid batteries that last about 6.5 h each under normal conditions.

5.3. Novacor®

The Novacor (World Heart Corporation, Oakland, CA) device is similar to the Heartmate XVE in its overall design and its implantation technique (Fig. 8). It was first FDA approved as a bridge to transplant in 1998. It is a positive displacement pump that serves only as an LVAD. Its pusher plate

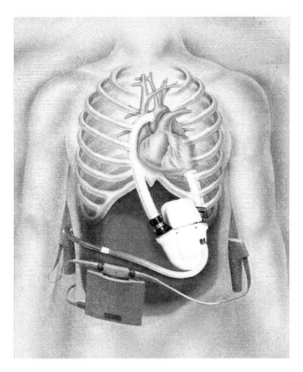

Fig. 8. The Novacor VAD.

mechanism is unique in that it has a dual chamber design that minimizes torque, which improves device longevity. Patients have been supported on their original device for over 4 years. The pump stroke volume is 70 ml and it can provide up to 10 l/min. Unlike the Heartmate, the blood-contacting surface of the pumping chamber is smooth and thrombogenic requiring systemic anticoagulation and antiplatelet therapy. Like the Heartmate XVE, the Novacor device is portable, wearable, and patients may be discharged home on this device. Because of its intracorporeal location, it can only be used in patients with BSA >1.7 m^2.

6. SECOND-GENERATION DEVICES: AXIAL FLOW PUMPS

Major advantages of the axial flow pumps include small size, lower power consumption, durability, and lack of valves. These features broaden the range of patient sizes in which the device can be implanted. They also appear to be more infection resistant than the positive displacement pumps. Previous concerns regarding the lack of pulsatile flow and the potential for hemolysis have not been clinically realized.

6.1. Debakey VAD®

The DeBakey VAD (Micromed Technology Inc., Houston, TX) (Fig. 9) was developed in a joint venture among Baylor College of Medicine, MicroMed Technology, Inc., and NASA *(7, 18–21)*. The Debakey VAD received the CE Mark in 2001 and is currently in US pivotal trials for

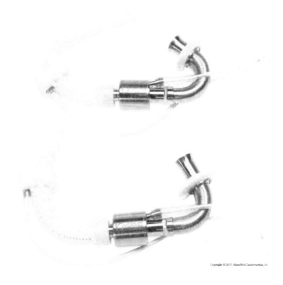

Fig. 9. The Micromed – DeBakey axial flow pump.

BTT and DT. Like other axial flow pumps, the DeBakey VAD is compact, measures 1.2 by 3 in., and weighs 95 g. The pump contains an inducer impeller, actuated by an electromagnet, and is the only moving part of the system. It is supported at both ends by double pivot bearings. The inducer impeller has three blades with eight magnets hermetically sealed in each blade. Blood flowing through the pump first travels through a flow straightener, followed by the inducer impeller, and finally through a diffuser before exiting the device. The diffuser redirects the tangential blood flow to axial flow, thus imparting pressure to the blood. Like all impeller pumps, flow is both preload and afterload dependent. It spins at 7500–12,500 rpm and is capable of generating flow in excess of 10 l/min. At 10,000 rpm it requires less than 10 W of power. The tip of the curved titanium inflow cannula is inserted into the LV apex, and a Dacron outflow graft is sewn to the ascending aorta. An ultrasonic flow probe is positioned on the outflow graft to quantify flow rates.

6.2. Heartmate II®

The Heartmate II (Thoratec Corporation, Pleasanton, CA) (Fig. 10) is an axial flow pump developed through a collaboration between Nimbus and the University of Pittsburgh (22, 23). The rpm range is from 6000 to 15,000, and flows are as high as 10 l/min. Like the Debakey VAD, the inflow cannula is joined at the apex of the LV and the outflow to the aorta. The pump is small (124 ml) and connects to its controller via a percutaneous cable. The spinning rotor has three curved blades and is energized by a magnet-coupling force. A control algorithm senses the volume status of the ventricle and adjusts impellar speed accordingly. The Heartmate II is currently

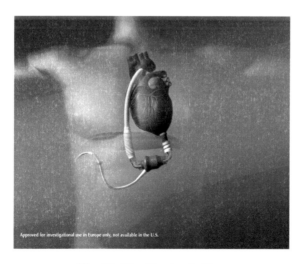

Approved for investigational use in Europe only, not available in the U.S.

Fig. 10. The Heartmate II.

undergoing Phase II pivotal trials in the United States for BTT and DT. The blood-contacting surface of the Heartmate II is a hybrid between the textured surface of the original Heartmate as well as a smooth titanium surface to minimize thromboembolization.

6.3. Jarvik 2000®

Held in the hand, the Jarvik 2000 pump (Fig. 11) is about the size of a C battery and weighs only 90 g. It is only 25 mm in diameter and 55 mm in length. It is an intracorporeal device that has no true inflow cannula since the impeller lies within the ventricular cavity. Within its welded titanium shell sits a direct-current motor, a rotor supported by two ceramic bearings, and a small, spinning titanium impeller that pumps blood from the heart up to 7 l/min. The impeller consists of a neodymium–iron–boron magnet and two hydrodynamic titanium blades on its surface. The blood-contacting surface comprises a smooth mirror finish of titanium. The outflow consists of a 16 mm Dacron graft. The device can be used as either an LVAD or RVAD. As an LVAD, it can be implanted either via a sternotomy or a left thoracotomy. In the latter case, the outflow anastomosis is made to the descending aorta. The device received the CE Mark in 2005 both as BTT and DT. It is currently undergoing BTT trials in the United States. The DT version used in Europe is implanted with the driveline connection on a skull-based pedestal to lower the incidence of infection.

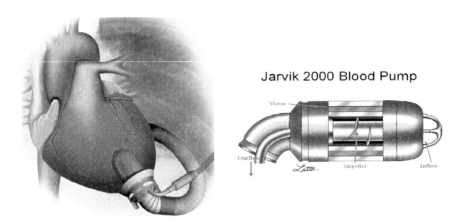

Fig. 11. The Jarvik axial flow pump.

7. THIRD-GENERATION DEVICES: MAGLEV TECHNOLOGY

The third-generation blood pumps are currently under various stages of development and are characterized by magnetically levitated systems ("maglev") to improve durability (24, 25). There are three categories of maglev technology: (1) An external motor-driven system (Terumo Duraheart®), (2) the direct-drive motor-driven system (Berlinheart Incor®), and (3) the bearingless motor system (Levitronix Centrimag®). Because the technology is more complex, the pumps are larger than the second-generation devices *(24)*.

8. TOTAL ARTIFICIAL HEARTS (TAH)

Only two types of TAH (Fig. 12) have been implanted in humans: The Cardiowest® (Syncardia Systems, Tucson, AZ) and the Abiocor® (Abiomed Inc, Danvers, MA) *(26)*. TAHs provide biventricular circulation in one device which not only provides right ventricular support "prophylaxis" but broadens patient applicability. TAHs can be implanted in patients with many types of cardiac pathology that complicate LVAD therapy such as aortic insufficiency, mitral stenosis, LV thrombus, calcified LV aneurysms, severe biventricular failure, ventricular septal defects, atrial septal defects, amyloidosis, cancer survivors on cardiotoxic agents, diffuse cardiac tumors, and failed heart transplants *(26)*. The primary disadvantage of the TAH is that there is no backup system in place (i.e., the native heart) in case device failure occurs. The CardioWest TAH is approved only for BTT; the Abiocor TAH is only investigational as a DT device.

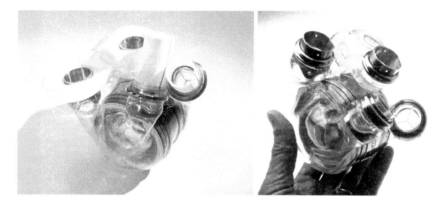

Fig. 12. Total artificial hearts (Cardiowest and Abiocor).

The Abiocor is driven by an internal motor using hydraulic-coupled chambers so that while one side is ejecting, the other side is filling. It is completely implantable and is powered by a transcutaneous energy transmission system that consists of internal and external coils that transmit power across the skin. The Abiocor consists of an internal thoracic unit, rechargeable battery, miniaturized electronics, and an external battery pack. All blood-contacting surfaces, including the two blood pumps (stroke volume of 60 ml) and the four trileaflet valves (24-mm internal diameter) are fabricated from polyurethane (Angioflex®, Abiomed Inc, Danvers, MA). An atrial balance chamber is present and allows for the differences in right- and left-sided stroke volumes (27).

The Cardiowest TAH (28, 29) was first implanted by Dr. DeVries in 1982. The patient, Barney Clark, survived for 112 days (30). The Cardiowest TAH was approved by the FDA as a BTT in 2004 and is the only such device available in the United States. DT implants are being performed in Europe. The pump is pneumatically driven and has a pair of ventricles made of polyurethane. There are four Medtronic-hall mechanical valves to maintain unidirectional flow. Each ventricle contains an air sac and a blood sac, and these sacs are separated by a four-layered polyurethane membrane. Air is driven into each air sac via percutaneous lines, and the forced air causes the air sac to expand and the blood sac to be compressed during systole. The reverse process occurs for diastole. The drivelines attach to a large external console although a portable driver is available in Europe. The maximum stroke volume is 70 ml and the maximum output is greater than 9 l/min[26].

9. PATIENT AND DEVICE SELECTION

MCS is indicated when circulatory failure persists despite maximal medical therapy. Maximal therapy is generally defined by high-dose inotropic/vasopressor support and the use of either mechanical ventilation and/or IABP. The hemodynamic profile includes a cardiac index of <2.0 l/min/m^2, a pulmonary capillary wedge pressure of >20 mmHg, and a systolic blood pressure of <80 mmHg. The primary concerns at the time of potential implant are the morbidity and mortality of device implantation and the anticipated length of support (31). In acute situations, percutaneous devices are preferable since the time to support is the shortest and the morbidity of the procedure least. Exclusion criteria include irreversible pulmonary, hepatic, neurologic, or renal failure. Risk factors for mortality include urine output less than 30 ml/h, central venous pressure greater than 16 mmHg, mechanical ventilation, prothrombin time greater than 16 s, a redo sternotomy, and a white blood cell count greater than 15,000 (32). A scoring system has been developed that incorporates some of these clinical criteria (Table 2). Others have also found that respiratory failure due to sepsis, right heart failure, age >65 years, acute postcardiotomy, and acute infarction portend poor survival (33).

An important decision at the time of device implant is whether the patient needs left ventricular or biventricular support. Approximately 10–20% of patients require biventricular support and such patients have poorer outcomes than those who only require LVAD therapy. Right ventricular failure dramatically increases operative mortality when it complicates LVAD implantation with mortality rates as high as 50% (34). In the setting of acute circulatory collapse from left heart disease, a biventricular device is generally required because multiorgan system failure is present. This decision is

Table 2
Predicting survival after LVAD therapy

Revised system	
Variable	Score
Ventilation	4
Redo surgery	2
Previous LVAD insertion	2
CVP > 16 mmHg	1
PT > 16 s	1
Score	Mortality
>5	47%
<5	9%
Original system	
Variable	Score
Urine output < 30 ml/h	3
Ventilation	2
CVP A> 16 mmHg	2
PT > 16 s	2
Redo surgery	1

particularly relevant when the preoperative central venous pressure is greater than 20 mmHg suggesting concomitant right ventricular failure. Even more ominous is when a high central venous pressure is accompanied by low or normal pulmonary arterial pressures suggesting both diastolic and systolic right ventricular dysfunction. Other predictors for post-LVAD right ventricular dysfunction include large RV volumes, decreased RV stroke work, a transpulmonary gradient of 15 mmHg, and less than a drop of 10 mmHg in the mean pulmonary arterial pressure after LVAD insertion (35). In patients without obvious preoperative indications for RVAD support, intraoperative indications may arise as is often the case when a patient receives numerous transfusions. Transfusions are associated with cytokine release, diffuse inflammation, and rapid volume overload which may result in pulmonary hypertension and consequent right ventricular failure. On rare occasions, only RVAD support may be required as in the case of isolated right ventricular infarction in the absence of significant left ventricular dysfunction. It should be noted that biventricular or RVAD-only support are only indicated as BTT or BTR, not for DT.

10. CLINICAL EXPERIENCES

10.1. Acute Cardiogenic Shock

Acute cardiogenic shock may occur after a range of insults, including myocardial infarction, acute myocarditis, and pregnancy. Any of the devices discussed under the short-term support section are appropriate in this situation. Percutaneous devices are preferable because in contrast to surgically implanted devices, they can be placed quickly and less invasively. In a recent study by Burkhoff and colleagues, the feasibility, safety, and hemodynamic impact of the Tandemheart percutaneous LVAD was investigated in 13 patients presenting with acute cardiogenic shock *(36)*. The VAD was successfully placed in all 13 patients, and the mean duration of support was 60 ± 44 h. During support, cardiac index increased from 2.09 ± 0.64 at baseline to 2.53 ± 0.65 ($P = 0.02$), mean blood pressure increased from 70.6 ± 11.1 to 81.7 ± 14.6 ($P = 0.01$), and wedge pressure decreased from 27.2 ± 12.2 to 16.5 ± 4.8 ($P=0.01$). Ten patients survived to device explant, six of whom were bridged to another therapy. Seven patients survived to hospital discharge and were all alive at 6 months. The two most common adverse events were distal leg ischemia ($n = 3$) and bleeding from the cannulation site ($n = 4$). There have also been several reports of the successful treatment of acute fulminant myocarditis with surgically placed MCS devices. In a report from UCLA, four moribund patients with acute myocarditis were supported with the Abiomed BVS 5000 system. Two patients received immunotherapy with OKT3. Biventricular assist was used in three patients and left ventricular assist was used only in one. All four patients were weaned from their devices after a mean support time of 8.3 days (7–11) and were successfully discharged home *(37)*.

10.2. Postcardiotomy Cardiogenic Shock

Patients who cannot be weaned from cardiopulmonary bypass are commonly considered for MCS. Most commonly, PCCS support is anticipated because the patient arrives in the operating room in cardiogenic shock but may be unanticipated when there is prolonged cross clamp time and/or inadequate myocardial protection. Patients experiencing PCCS are more likely to require biventricular support because of the severity of the insult. Most of the published experience with PCCS support involves the use of the Abiomed BVS 5000 system, a popular MCS device for community hospitals because of cost and ease of insertion. A prospective multicenter study in the early 1990s established the efficacy and safety of the BVS 5000 for PCCS *(38)*. In this small cohort of 31 patients, 55% were successfully weaned from support and 29% were discharged. Postoperative bleeding was common occurring in 76%. Eight patients were NYHA I or II at 1-year follow-up. Cardiac arrest before VAD support, in particular, was a poor prognostic indicator. In a later retrospective review from Hahnemann University Hospital, 45 patients in cardiogenic shock were supported with the BVS 5000 during a 6-year period *(39)*. Devices were inserted for postcardiotomy shock in most patients; 20% had precardiotomy shock. The average duration of support was 8.3 days (range 1–31 days). Overall, half of the patients were eventually weaned from support and a third discharged from the hospital. The most common complications were bleeding and neurologic events. The investigators found that the outcomes could be improved by the establishment of a VAD insertion algorithm, which emphasizes the timely insertion of ventricular assistance. In summary, PCCS is a rare event (0.3% from the Society of Thoracic Surgeons database 1995–2004) but can be successfully treated with MCS devices. Over half of patients can be expected to survive until discharge and MCS devices have significantly improved outcomes over the past decade.

10.3. Bridge to Decision and Bridge to Bridge

Many patients who undergo insertion of a short-term VAD for cardiogenic shock or PCCS are in extremis at the time of initial evaluation, and therefore their neurologic status and/or candidacy for heart transplantation are unknown. Ideally, a simple and less invasive short-term device is placed to allow for a period of assessment, i.e., bridge to decision. These devices include extracorporeal membrane oxygenators (ECMO), percutaneous VADs, and even the Abiomed BVS system. In the case of irreversible neurologic damage or poor candidacy for heart transplantation, support can be terminated in the post-VAD implant period. In the case of myocardial recovery, such devices can be readily explanted. For those who are transplant candidates but myocardial recovery does not occur, the devices can be used to BTT or undergo conversion to a more long-term device, i.e., as a bridge to bridge. Hoefer et al. recently described their experience using ECMO as a bridge to bridge *(40)*. One hundred thirty-one patients were supported with ECMO over a 10-year period. After further evaluation and management, 28 patients ultimately underwent ECMO to VAD conversion. Half of these patients were long-term survivors at a mean follow-up of 39 months. The authors found that previous cardiopulmonary resuscitation, elevated lactate levels, and impaired liver function predicted poor post-VAD mortality despite pre-VAD ECMO support.

10.4. Bridge to Transplantation (BTT)

The vast majority of long-term VADs are currently placed as a BTT and most of the experience regarding long-term MCS comes from BTT trials. The International Society of Heart Lung Transplantation (ISHLT) MCS device database shows that 75% of devices were placed for BTT, 12% for DT, and 5% for BTR *(41)*. The growth of heart transplantation and VAD therapy have been synergistic. The proportion of patients supported by mechanical devices at the time of transplantation has increased from 3% in 1990 to over 28% in 2004 *(42)*. In one of the earliest reports of using VADs to BTT, Frazier and colleagues *(43)* reported that 65% of 34 patients bridged with the Heartmate IP successfully underwent heart transplantation and 80% were discharged from the hospital. In contrast, of six nonrandom-ized controls who did not undergo VAD placement for logistical reasons, only three underwent heart transplantation and none of these patients sur-vived. Complications in the BTT patients included bleeding, infection, and right heart failure. Importantly, right heart failure was significantly associ-ated with an adverse outcome. In larger subsequent report of 280 transplant candidates from 24 centers with medically refractory heart failure, the Heart-mate VE showed a marked survival benefit when compared to a historical control group of 48 patients who did not undergo LVAD placement (Figs. 13 and 14). The two groups were similar with respect to many preoperative variables although the VAD group was significantly more hypotensive and had worse cardiac function. Seventy-one percent of the VAD patients sur-vived to transplant in contrast to 33% of the non-VAD group (*P*<0.0001). Post-transplant survival was also superior in patients supported with VADs compared to historically similar but non-VAD supported transplanted patients *(44)*.

VAD implantation allows time for optimization of organ systems and nutritional status prior to transplantation. In patients who are bridged to transplantation, the best outcome is achieved if the patients are supported for at least one month after VAD insertion to allow for physical, nutritional, and end-organ recovery. Ashton and colleagues reported on their analysis of patients supported either less than one month or greater than one month before undergoing transplantation *(45)*. They found that patients supported

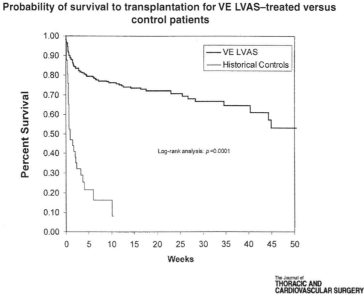

Probability of survival to transplantation for VE LVAS–treated versus control patients

The Journal of THORACIC AND CARDIOVASCULAR SURGERY

Fig. 13A. Benefit of LVAD support prior to heart transplantation *(44)*.

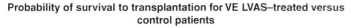

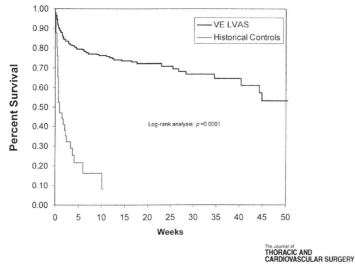

Fig. 13B. Post-transplant benefit of pretransplant LVAD support *(44)*.

REMATCH TRIAL

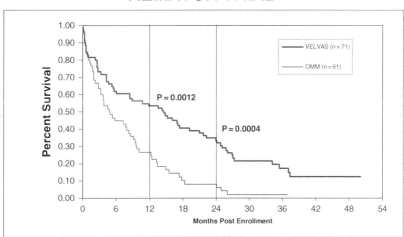

Class IV heart failure after at least 90 days of maximal medical therapy and/or inotrope dependent.

Not eligible for cardiac transplantation.

Fig. 14. REMATCH Trial *(63)*.

for less than one month had a threefold greater perioperative mortality compared with patients supported more than 30 days ($P = 0.031$). These findings have been supported by other investigators and other VADs, such as the Novacor *(46–48)*.

There is a growing experience with the use of second-generation devices as BTT. In 2003, Goldstein and colleagues reported on the worldwide experience with the MicroMed DeBakey VAD as a bridge to transplantation *(49)*. One hundred and fifty patients underwent implantation with this device from 1998 to 2002. Fifty-five percent were bridged to either transplant or recovery or still supported; 45% had died. There was a low rate of device infection (0.16 per patient-year) and pump failure (0.13 per patient-year). Of concern was a 0.61 incidence per patient-year of pump thrombus.

The Heartmate II experience has been more encouraging. One hundred and thirty-three patients at 26 centers were enrolled in less than a year. Seventy-five percent of the cohort met the trial's primary endpoint of cardiac transplantation or survival at 180 days while remaining eligible for transplantation. In addition, secondary endpoints, including frequency of adverse events, functional status, and quality of life, were improved. The mean support duration was 169 days, with one patient supported by the device for 600 days. Fifty-one percent were transplanted and three additional patients recovered sufficient function of their natural heart to have the device removed. Twenty-two percent were still being supported by the device at 180 days or longer and remained eligible for transplantation; 25% did not meet the primary endpoint, including 25 patients who died while being supported on the device. There were no reported mechanical pump failures, no pocket infections, and only 18 percutaneous lead infections. Bleeding and stroke were also decreased when compared to the Heartmate XVE experience. The Jarvik device also appears to be effective as a BTT *(50)*.

The TAH can also be considered when there is biventricular failure and the patient needs to be BTT. In a nonrandomized prospective study of 81 patients in five centers using CardioWest TAH *(51)*, survival to transplant was 79% compared to 46% for historical controls ($P<0.001$). Survival rates of 1- and 5-year after transplant for those supported with the TAH were 86 and 64%, respectively. These results compare favorably with the results of BTT with LVAD therapy and confirm the superiority of MCS in bridging the most ill patients to transplantation.

10.5. Bridge to Recovery

BTR is considered when the primary myocardial insult is felt to be acute, transient, and reversible, e.g., myocardial ischemia, myocarditis, or post-transplant rejection. BTR may also be employed to provide circulatory support to facilitate the pharmacologic treatment of a more chronic underlying disorder such as idiopathic dilated cardiomyopathy. Significant biochemical, neurohormonal, and structural improvements occur with chronic VAD support *(52–56)*. For example, increased beta-adrenergic responsiveness, normalization of ryanodine phosphorylation, and greater beta-adrenergic receptor density have been documented in human left and right ventricular trabeculae after LVAD support *(57)*. However, in most published experiences, only a minority of patients (5–10%) who require circulatory assistance are weanable from support *(58, 59)*. Criteria that have been used to predict explantation success include brief heart failure duration, nonischemic etiology, and spontaneous significant improvements in myocardial performance assessed during routine surveillance echocardiography during full VAD support. A number of weaning protocols to predict explantation success have been proposed that involve hemodynamic and echocardiographic assessments during exercise and/or inotropic challenge *(60)*. An ejection fraction >45%, an LVEDD <55 mm, normal resting hemodynamics, and augmentation of cardiac output with either exercise or dobutamine while VAD support is transiently decreased are predictive of post-VAD explant transplant-free survival *(61)*.

Pharmacologic management during VAD weaning should consist of contemporary heart failure therapy including renin–angiotensin antagonists, beta-blockers, and aldosterone antagonists. Several investigators have examined the role of a variety of other novel pharmacological interventions designed to accelerate or improve this process. Clenbuterol, a beta 2-adrenergic receptor agonist, has been reported to induce myocardial hypertrophy, prevent myocardial atrophy, and improve intracellular calcium handling. In a recent single center report from Great Britain, 11 of 15 patients with nonischemic dilated cardiomyopathy that required LVAD support met explantation criteria after being treated with contemporary heart failure neurohormonal antagonists and clenbuterol. Four-year survival was 88.9% with nearly normal quality of life scores and oxygen consumption. Stem cell and gene therapies can also be provided during VAD support in hopes of myocardial recovery and preliminary studies are being conducted *(62)*.

10.6. Destination Therapy (DT)

With the success of BTT but the increase in waiting times for transplantation, the role of MCS devices as an alternative to transplantation has emerged as a reasonable option for patients with end-stage heart failure. DT is the institution of MCS devices with the goal of permanent implantation. The landmark REMATCH trial, published in 2001, established the superiority of LVAD support versus medical therapy in patients with end-stage heart failure patients who were not candidates for transplantation *(63)*. The 129 heart failure patients studied in this trial were quite ill with NYHA IV symptoms, average ejection fractions of 17%, and were not transplant candidates because of advanced age and other significant comorbidity. These patients were the most ill ever enrolled in a heart failure trial: 70% were inotrope dependent (Table 3). The survival at 1 year was 52% in the LVAD group versus 25% in the OMM group ($P = 0.002$). At 2 years, survival was 23% in the LVAD group versus 8% in the OMM group ($P = 0.09$) (Fig. 15). Quality of life was also significantly improved in the LVAD group. Survival improved over the course of the trial suggesting that experience with patient selection and perioperative management improved outcomes *(64)*. Adverse events did occur 2.35 times more frequently in the LVAD group. Most of these adverse events were infection, bleeding, and device malfunction.

Table 3
Comparisons between study subjects in various heart failure trials

	Consensus	*VMAC*	*Copernicus*	*First*	*Rematch (po)*	*Rematch (IV ino)*
SBP (mmHg)	119	121	125	107	107	100
LVEF (%)		26	20	19	17	17
Na (mmol/l)	138	137		138	137	134
6-month mortality (%)	29	23	10	37	39	61

SBP, systolic blood pressure; LVEF, left ventricular ejection fraction; Na, serum sodium.

Since the REMATCH trial, DT morbidity and mortality have improved. In addition, death due to sepsis has been significantly lower in the post-

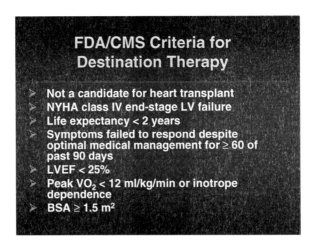

Fig. 15. Criteria for destination therapy.

REMATCH era *(65)*. In a review of 280 post-REMATCH DT patients treated from November 2001 to December 2005, overall in-hospital mortality was 27% and the 1-year survival was 56%. Most patients died from sepsis, right heart failure, or multiorgan system failure. Determinants of in-hospital mortality included nutritional status, hematologic abnormalities, right ventricular or end-organ dysfunction, and lack of inotropic support. Using a scoring system with risk factors developed from a multivariate analysis, low risk patients (<9) had an excellent 1-year survival of 81.2%, which approaches 1-year post-transplant survival. In contrast, those patients with high risk scores (17–19) had a poor 1-year survival of 27.8% *(66)*.

DT is now FDA approved for the management of end-stage heart failure patients who are not transplant candidates. However, it should be noted that benefits may not be uniform among patient groups since those who are not inotrope dependent at the time of implant may not have the same improvements in quality of life experienced by the inotrope-dependent patients *(67)*. The Center for Medicaid and Medicare (CMS) currently provides reimbursement for DT in those centers that have successfully implanted ten ventricular assist devices either as a bridge to transplant or as DT within a 3-year period. The current CMS and FDA-approved indications for DT therapy are consistent with the original REMATCH criteria (Fig. 15). Only the Heartmate XVE is approved for this indication. Other devices are under investigation for this indication and include the Novacor device, Heartmate II, and the Debakey VAD.

Cost has been raised as a significant barrier to the widespread adoption of DT as a practical therapeutic option to end-stage heart disease. In one analysis from the REMATCH trial, implant-related hospital costs were $210,187 ± 193,295 although mean costs varied significantly between survivors and nonsurvivors ($159,271 ± 106,423 versus $315,015 ± 278,713). Sepsis, pump housing infection, and perioperative bleeding were the major determinants of implantation cost *(68)*. As anticipated, these costs appear to be decreasing: analysis from the post-REMATCH era suggests the mean cost is now approximately $150,000 *(69)*. These economic costs appear to be comparable to other forms of therapy, that are well accepted, including heart transplantation (Table 4) *(70)*. However, other authors suggest from limited data that VADs are not cost-effective *(71)*.

10.7. Complications

Infection is one of the most common causes of morbidity and mortality following VAD placement: in REMATCH, sepsis resulted in 41% of the deaths and almost a third of patients developed an LVAD infection within the first 3 months of surgery. Other BTT trials have also reported a high incidence of infection *(72)*. In the ISHLT database, the incidence of postoperative infection was 32.5% *(41)*. VAD infections can involve the superficial

Table 4
Cost-effectiveness of destination therapy *(70)*

Treatment	Cost–utility ratio ($/QALY)
ACEi (SOLVD)	115
Cholesterol testing/diet	330
Pacemaker	1650
CABG (left main disease)	3135
Home hemodialysis	25,890
Heart transplantation	37,000
ICD (SCD-HeFT)	41,530
LVAD	91,000–126,000
Neurosurgery for malignant brain tumor	161,170

driveline, the pump pocket, the mediastinum, or the internal components of the pump (Endovaditis). The pathophysiology of the infection includes a predilection for organisms that can form a biofilm, which is a physical barrier to leukocytes, antibodies, complement, and antibiotics *(73)*. These organisms include *Staphylococcus*, *Pseudomonas*, *Enterococcus*, and *Candida (74, 75)*. Biofilms are composed of cells, which make up 15% of their volume, and a matrix, which makes up 85% of the volume. Biofilms also play an important role in the spread of antibiotic resistance. Improvements in device design and clinical management have begun to address these issues *(74)*. VAD implantation is also associated with defects of cellular immunity by inducing aberrant activation of T cells, resulting in apoptosis of CD4 cells *(76–78)*. This heightened state of T cell activation also appears to lead to B cell hyperreactivity and the development of HLA-antigen allosensitization *(79)*. Other factors, including platelet and red cell transfusion and patient-related factors may also contribute to post-VAD allosensitization. This issue can be particularly vexing when the VAD is used as a BTT.

Risk factors for device infection include lengthy hospitalization; malnutrition; cardiac, renal, hepatic, immunologic dysfunction; postoperative bleeding; long operative time, particularly for redo surgery; invasive lines; transcutaneous sites for drivelines and device cannulae; preexisting infections; and mechanical ventilation. Treatment strategies for infection depend upon the components involved, but systemic antibiotics remain the cornerstone of management. Driveline infections can be managed conservatively with local wound measures but may require debridement and/or surgical repositioning. Pocket infections usually require surgical drainage and/or device replacement. Medically refractory VAD infections require replacement of the device or specific components.

Thromboembolism is a constant threat in patients treated with assist devices. The more biocompatible the surface and the fewer areas of relative blood stasis, the less likely thromboembolism will occur. The Heartmate device has been associated with one of the lowest thromboemoblic rates due to its unique blood-contacting surface; only aspirin therapy is recommended. Other devices such as the Thoratec PVAD require systemic anticoagulation with warfarin as well as concomitant aspirin therapy. Despite these anticoagulation strategies, stroke remains a significant complication. In the REMATCH study, 16% of the LVAD patients had strokes with an annualized stroke rate of 0.19. The mean time to stroke was approximately 222 days; surprisingly, previous stroke, age, and sepsis were not predictors of stroke in these patients. In contrast, the rate was 0.052 in the medical, non-LVAD arm. Yet, LVAD therapy was associated with a 44% decrease in the rate of stroke or death when compared to the optimal medical therapy arm *(80)*.

The risk of bleeding after VAD placement has been estimated to be as high as 50%. Preoperative coagulopathies and hematologic abnormalities, malnutrition, azotemia, warfarin, and antiplatelet therapy, liver dysfunction, and prior cardiac surgery all contribute to bleeding *(81)*. Furthermore, blood transfusions predispose to infection, respiratory failure, right heart dysfunction, allosensitization, and viral transmission. To limit bleeding, some surgeons use bioglue at inflow and outflow suture lines, a common difficult site to control intraoperative bleeding. Aprotinin can be considered to achieve hemostasis for VAD implants but concerns have been raised about its association with renal failure and mortality. Monitoring of anticoagulation status is critical and some centers have advocated the use of thromboelastograms rather than activated clotting times or partial thromboplastin times. Bleeding is also complicated by chronic hemolysis. Mechanical hemolysis occurs through two primary mechanisms: (1) thermal injury to red cells from heat generated from friction within the device and (2) the high shear forces associated with rotation of the impeller blades and rotating seals.

Device failure is an inevitable limitation of contemporary VAD therapy. In REMATCH, the rate of mechanical failure of the Heartmate was 35% at 2 years *(63)*. Each device has its own idiosyncratic incidence and mode of failure although second and third-generation devices are clearly more durable. For the Heartmate LVAD, inflow valve failure and mechanical bearing wear have been the primary mechanisms of device failure. Specific clinical strategies may improve the "wear-and-tear" of VADs, particularly the displacement pumps. Minimizing total VAD "beats" can be accomplished by placing the pump in low fixed rate modes when the patient is sleeping or inactive. Controlling VAD afterload with antihypertensive therapy is also important, since high blood pressure increases early intraVAD ejection pressure and decreases inflow valve durability.

Device dysfunction can be detected in a number of ways. A simple change in the cadence and sounds of the VAD may suggest impending pump failure from bearing wear or valvular insufficiency. Routine analysis of air vent filters can detect small amounts of metal that herald the breakdown of ball bearings. Interrogation of the device for waveform analysis can also be used to assess pump performance. Inflow valve insufficiency may cause a rise in device rate and output, since preload is artificially augmented. Ultimately, device function is followed with echocardiography. Echocardiography can be used to assess adequacy of ventricular decompression, aortic valve opening, intracardiac thrombus, positioning of the inflow cannula, flow velocity across the inflow cannula, and right ventricular size and function. The development of increased left ventricular size, aortic valve opening, and VAD systolic flow retrograde into the left ventricle through the inflow cannula is diagnostic of inflow valvular insufficiency. Cardiac catheterization can also be used to obtain hemodynamics that are diagnostic of either outflow valve/graft obstruction and/or inflow valvular insufficiency. Often, both echocardiography and invasive hemodynamic studies may be required to specifically diagnose the nature of device dysfunction *(82, 83)*. Many patients may only require heightened surveillance if device dysfunction occurs but some ultimately require device or valve replacement.

Psychologic issues may be of concern after VAD implantation. Although quality of life is improved after VAD therapy in patients awaiting transplant or in the context of DT, there is a psychologic adjustment that must be made and may be comparable to patients who have had internal cardiac defibrillators. However, research of the psychologic aspects of VAD therapy has been limited to date *(84–86)*. Surprisingly, post-traumatic stress disorder (PTSD) has not been described in patients who have undergone VAD implantation but rather in their spouses *(87)*. In one particular survey, 26% of spouses, but none of the patients, met criteria for PTSD. Spousal fears often revolved around device-related problems in contrast to the patients who were less worried. Surprisingly, the noise of the device was not an issue.

11. CONCLUSIONS

Advanced heart failure affects close to 10% of all patients with heart failure due to systolic dysfunction, and in many, persistent symptoms and disease progression occur despite optimal medical and device therapy. Heart transplantation, the best currently available solution for the appropriate patient, is unfortunately limited by donor availability. Mechanical circulatory support (MCS) serves an important role in advanced heart failure. Such devices replace or supplement the native cardiac output and consist of ventricular assist devices (VADs) and total artificial hearts (TAHs). There are approximately 30 devices either in use or in preclinical phase and have evolving clinical applications including postcardiotomy circulatory support (PCCS), bridge to transplantation (BTT), bridge to recovery (BTR), and destination therapy (DT). Newly evolving concepts are the use of devices as a bridge to bridge or bridge to decision. Overall, MCS is emerging as an important treatment option for acute and chronic heart failure refractory to medical therapy.

REFERENCES

1. Hunt, S.A., et al., ACC/AHA Guidelines for the Evaluation and Management of Chronic Heart Failure in the Adult: Executive Summary A Report of the American College of Cardiology/American Heart Association Task Force on Practice Guidelines (Committee to Revise the 1995 Guidelines for the Evaluation and Management of Heart Failure): Developed in Collaboration With the International Society for Heart and Lung Transplantation; Endorsed by the Heart Failure Society of America. Circulation, 2001. 104(24):2996–3007.
2. Stevenson, L.W. and R.L. Kormos, Mechanical Cardiac Support 2000: Current applications and future trial design. J Thorac Cardiovasc Surg, 2001. 121(3):418–24.
3. Vitali, E., et al., Different clinical scenarios for circulatory mechanical support in acute and chronic heart failure. Am J Cardiol, 2005. 96(12A):34L–41L.
4. Moulopoulos, S.D., S.R. Topaz, and W.J. Kolff, Extracorporeal assistance to the circulation and intraaortic balloon pumping. Trans Am Soc Artif Intern Organs, 1962. 8: 85–9.
5. Kantrowitz, A., et al., Initial clinical experience with intraaortic balloon pumping in cardiogenic shock. JAMA, 1968. 203(2):113–8.
6. Allen, G.S., K.D. Murray, and D.B. Olsen, The importance of pulsatile and nonpulsatile flow in the design of blood pumps. Artif Organs, 1997. 21(8):922–8.
7. Song, X., et al., Axial flow blood pumps. Asaio J, 2003. 49(4):355–64.
8. Mudge, G.H., Jr., The management of mechanical hearts. Trans Am Clin Climatol Assoc, 2005. 116:283–91; discussion 292.
9. Pennington, D.G., et al., Long-term follow-up of postcardiotomy patients with profound cardiogenic shock treated with ventricular assist devices. Circulation, 1985. 72(3 Pt 2):II216–26.
10. Hill, J.D., et al., Bridge to cardiac transplantation: successful use of prosthetic biventricular support in a patient awaiting a donor heart. ASAIO Trans, 1986. 32(1):233–7.
11. Farrar, D.J., The thoratec ventricular assist device: a paracorporeal pump for treating acute and chronic heart failure. Semin Thorac Cardiovasc Surg, 2000. 12(3):243–50.
12. Thoratec, Heartmate XVE LVAS: Clinical Operation and Patient Management. 2006.
13. Rose, E.A., et al., Artificial circulatory support with textured interior surfaces. A counterintuitive approach to minimizing thromboembolism. Circulation, 1994. 90(5 Pt 2):II87–91.
14. Slater, J.P., et al., Low thromboembolic risk without anticoagulation using advanced-design left ventricular assist devices. Ann Thorac Surg, 1996. 62(5):1321–7; discussion 1328.
15. Long, J.W., Advanced mechanical circulatory support with the HeartMate left ventricular assist device in the year 2000. Ann Thorac Surg, 2001. 71(3 Suppl):S176–82; discussion S183–4.
16. Spanier, T., et al., Activation of coagulation and fibrinolytic pathways in patients with left ventricular assist devices. J Thorac Cardiovasc Surg, 1996. 112(4):1090–7.
17. Spanier, T.B., et al., Time-dependent cellular population of textured-surface left ventricular assist devices contributes to the development of a biphasic systemic procoagulant response. J Thorac Cardiovasc Surg, 1999. 118(3):404–13.
18. Tayama, E., et al., The DeBakey ventricular assist device: current status in 1997. Artif Organs, 1999. 23(12):1113–6.
19. Noon, G.P., et al., Development and clinical application of the MicroMed DeBakey VAD. Curr Opin Cardiol, 2000. 15(3):166–71.

20. Noon, G.P., et al., Clinical experience with the MicroMed DeBakey ventricular assist device. Ann Thorac Surg, 2001. 71(3 Suppl):S133–8; discussion S144–6.
21. SoRelle, R., First US implantation of DeBakey ventricular assist device. Circulation, 2000. 101(24):E9056–7.
22. Delgado, R. and M. Bergheim, HeartMate II left ventricular assist device: a new device for advanced heart failure. Expert Rev Med Dev, 2005. 2(5):529–32.
23. Amir, O., et al., A successful anticoagulation protocol for the first HeartMate II implantation in the United States. Tex Heart Inst J, 2005. 32(3):399–401.
24. Hoshi, H., T. Shinshi, and S. Takatani, Third-generation blood pumps with mechanical noncontact magnetic bearings. Artif Organs, 2006. 30(5):324–38.
25. Onuma, H., M. Murakami, and T. Masuzawa, Novel maglev pump with a combined magnetic bearing. Asaio J, 2005. 51(1):50–5.
26. Gray, N.A., Jr. and C.H. Selzman, Current status of the total artificial heart. Am Heart J, 2006. 152(1):4–10.
27. Dowling, R.D., et al., The AbioCor implantable replacement heart. Ann Thorac Surg, 2003. 75(6 Suppl):S93–9.
28. Smith, M.C., et al., CardioWest total artificial heart in a moribund adolescent with left ventricular thrombi. Ann Thorac Surg, 2005. 80(4):1490–2.
29. El-Banayosy, A., et al., CardioWest total artificial heart: Bad Oeynhausen experience. Ann Thorac Surg, 2005. 80(2):548–52.
30. DeVries, W.C., et al., Clinical use of the total artificial heart. N Engl J Med, 1984. 310(5):273–8.
31. Felker, G.M. and J.G. Rogers, Same bridge, new destinations rethinking paradigms for mechanical cardiac support in heart failure. J Am Coll Cardiol, 2006. 47(5): 930–2.
32. Oz, M.C., et al., Screening scale predicts patients successfully receiving long-term implantable left ventricular assist devices. Circulation, 1995. 92(9 Suppl):II169–73.
33. Deng, M.C., et al., Mechanical circulatory support for advanced heart failure: effect of patient selection on outcome. Circulation, 2001. 103(2):231–7.
34. Piccione, W., Jr., Mechanical circulatory assistance: changing indications and options. J Heart Lung Transplant, 1997. 16(6):S25–8.
35. Nakatani, S., et al., Prediction of right ventricular dysfunction after left ventricular assist device implantation. Circulation, 1996. 94(9 Suppl):II216–21.
36. Burkhoff, D., et al., Feasibility study of the use of the TandemHeart percutaneous ventricular assist device for treatment of cardiogenic shock. Catheter Cardiovasc Interv, 2006. 68(2):211–7.
37. Marelli, D., et al., Temporary mechanical support with the BVS 5000 assist device during treatment of acute myocarditis. J Card Surg, 1997. 12(1):55–9.
38. Guyton, R.A., et al., Postcardiotomy shock: clinical evaluation of the BVS 5000 Biventricular Support System. Ann Thorac Surg, 1993. 56(2):346–56.
39. Samuels, L.E., et al., Management of acute cardiac failure with mechanical assist: experience with the ABIOMED BVS 5000. Ann Thorac Surg, 2001. 71(3 Suppl):S67–72; discussion S82–5.
40. Hoefer, D., et al., Outcome evaluation of the bridge-to-bridge concept in patients with cardiogenic shock. Ann Thorac Surg, 2006. 82(1):28–33.
41. Deng, M.C., et al., Mechanical circulatory support device database of the International Society for Heart and Lung Transplantation: third annual report – 2005. J Heart Lung Transplant, 2005. 24(9):1182–7.
42. Jaski, B.E., et al., Cardiac transplant outcome of patients supported on left ventricular assist device vs. intravenous inotropic therapy. J Heart Lung Transplant, 2001. 20(4):449–56.
43. Frazier, O.H., et al., Multicenter clinical evaluation of the HeartMate 1000 IP left ventricular assist device. Ann Thorac Surg, 1992. 53(6):1080–90.

44. Frazier, O.H., et al., Multicenter clinical evaluation of the HeartMate vented electric left ventricular assist system in patients awaiting heart transplantation. J Thorac Cardiovasc Surg, 2001. 122(6):1186–95.

45. Ashton, R.C., Jr., et al., Duration of left ventricular assist device support affects transplant survival. J Heart Lung Transplant, 1996. 15(11):1151–7.

46. Aaronson, K.D., et al., Left ventricular assist device therapy improves utilization of donor hearts. J Am Coll Cardiol, 2002. 39(8):1247–54.

47. El-Banayosy, A., et al., Novacor left ventricular assist system versus Heartmate vented electric left ventricular assist system as a long-term mechanical circulatory support device in bridging patients: a prospective study. J Thorac Cardiovasc Surg, 2000. 119(3):581–7.

48. Navia, J.L., et al., Do left ventricular assist device (LVAD) bridge-to-transplantation outcomes predict the results of permanent LVAD implantation? Ann Thorac Surg, 2002. 74(6):2051–62; discussion 2062–3.

49. Goldstein, D.J., Worldwide experience with the MicroMed DeBakey ventricular assist device as a bridge to transplantation. Circulation, 2003. 108(Suppl 1):II272–7.

50. Frazier, O.H., et al., Use of the Jarvik 2000 left ventricular assist system as a bridge to heart transplantation or as destination therapy for patients with chronic heart failure. Ann Surg, 2003. 237(5):631–6; discussion 636–7.

51. Copeland, J.G., et al., Cardiac replacement with a total artificial heart as a bridge to transplantation. N Engl J Med, 2004. 351(9):859–67.

52. Bruckner, B.A., et al., Regression of fibrosis and hypertrophy in failing myocardium following mechanical circulatory support. J Heart Lung Transplant, 2001. 20(4): 457–64.

53. Baba, H.A., et al., Reversal of metallothionein expression is different throughout the human myocardium after prolonged left-ventricular mechanical support. J Heart Lung Transplant, 2000. 19(7):668–74.

54. McCarthy, P.M., et al., Structural and left ventricular histologic changes after implantable LVAD insertion. Ann Thorac Surg, 1995. 59(3):609–13.

55. Torre-Amione, G., et al., Decreased expression of tumor necrosis factor-alpha in failing human myocardium after mechanical circulatory support: A potential mechanism for cardiac recovery. Circulation, 1999. 100(11):1189–93.

56. Blaxall, B.C., et al., Differential gene expression and genomic patient stratification following left ventricular assist device support. J Am Coll Cardiol, 2003. 41(7): 1096–106.

57. Klotz, S., et al., Left ventricular assist device support normalizes left and right ventricular beta-adrenergic pathway properties. J Am Coll Cardiol, 2005. 45(5):668–76.

58. Simon, M.A., et al., Myocardial recovery using ventricular assist devices: prevalence, clinical characteristics, and outcomes. Circulation, 2005. 112(9 Suppl):I32–6.

59. Mancini, D.M., et al., Low incidence of myocardial recovery after left ventricular assist device implantation in patients with chronic heart failure. Circulation, 1998. 98(22):2383–9.

60. Khan, T., et al., Dobutamine stress echocardiography predicts myocardial improvement in patients supported by left ventricular assist devices (LVADs): hemodynamic and histologic evidence of improvement before LVAD explantation. J Heart Lung Transplant, 2003. 22(2):137–46.

61. Dandel, M., et al., Long-term results in patients with idiopathic dilated cardiomyopathy after weaning from left ventricular assist devices. Circulation, 2005. 112(9 Suppl): I37–45.

62. Dib, N., et al., Feasibility and safety of autologous myoblast transplantation in patients with ischemic cardiomyopathy. Cell Transplant, 2005. 14(1):11–9.

63. Rose, E.A., et al., Long-term mechanical left ventricular assistance for end-stage heart failure. N Engl J Med, 2001. 345(20):1435–43.

64. Park, S.J., et al., Left ventricular assist devices as destination therapy: a new look at survival. J Thorac Cardiovasc Surg, 2005. 129(1):9–17.
65. Long, J.W., et al., Long-term destination therapy with the HeartMate XVE left ventricular assist device: improved outcomes since the REMATCH study. Congest Heart Fail, 2005. 11(3):133–8.
66. Lietz, K., et al., Outcomes of left ventricular assist device implantation as destination therapy in the post-REMATCH era: implications for patient selection. Circulation, 2007. 116(5):497–505.
67. Stevenson, L.W., et al., Left ventricular assist device as destination for patients undergoing intravenous inotropic therapy: a subset analysis from REMATCH (Randomized Evaluation of Mechanical Assistance in Treatment of Chronic Heart Failure). Circulation, 2004. 110(8):975–81.
68. Oz, M.C., et al., Left ventricular assist devices as permanent heart failure therapy: the price of progress. Ann Surg, 2003. 238(4):577–83; discussion 583–5.
69. Miller, L.W., et al., Hospital costs for left ventricular assist devices for destination therapy: lower costs for implantation in the post-REMATCH era. J Heart Lung Transplant, 2006. 25(7):778–84.
70. McGregor, M., Implantable ventricular assist devices: is it time to introduce them in Canada? Can J Cardiol, 2000. 16(5):629–40.
71. Clegg, A.J., et al., The clinical and cost-effectiveness of left ventricular assist devices for end-stage heart failure: a systematic review and economic evaluation. Health Technol Assess, 2005. 9(45):1–148.
72. Minami, K., et al., Morbidity and outcome after mechanical ventricular support using Thoratec, Novacor, and HeartMate for bridging to heart transplantation. Artif Organs, 2000. 24(6):421–6.
73. Holman, W.L., et al., Infection in ventricular assist devices: prevention and treatment. Ann Thorac Surg, 2003. 75(6 Suppl):S48–57.
74. Padera, R.F., Infection in ventricular assist devices: the role of biofilm. Cardiovasc Pathol, 2006. 15(5):264–70.
75. Costerton, J.W., L. Montanaro, and C.R. Arciola, Biofilm in implant infections: its production and regulation. Int J Artif Organs, 2005. 28(11):1062–8.
76. Chinn, R., et al., Multicenter experience: prevention and management of left ventricular assist device infections. Asaio J, 2005. 51(4):461–70.
77. Itescu, S., et al., Immunobiology of left ventricular assist devices. Prog Cardiovasc Dis, 2000. 43(1):67–80.
78. Ankersmit, H.J., et al., Activation-induced T-cell death and immune dysfunction after implantation of left-ventricular assist device. Lancet, 1999. 354(9178):550–5.
79. Gonzalez-Stawinski, G.V., et al., Early and midterm risk of coronary allograft vasculopathy in patients bridged to orthotopic heart transplantation with ventricular assist devices. Transplantation, 2005. 79(9):1175–9.
80. Lazar, R.M., et al., Neurological events during long-term mechanical circulatory support for heart failure: the Randomized Evaluation of Mechanical Assistance for the Treatment of Congestive Heart Failure (REMATCH) experience. Circulation, 2004. 109(20):2423–7.
81. Goldstein, D.J. and R.B. Beauford, Left ventricular assist devices and bleeding: adding insult to injury. Ann Thorac Surg, 2003. 75(6 Suppl):S42–7.
82. Horton, S.C., et al., Left ventricular assist device malfunction: an approach to diagnosis by echocardiography. J Am Coll Cardiol, 2005. 45(9):1435–40.
83. Horton, S.C., et al., Left ventricular assist device malfunction: a systematic approach to diagnosis. J Am Coll Cardiol, 2004. 43(9):1574–83.
84. Ruzevich, S.A., et al., Retrospective analysis of the psychologic effects of mechanical circulatory support. J Heart Transplant, 1990. 9(3 Pt 1):209–12.

85. Dew, M.A., et al., Life quality in the era of bridging to cardiac transplantation. Bridge patients in an outpatient setting. Asaio J, 1993. 39(2):145–52.
86. Petrucci, R., et al., Cardiac ventricular support. Considerations for psychiatry. Psychosomatics, 1999. 40(4):298–303.
87. Bunzel, B., et al., Mechanical circulatory support as a bridge to heart transplantation: what remains? Long-term emotional sequelae in patients and spouses. J Heart Lung Transplant, 2007. 26(4):384–9.

14   Device Therapy for Left Ventricular Dysfunction

Clyde W. Yancy, MD

CONTENTS

Abstract

Pharmacotherapeutic interventions are proven to reduce symptoms and improve survival in patients with heart failure due to left ventricular dysfunction. The primary target of these medical interventions has been reverse remodeling. Creating a smaller ventricular cavity with improved contractility that is more conical and less spherical in shape has represented a reasonable surrogate of efficacy for effective drug interventions. This chapter reviews the medical devices that are designed to "reverse remodel" the heart, including tethers, socks, and cardiac support devices.

Key Words: Heart failure; Medical device; Remodeling; Cardiac support.

1. INTRODUCTION

Elucidation of causative pathophysiological mechanisms of left ventricular dysfunction has yielded an array of pharmacotherapeutic interventions that have profoundly improved the natural history of left ventricular

From: *Contemporary Cardiology: Device Therapy in Heart Failure*
Edited by: W.H. Maisel, DOI 10.1007/978-1-59745-424-7_14
© Humana Press, a part of Springer Science+Business Media, LLC 2010

dysfunction and in turn improved outcomes for chronic heart failure. The target of these pharmacotherapeutic interventions has been reverse remodeling. Creating a smaller ventricular cavity with improved contractility that is more conical and less spherical in shape has represented a reasonable surrogate of efficacy for effective drug interventions *(1)*. Certain implantable device therapies have also been identified that are indeed helpful, especially implantable defibrillators, cardiac resynchronization pacemakers [CRT], or a combination of both *(2, 3)*. With regard to the use of a CRT device, the presumed mechanism of benefit is remarkably similar to that of pharmacotherapy, i.e., reverse remodeling. This consistency of ventricular remodeling as a major pathophysiological consideration in the genesis of left ventricular dysfunction and in turn the reversal of LV remodeling as a useful intervention has prompted investigation into other modalities that might effect reverse remodeling and improve either symptoms or the natural history of heart failure.

At a fundamental level, remodeling of the left ventricle is a reflection of an increase in cardiac myocyte length resulting from sarcomere growth in series that is facilitated by an exaggerated neurohormonal milieu. This process is typically initiated by an inciting event – either acute as in a myocardial infarction or chronic as in a dilated cardiomyopathy. The response to this injury is then reflected in alterations in myocyte biology, gross myocardial changes, changes in the extracellular matrix, and alterations in left ventricular chamber geometry *(4)*. Mann has outlined this cascade of changes and has further aligned these changes with subsequent "mechanical disadvantages" that negatively impact left ventricular function including increased wall stress, afterload mismatch, increased myocardial oxygen consumption, functional mitral insufficiency, and maladaptive gene expression *(4)*. Force and others have suggested that myocyte stretch activates a biological cascade of events that further contributes to ventricular remodeling. Certain humoral factors are released via "stretch-activated sensors" and include angiotensin II, interleukin-6, insulin-like growth factor, and possibly endothelin-1. Other pathways that are stimulated by myocyte stretch include stretch-activated ion channels, integrins, protein kinase C, calcineurin, and calcium/calmodulin-dependent protein kinases *(5)*. Taken together these and other described responses to stretch create a growth signal that stimulates myocyte enlargement which in turn contributes to chamber dilation and a decline in ventricular function. If left unchecked, this elaborate cascade of events results in progressive left ventricular dysfunction and worsening heart failure with the expected morbidity and mortality. A conceptualization of the stretch-activated growth response is displayed in Fig. 1 *(5)*.

The aforementioned medical and device therapies reverse left ventricular remodeling but do not completely restore left ventricular size and function. While certain biological therapeutic interventions are under active investigation and may yield great promise, recent attention has been focused on newer device platforms that might be of benefit that once again target ventricular

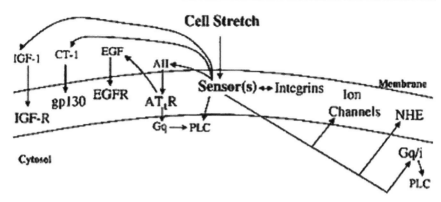

Fig. 1. Model of stretch-induced signal transduction in the heart. Stretch activates signaling pathways via two parallel mechanisms: the release of autocrine or paracrine growth factors (*left*) and direct activation of specific signal transduction pathways (*right*). The pathways that are directly activated after stretch include integrins, stretch-activated ion channels (SACs), Na+/H+ exchanger (NHE), heterotrimeric G proteins of the Gq and Gi class, and possibly phospholipase C (PLC). The autocrine/paracrine factors believed to be of most importance include angiotensin II, cytokines of the interleukin-6 (IL-6) family, insulin-like growth factor-1 (IGF-1), and possibly endothelin-1 (ET-1), all of which act via specific cell surface receptors. (Adapted with permission *(5)*).

remodeling. With an intent to reshape the ventricle as a focus of intervention, the goal has been to either decrease the left ventricular cavity and/or attenuate mitral insufficiency (if functional mitral insufficiency is present). Focusing on the LV cavity first, attempts have been made to change LV size and geometry via direct surgical intervention or through extrinsic or intrinsic device applications. To accomplish this, a variety of tethers and restraining devices have been evaluated. Focusing on the mitral valve, a number of efforts have been evaluated that include direct surgical "repair" of functional MR using clips or rings and more recently percutaneous deployment of mitral valve clips. Table 1 lists a summary of candidate devices that target LV remodeling.

A number of additional device therapies have been used to treat LV dysfunction. The use of a left ventricular assist device has been the gold standard as a bridge to transplantation and is also indicated as appropriate for "destination" or permanent therapy *(6–8)*. Recently developed smaller platforms are now deemed appropriate as a bridge to transplantation and will likely become appropriate as destination therapy *(9)*. As the morbidity and costs of prolonged left ventricular mechanical support becomes more practical and patient selection schemes improve, the use of these devices will increase and in fact, smaller, more durable LV assist devices will likely challenge many of the current device therapies that are currently under investigation. Though the total artificial heart represents a "device," it is not yet a practical option

Table 1
Device therapy for LV remodeling

I. Left ventricular cavity
   a. Intrinsic devices
      i. Tethers
      ii. Cords
   b. Extrinsic devices
      i. Socks
      ii. Cardiac restraint devices
II. Mitral valve
   a. Surgical approaches
      i. Ring repair
      ii. Clips or partial closure
   b. Percutaneous approaches
      i. Clips

for the ordinary patient with heart failure, even with advanced disease, and in large measure remains either experimental or appropriate only for use in extreme circumstances *(10)*. Similarly, one might consider coronary artery conduits as "devices" and consider higher risk coronary artery bypass grafting as "device therapy" for advanced left ventricular failure with underlying left ventricular remodeling.

2. HISTORY OF LEFT VENTRICULAR REMODELING SURGERY

The history of left ventricular remodeling surgery encompasses several approaches – left ventricular aneurysmectomy, surgical restoration of left ventricular size, and partial left ventriculectomy. Both left ventricular aneurysmectomy and left ventricular restoration target the pathological remodeling that occurs after myocardial infarction which yields a left ventricular scar defined by a region of the left ventricle that is either akinetic or frankly dyskinetic. Simple resection of the left ventricular aneurysm led to a more refined procedure that involved left ventricular restoration using an endoventricular patch *(11)*. Either circumstance results in a less spherical ventricle with at least the potential to realize an improvement in left ventricular contractility. Postoperative studies are consistent with improvements in myocardial oxygen consumption, myocardial efficiency, and an improved neurohormonal milieu *(12)*. This procedure relies heavily on the skill of the surgeon to reconstruct the ventricle. However, a multicenter study, Reconstructive Endoventricular Surgery Returning Torsion Original Radius Elliptical Shape to the Left Ventricle [RESTORE] has been completed *(13)*. In this ~1200 patient study, all patients underwent left ventricular restoration along with myocardial revascularization and/or mitral valve repair; in most cases, the data were promising. The 30-day mortality was 5.3%. Ejection fraction increased from 29.6 to 39% (*P*<0.001) and the LV end-systolic volume index decreased as well. Survival at 5 years was ~70% and freedom from hospitalization for heart failure was nearly 80%. Preoperatively 67% of patients were in NYHA class III or IV but postoperatively, 85% were in NYHA class I or II *(13)*. These findings are encouraging but without a control group it is unclear whether or not this is better than standard medical therapy.

The Batista operation brought surgical targeting of left ventricular remodeling into the mainstream thought process of heart failure therapy. Dr. Batista pioneered a radical approach which was simply to resect the posterolateral left ventricular wall in patients with advanced heart failure in order to reduce the radius of the left ventricle and in turn to reduce wall stress *(14, 15)*. This provocative approach was rapidly acknowledged as a potential breakthrough but attempts to replicate the early results in US-based populations failed and this approach is no longer considered appropriate therapy for advanced heart failure *(16)*. Nevertheless, these direct surgical approaches laid the foundation for newer novel surgical approaches that might accomplish reverse remodeling of the failing left ventricle.

The focus of the remainder of this chapter will be to highlight the devices that are specifically targeting LV remodeling. Discussions regarding implantable ICD with or without CRT (Chapters 6 and 7), LVADs (Chapter 13), and the use of artificial hearts (Chapter 13) are discussed in other chapters in this book.

3. LEFT VENTRICULAR DEVICE THERAPIES

The core hypothesis that is challenged by these devices is that decreasing left ventricular size matters in LV remodeling/heart failure and the method used to effect a decrease in size is not pertinent. As noted above, remodeling is defined as progressive enlargement of the left ventricle driven by an increase in wall stress, facilitated by an exaggerated neurohormonal environment, with a corresponding transition to a more spherical shape followed by worsening left ventricular systolic dysfunction. The premise of this concept is grounded in the law of LaPlace:

Wall stress ~ constant (LV diameter)*r*(LV pressure)/2 (LV wall thickness)

When left ventricular remodeling is targeted by medical therapies, the gradual withdrawal of the consequences of deleterious neurohormonal stimulation allows for a favorable change in LV geometry and a corresponding improvement in ventricular function. The *sine qua non* of reverse remodeling is both a smaller ventricular cavity and an improvement in contractility – usually measured as an improved left ventricular ejection fraction. It is not entirely clear whether simply changing the shape of the ventricle is sufficient, or if withdrawing the stimulus for dilation, plus altering the neurohormonal and ultrastructural milieu while changing the shape is most important.

3.1. Tethers

Several iterations of LV tethers have been evaluated. In principle, the idea is to affix a semi-rigid device from the septum to the LV posterior or lateral wall that tethers or prevents the ventricle from further expansion or perhaps even decreases its size. How many tethers are required and the physical characteristics of those tethers remain active questions. As well, both the thrombogenicity of the tethers and any predisposition to ventricular arrhythmias from ventricular affixation remains a question with these devices.

The Coapsys Annuloplasty System® (Myocor, Minneapolis, MN) is a prototype-tethering device. It is a single cord that is surgically placed and affixes the septum and left ventricular lateral wall in order to decrease the septal-LV lateral dimension just below the mitral valve (*17, 18*). The intent is to both decrease ventricular size and improve mitral valve leaflet coaptation. The RESTORE-MV (Randomized Evaluation of a Surgical Treatment for Off-pump Repair of Mitral Valve) study evaluates this device. All patients in this study have ischemic heart disease and mitral insufficiency but not necessarily heart failure and are randomized to CABG with an undersized annuloplasty vs. CABG with the Coapsys system (*19*). These data should serve to put the use of this device in some context. See the Coapsys Annuloplasty System® in Fig. 2.

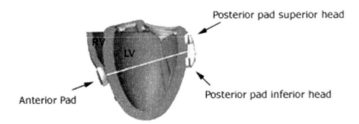

Fig. 2. The Coapsys devices are implanted so that the two pads are located on the surface of the heart with the chord passing across the left ventricle. The posterior pad of each device has a superior (*top*) and inferior (*bottom*) head. During the implant procedure, the pads are pulled toward each other to decrease the distance between the mitral valve leaflets and reshape the left ventricle.

3.2. Socks

The use of extrinsic devices to stabilize the size of the left ventricle has been a very provocative area of research with some promise of efficacy. Again, several iterations of this strategy have been evaluated but in principle, a surgeon applies the equivalent of a sock to the free wall of the left ventricle. The characteristics of the sock are designed to exert a low level of extrinsic pressure against the LV resulting in a gradual decrement in LV size. Very provocative animal work has suggested that certain restraint devices decrease genetic signals that promote growth and remodeling, i.e., fetal gene programs are downregulated. These observations are encouraging and suggest that rather than simply making the ventricle smaller, cardiac restraint devices may serve to change an important pathophysiological component of LV remodeling.

A key pathophysiological consideration for any surgical approach that impacts a change in LV geometry is whether or not the reconfigured left ventricle is affected by a similar decrease in both LV systolic and diastolic wall stress. A reduction in LV size has been associated with a prompt reduction in LV end-systolic pressure but remarkably, the reduction in LV diastolic pressures does not follow proportionately *(20)*. This dissimilar response affecting systolic and diastolic function is an important observation. A persistent elevation of LVEDP despite the smaller geometry may actually lead to an increase in LV wall stress which would stimulate growth signals and result in further LV remodeling.

Yet another important consideration is the morbidity and mortality of the surgical intervention. Patients with advanced HF are at higher risk when exposed to routine surgical procedures and procedures designed to modify ventricular geometry constitute at least intermediate if not higher risk procedures. Thus any benefit of the intended procedure must be juxtaposed against the observed surgical risk – both morbidity and mortality. Like the tethers described above, placement of an extrinsic cardiac restraint device represents the presence of a foreign body in or near the heart. Thus thrombogenicity, the propensity for ventricular and/or atrial arrhythmias, and direct inflammatory responses must be considered in understanding the risk benefit of these devices.

3.3. Cardiac Support Devices

Among the cardiac restraint devices, the ACORN CorCap® device has undergone the most extensive study *(21–26)*. See Fig. 3. This is a proprietary device that utilizes a biocompatible mesh that is affixed to the left ventricle. The device is not intended to evoke an abrupt change in ventricular size and shape but rather to exert a modest restraining force that over time not only decreases left ventricular cavity size but also reverses ultrastructural markers of cardiac remodeling. Animal models confirmed a decrease in LV size and improved LV function at the macro level and a reduction in stretch proteins, hypertrophy, and apoptosis at the micro level *(27–29)*. The cardiac support device also improved calcium cycling within the sarcoplasmic reticulum and up-regulated mRNA gene expression for the alpha-myosin

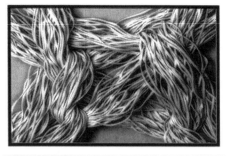

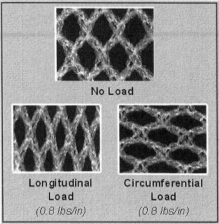

Fig. 3. The CorCap™ Cardiac Support Device is constructed from a multifilament yam/knit fabric. There are four key design features: (**a**) "optimal" compliance, (**b**) bidirectional properties designed to reshape the heart into an ellipsoid, (**c**) a 31-microfiber construction, and (**d**) long-term biocompatibility. The materials are used in other implantable devices.

heavy gene. In animals treated with the cardiac support device, plasma norepinephrine levels were reduced from pre-treatment to post-treatment *(30)*. These findings taken in aggregate would strongly suggest a reverse remodeling mechanism of action for this cardiac support device.

A pivotal trial was completed using the ACORN CorCap Cardiac Support Device. Patients with moderate to severe heart failure were recruited and then stratified into those who had clinically significant mitral insufficiency and had an indication for mitral valve surgery and those who did not require mitral valve surgery. Within each of these two broad strata, patients were then randomized the CorCap® device (with or without mitral valve surgery depending on the strata) plus medical therapy vs. medical therapy alone. Thus, four groups of patients were recruited. A composite endpoint was constructed that included change in NYHA class, freedom from cardiac procedures, and mortality. The primary endpoint was reached and proven to be statistically better than reference therapy. However, interpretation of the primary endpoint of this trial has been challenging; fewer cardiac procedures were required in the intervention group but both major and minor interventions were included. In this unblinded trial, therefore, bias cannot be fully addressed. A mortality benefit was not achieved and though NYHA class improved, not all patients had both a baseline and intervention assessment of NYHA class so this endpoint was similarly difficult to interpret. The objective of the cardiac support device was to effect reverse remodeling. The data demonstrated clear evidence of a decrement in the size of the LV cavity but there was no clear evidence of an improvement in contractility. Sphericity index did improve. This promising device is not yet approved by the FDA and remains under active investigation.

In a subgroup of 193 patients in the original pivotal trial for the CorCap® device, 102 patients had mitral valve surgery alone and 91 had both the cardiac support device and mitral valve surgery. Acker reported that the addition of the cardiac support device led to greater decreases in left ventricular end-diastolic volume and left ventricular end-systolic volume, a more elliptical shape, and a trend toward a reduction in major cardiac procedures and an improvement in quality of life. This novel application of a cardiac support device in conjunction with mitral valve surgery for functional mitral insufficiency is provocative and merits further evaluation *(25)*.

A second such device is also under active study. The Paracor® device is a similar cardiac restraint device that is made of a nitinol mesh that conforms to the left ventricle and does not require suturing to the epicardial surface. It does not require an extensive operation. A randomized trial is ongoing. See Fig. 4 *(31)*.

3.4. Mitral Valve Interventions

Aggressive medical therapy for advanced heart failure on occasion incorporates manipulation of invasively determined hemodynamic measures with the skilled administration of high-dose parenteral therapy followed then by oral vasodilator therapy. This approach, known as "tailored therapy," has been shown to be of benefit in tertiary care centers that evaluate heart transplant candidates. A key marker of benefit of this aggressive medical approach has been to observe a reduction in mitral insufficiency. Use of CRT as noted above, also appears to be especially effective when there is a reduction in mitral insufficiency from baseline to post intervention. These observations would suggest that the presence of significant functional mitral insufficiency in the setting of advanced heart failure is a reasonable target of therapy.

Surgical modification of the mitral valve for important mitral insufficiency is a well known and frequently utilized intervention for mitral valve disease. This becomes germane to the current discussion when the mitral valve disease occurs concomitantly with left ventricular dysfunction, i.e., functional

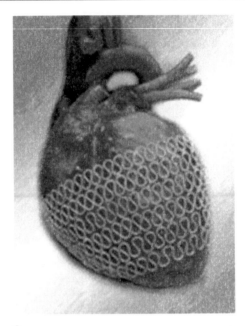

Fig. 4. The Paracor® Device is shown. It is a cardiac restraint device made of a nitinol mesh that conforms to the left ventricle.

or secondary mitral regurgitation (MR). The traditional teaching has been to refrain from mitral valve surgery for primary valve disorders in the setting of a dilated left ventricle. Given the change in geometry (eccentric hypertrophy) imparted by a chronically volume-loaded left ventricle (due to mitral insufficiency), correction of MR (a low-impedance circuit) would lead to an abrupt increase in afterload (a high-impedance circuit) in a poorly conditioned ventricle and the patient would likely fare quite poorly. However, when mitral insufficiency is a functional event that is due to LV cavity dilation and chronically elevated LV end-diastolic pressure, it appears that mitral valve repair, not replacement, can be done with reasonable safety. There remains debate as to whether this approach leads to reverse remodeling and improved outcomes. The work of Bolling et al. created early enthusiasm for this approach. Using a dramatically undersized mitral valve ring, a significant reduction in MR was achieved with an acceptable perioperative mortality rate and similar observational outcomes when compared to transplantation *(32)*. However, longer term survival was not ideal and recurrence of significant MR has been noted to be as high as 30% at 6 months *(33, 34)*. Moreover, reverse remodeling does not consistently occur after mitral valve repair of functional MR. The procedure is not without risk including an overt risk of death and candidate selection, though imprecise, must be done cautiously. Though not subjected to the rigor of randomized controlled clinical trials, more recent evaluations of this approach have demonstrated only similar outcomes when compared to medically treated patients with a similar substrate.

At best, intervention on the mitral valve in the setting of heart failure should be considered an unproven and still investigational procedure to be done by surgeons skilled in this approach and accompanied by optimized medical therapy for chronic heart failure including implantable ICD with or without CRT.

Given that some of the risk of mitral valve repair has been the perioperative morbidity and mortality, much enthusiasm has arisen as of late with the advent of a percutaneous approach which allows for clipping of the mitral valve, i.e., a clip is affixed to the anterior and posterior mitral valve leaflets effecting a markedly smaller orifice area and a reduction in mitral insufficiency. These procedures are done via a transseptal puncture and with transesophageal guidance. The EVEREST I (Endovascular Valve Edge to Edge Repair Study) evaluated the clinical results of percutaneous mitral valve repair. Of 27 patients 24 underwent percutaneous mitral valve clips with 6-month follow-up. All patients had moderately severe to severe mitral insufficiency with an ejection fraction <60% but >30%. There were four major adverse events including one stroke and three detachments of the clip requiring elective valve surgery. Three other patients required surgical mitral valve procedures. The remaining patients were free from further surgery and 13 had sustained reductions in mitral insufficiency (35). These results are encouraging but not yet definitive. These procedures remain under

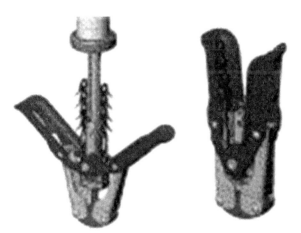

Fig. 5. Schematic drawing of the components of the clip. On the inner portion of the clip is a U-shaped gripper that matches up to each arm and helps to stabilize the leaflets from the atrial aspect as they are captured during closure of the clip arms. Leaflet tissue is secured between the closed arms and each side of the gripper, and the clip is then closed and locked to effect and maintain coaptation of the two leaflets.

the realm of active clinical investigation and have not yet recruited patients with overt heart failure. However, it is entirely plausible that a positive proof of concept study would immediately yield an inquiry into whether or not such an approach would work for those patients with heart failure and functional MR. See Fig. 5.

4. A REGULATORY PERSPECTIVE

The evaluation of a new device platform for heart failure carries with it certain confounding variables that further hamper device development. As the standard of care for heart failure improves, the benchmark against which a new device must be measured must change. Theoretically, a randomized controlled clinical trial would be ideal but in this clinical domain, a trial cannot be blinded and thus investigator bias cannot be completely removed. Moreover, patients are sometimes reluctant to participate in such trials, particularly if the device is perceived to be the better therapy; if the patient is relegated to medical therapy, they may be less engaged, less compliant, and less appropriate as a comparator. Given that a surgical approach is required to deploy nearly all of these devices, any clinical trial design must account for the perioperative morbidity and mortality in the longitudinal assessment of efficacy. This is yet another obstacle as undoubtedly a learning curve exists for all new devices and a high morbidity/mortality signal seen early in product development may become more muted longitudinally.

A novel approach to facilitate device development has been the willingness by the FDA and its European counterpart to accept a single arm study. One standard against which such a study must be judged is known as "objective performance criteria" or OPC. Either for the determination of efficacy or evaluation of risk, contemporary databases (e.g., registries) with similar patient cohorts can be accessed to determine the expected outcome using medical therapy or the usual perioperative risk for a similar type procedure. Though this is an intuitive and inherently reasonable strategy, the identification of contemporary data sets, especially of sufficient size can be quite challenging. Once a mean response or risk rate is determined, confidence intervals must then be assigned. The intent would be for a single arm study to meet the OPC for efficacy (i.e., at or above the lower 95% confidence interval) and safety (i.e., not above the predetermined upper 95% confidence interval for risk). Therefore, setting the confidence intervals wide facilitates a positive single arm study but allows for marginal efficacy and higher risk while setting a more narrow confidence interval establishes a threshold that may not be attainable with a new device application where the patient population studied may be different from that used to set the OPC and confidence intervals. Designing an ideal registration trial for a device indication remains a work in progress both for regulatory bodies and investigators but one that is necessary if the true benefit and risk of novel devices and procedures are to be clearly identified.

5. CONCLUSIONS

Based on a review of the available data, current device platforms that target LV remodeling are encouraging but have not yet been shown to be of benefit and cannot be suggested as standard treatment options. Though remodeling is a key component of the progression of left ventricular dysfunction, it is clear that remodeling is a very complex biological response to ventricular injury and many responses are at play. It is evident that the way in which remodeling is addressed, i.e., reversed, does matter and simply effecting a decrease in left ventricular chamber size may not be sufficient. It is plausible that a novel iteration of one or more of the described techniques may yield a significant signal of clinical efficacy but any further development of these platforms will eventually be compared to emerging biological strategies and/or even smaller more durable left ventricular assist devices. Moreover, as medical therapy for left ventricular dysfunction continues to improve and with greater adherence to guideline prompted evidence-based care, the niche for these LV remodeling devices is likely to become smaller. Designing an appropriate and scientifically valid/rigorous clinical trial is a major obstacle as the comparator groups, study endpoints, and sample size represent major challenges and in some cases may reflect prohibitive impediments to study completion. Nevertheless, the need for more treatment options for advanced heart failure is real and the emergence of safe and effective devices that target left ventricular remodeling represents an important opportunity to advance the care for these patients.

REFERENCES

1. Cohn JN. New therapeutic strategies for heart failure: left ventricular remodeling as a target. *J Card Fail* 2004; 10(6 Suppl):S200–S201.
2. Bardy GH, Lee KL, Mark DB, Poole JE, Packer DL, Boineau R, et al. Amiodarone or an implantable cardioverter-defibrillator for congestive heart failure. *N Engl J Med* 2005; 352(3):225–237.
3. Bristow MR, Feldman AM, Saxon LA. Heart failure management using implantable devices for ventricular resynchronization: Comparison of Medical Therapy, Pacing, and Defibrillation in Chronic Heart Failure (COMPANION) trial. COMPANION Steering Committee and COMPANION Clinical Investigators. *J Card Fail* 2000; 6(3):276–285.
4. Mann DL. Basic mechanisms of left ventricular remodeling: the contribution of wall stress. *J Card Fail* 2004; 10(6 Suppl):S202–S206.
5. Force T, Michael A, Kilter H, Haq S. Stretch-activated pathways and left ventricular remodeling. *J Card Fail* 2002; 8(6 Suppl):S351–S358.
6. Lietz K, Long JW, Kfoury AG, Slaughter MS, Silver MA, Milano CA, et al. Outcomes of left ventricular assist device implantation as destination therapy in the post-REMATCH era: implications for patient selection. *Circulation* 2007; 116(5):497–505.
7. Long JW, Kfoury AG, Slaughter MS, Silver M, Milano C, Rogers J, et al. Long-term destination therapy with the HeartMate XVE left ventricular assist device: improved outcomes since the REMATCH study. *Congest Heart Fail* 2005; 11(3):133–138.
8. Stevenson LW, Miller LW, Svigne-Nickens P, Ascheim DD, Parides MK, Renlund DG, et al. Left ventricular assist device as destination for patients undergoing intravenous

inotropic therapy: a subset analysis from REMATCH (Randomized Evaluation of Mechanical Assistance in Treatment of Chronic Heart Failure). *Circulation* 2004; 110(8):975–981.

9. Miller LW, Pagani FD, Russell SD, John R, Boyle AJ, Aaronson KD, et al. Use of a continuous-flow device in patients awaiting heart transplantation. *N Engl J Med* 2007; 357(9):885–896.

10. Nose Y. FDA approval of totally implantable permanent total artificial heart for humanitarian use. *Artif Organs* 2007; 31(1):1–3.

11. Acker MA. Surgical therapies for heart failure. *J Card Fail* 2004; 10(6 Suppl): S220–S224.

12. De BM, Alfieri O. Surgical methods to reverse left ventricular remodeling. *Curr Heart Fail Rep* 2007; 4(4):214–220.

13. Athanasuleas CL, Buckberg GD, Stanley AW, Siler W, Dor V, Di DM, et al. Surgical ventricular restoration in the treatment of congestive heart failure due to post-infarction ventricular dilation. *J Am Coll Cardiol* 2004; 44(7):1439–1445.

14. Batista RJ, Verde J, Nery P, Bocchino L, Takeshita N, Bhayana JN, et al. Partial left ventriculectomy to treat end-stage heart disease. *Ann Thorac Surg* 1997; 64(3): 634–638.

15. Batista RJ, Santos JL, Takeshita N, Bocchino L, Lima PN, Cunha MA. Partial left ventriculectomy to improve left ventricular function in end-stage heart disease. *J Card Surg* 1996; 11(2):96–97.

16. Mccarthy JF, McCarthy PM, Starling RC, Smedira NG, Scalia GM, Wong J, et al. Partial left ventriculectomy and mitral valve repair for end-stage congestive heart failure. *Eur J Cardiothorac Surg* 1998; 13(4):337–343.

17. Carraway EA, Rayburn BK. Device therapy for remodeling in congestive heart failure. *Curr Heart Fail Rep* 2007; 4(1):53–58.

18. Hamner C, Ruth G, Raffe M, Schoen FJ, Schaff H. Safety and biocompatibility of the Myosplint system – a passive implantable device that alters ventricular geometry for the treatment of heart failure. *ASAIO J* 2004; 50(5):438–443.

19. Grossi EA, Saunders PC, Woo YJ, Gangahar DM, Laschinger JC, Kress DC, et al. Intraoperative effects of the coapsys annuloplasty system in a randomized evaluation (RESTOR-MV) of functional ischemic mitral regurgitation. *Ann Thorac Surg* 2005; 80(5):1706–1711.

20. Burkhoff D, Wechsler AS. Surgical ventricular remodeling: a balancing act on systolic and diastolic properties. *J Thorac Cardiovasc Surg* 2006; 132(3):459–463.

21. Sabbah HN. Global left ventricular remodeling with the Acorn Cardiac Support Device: hemodynamic and angiographic findings in dogs with heart failure. *Heart Fail Rev* 2005; 10(2):109–115.

22. Sabbah HN, Sharov VG, Gupta RC, Mishra S, Rastogi S, Undrovinas AI, et al. Reversal of chronic molecular and cellular abnormalities due to heart failure by passive mechanical ventricular containment. *Circ Res* 2003; 93(11):1095–1101.

23. Starling RC, Jessup M, Oh JK, Sabbah HN, Acker MA, Mann DL, et al. Sustained benefits of the CorCap Cardiac Support Device on left ventricular remodeling: three year follow-up results from the Acorn clinical trial. *Ann Thorac Surg* 2007; 84(4): 1236–1242.

24. Mann DL, Acker MA, Jessup M, Sabbah HN, Starling RC, Kubo SH. Clinical evaluation of the CorCap Cardiac Support Device in patients with dilated cardiomyopathy. *Ann Thorac Surg* 2007; 84(4):1226–1235.

25. Acker MA, Bolling S, Shemin R, Kirklin J, Oh JK, Mann DL, et al. Mitral valve surgery in heart failure: insights from the Acorn Clinical Trial. *J Thorac Cardiovasc Surg* 2006; 132(3):568–77, 577.

26. Mann DL, Acker MA, Jessup M, Sabbah HN, Starling RC, Kubo SH. Rationale, design, and methods for a pivotal randomized clinical trial for the assessment of a cardiac

support device in patients with New York health association class III–IV heart failure. *J Card* Fail 2004; 10(3):185–192.

27. Sabbah HN. Global left ventricular remodeling with the Acorn Cardiac Support Device: hemodynamic and angiographic findings in dogs with heart failure. *Heart Fail Rev* 2005; 10(2):109–115.

28. Rastogi S, Gupta RC, Mishra S, Morita H, Tanhehco EJ, Sabbah HN. Long-term therapy with the acorn cardiac support device normalizes gene expression of growth factors and gelatinases in dogs with heart failure. *J Heart Lung Transplant* 2005; 24(10):1619–1625.

29. Sabbah HN, Sharov VG, Gupta RC, Mishra S, Rastogi S, Undrovinas AI, et al. Reversal of chronic molecular and cellular abnormalities due to heart failure by passive mechanical ventricular containment. *Circ Res* 2003; 93(11):1095–1101.

30. Sabbah HN. Effects of cardiac support device on reverse remodeling: molecular, biochemical, and structural mechanisms. *J Card Fail* 2004; 10(6 Suppl):S207–S214.

31. Magovern JA. Experimental and clinical studies with the Paracor cardiac restraint device. *Semin Thorac Cardiovasc Surg* 2005; 17(4):364–368.

32. Bolling SF, Pagani FD, Deeb GM, Bach DS. Intermediate-term outcome of mitral reconstruction in cardiomyopathy. *J Thorac Cardiovasc Surg* 1998; 115(2):381–386.

33. Wu AH, Aaronson KD, Bolling SF, Pagani FD, Welch K, Koelling TM. Impact of mitral valve annuloplasty on mortality risk in patients with mitral regurgitation and left ventricular systolic dysfunction. *J Am Coll Cardiol* 2005; 45(3):381–387.

34. McGee EC, Gillinov AM, Blackstone EH, Rajeswaran J, Cohen G, Najam F, et al. Recurrent mitral regurgitation after annuloplasty for functional ischemic mitral regurgitation. *J Thorac Cardiovasc Surg* 2004; 128(6):916–924.

35. Feldman T, Wasserman HS, Herrmann HC, Gray W, Block PC, Whitlow P, et al. Percutaneous mitral valve repair using the edge-to-edge technique: six-month results of the EVEREST Phase I Clinical Trial. *J Am Coll Cardiol* 2005; 46(11):2134–2140.

Subject Index

From: *Contemporary Cardiology: Device Therapy in Heart Failure*
Edited by: W.H. Maisel, DOI 10.1007/978-1-59745-424-7
© Humana Press, a part of Springer Science+Business Media, LLC 2010